Dermatopathology

Editor

MICHAEL T. TETZLAFF

SURGICAL PATHOLOGY CLINICS

www.surgpath.theclinics.com

Consulting Editor
JASON L. HORNICK

June 2021 • Volume 14 • Number 2

ELSEVIER

1600 John F. Kennedy Boulevard • Suite 1800 • Philadelphia, Pennsylvania, 19103-2899

http://www.theclinics.com

SURGICAL PATHOLOGY CLINICS Volume 14, Number 2
June 2021 ISSN 1875-9181, ISBN-13: 978-0-323-79347-6

Editor: Katerina Heidhausen
Developmental Editor: Diana Ang

Surgical Pathology Clinics (ISSN 1875-9181) is published quarterly by Elsevier Inc., 360 Park Avenue South, New York, NY 10010. Months of issue are March, June, September, and December. Business and Editorial Office: Elsevier Inc., 1600 John F. Kennedy Blvd., Ste. 1800, Philadelphia, PA 19103-2899. Accounting and Circulation Offices: Elsevier Inc., 3251 Riverport Lane, Maryland Heights, MO 63043. Periodicals postage paid at New York, NY and at additional mailing offices. Subscription prices are $228.00 per year (US individuals), $358.00 per year (US institutions), $100.00 per year (US students/residents), $283.00 per year (Canadian individuals), $383.00 per year (Canadian Institutions), $274.00 per year (foreign individuals), $383.00 per year (foreign institutions), and $120.00 per year (international students/residents), $100.00 per year (Canadian students/residents). Foreign air speed delivery is included in all *Clinics'* subscription prices. All prices are subject to change without notice. **POSTMASTER:** Send address changes to *Surgical Pathology Clinics*, Elsevier, 3251 Riverport Lane, Maryland Heights, MO 63043. **Customer Service: 1-800-654-2452 (US). From outside the United States, call 1-314-447-8871. Fax: 1-314-447-8029. E-mail: JournalsCustomerServiceusa@elsevier.com (for print support)** and **JournalsOnlineSupport-usa@elsevier.com (for online support)**.

Reprints. For copies of 100 or more, of articles in this publication, please contact the Commercial Reprints Department, Elsevier Inc., 360 Park Avenue South, New York, NY 10010-1710. Tel. 212-633-3874; Fax: 212-633-3820; E-mail: reprints@elsevier.com.

Surgical Pathology Clinics of North America is covered in *MEDLINE/PubMed (Index Medicus)*.

Contributors

CONSULTING EDITOR

JASON L. HORNICK, MD, PhD
Director of Surgical Pathology and
Immunohistochemistry, Brigham and Women's
Hospital, Professor of Pathology, Harvard
Medical School, Boston, Massachusetts, USA

EDITOR

MICHAEL T. TETZLAFF, MD, PhD
Professor, Departments of Pathology and
Dermatology, Dermatopathology and Oral
Pathology Unit, University of California, San
Francisco, San Francisco, California, USA

AUTHORS

SEPIDEH ASADBEIGI, MD
Department of Dermatology, Feinberg School
of Medicine, Northwestern University,
Chicago, Illinois, USA

SARAH BENTON, BA
Department of Dermatology, Feinberg School
of Medicine, Northwestern University,
Chicago, Illinois, USA

STEVEN D. BILLINGS, MD
Co-Director, Dermatopathology Section,
Department of Pathology, Cleveland Clinic,
Cleveland, Ohio, USA

CAROLE BITAR, MD
Department of Pathology, University of
Michigan, Ann Arbor, Michigan, USA

THOMAS BRENN, MD, PhD, FRCPath
Professor, Departments of Pathology and
Laboratory Medicine, and Medicine, Arnie
Charbonneau Cancer Institute, Cumming
School of Medicine, University of Calgary,
Calgary, Alberta, Canada

KLAUS J. BUSAM, MD
Department of Pathology, Memorial Sloan
Kettering Cancer Center, New York, New York,
USA

MAY P. CHAN, MD
Department of Pathology, University of
Michigan, Ann Arbor, Michigan, USA

SUSAN Y. CHON, MD
Professor, Department of Dermatology, The
University of Texas MD Anderson Cancer
Center, Houston, Texas, USA

EMILY Y. CHU, MD, PhD
Associate Professor, Department of
Dermatology, University of Pennsylvania,
Philadelphia, Pennsylvania, USA

JONATHAN L. CURRY, MD
Professor, Departments of Pathology, and
Translational Molecular Pathology, and
Dermatology, The University of Texas MD
Anderson Cancer Center, Houston, Texas,
USA

MOHAMMED DANY, MD, PhD
Resident Physician, Department of
Dermatology, Hospital of the University of
Pennsylvania, University of Pennsylvania,
Philadelphia, Pennsylvania, USA

JOSEPHINE K. DERMAWAN, MD, PhD
Bone and Soft Tissue Fellow, Department of
Pathology, Cleveland Clinic, Cleveland, Ohio,
USA

ANDREW S. FISCHER, MD
Dermatopathology Fellow, Department of
Dermatology, Hospital of the University of
Pennsylvania, University of Pennsylvania,
Philadelphia, Pennsylvania, USA

JEFF R. GEHLHAUSEN, MD, PhD
Dermatology Resident, PGY-3, Department of
Dermatology, Yale University, New Haven,
Connecticut, USA

PEDRAM GERAMI, MD
Department of Dermatology, Robert H. Lurie
Cancer Center, Feinberg School of Medicine,
Northwestern University, Chicago, Illinois, USA

PAUL W. HARMS, MD, PhD
Departments of Dermatology and Pathology,
University of Michigan, Ann Arbor, Michigan,
USA

WOLFGANG HARTSCHUH, MD
Professor, Department of Dermatology,
University Medical Center, Ruprecht-Karls-
University, Heidelberg, Germany

GRACE HILE, MD
Department of Dermatology, University of
Michigan, Ann Arbor, Michigan, USA

AURIS HUEN, MD, PharmD
Assistant Professor, Department of
Dermatology, The University of Texas MD
Anderson Cancer Center, Houston, Texas,
USA

SWAMINATHAN P. IYER, MD
Professor, Department of Lymphoma/
Myeloma, The University of Texas MD
Anderson Cancer Center, Houston, Texas,
USA

ACHIM A. JUNGBLUTH, MD
Department of Pathology, Memorial Sloan
Kettering Cancer Center, New York, New York,
USA

DANIEL KIM, BS
Department of Dermatology, Feinberg School
of Medicine, Northwestern University,
Chicago, Illinois, USA

CHRISTINE J. KO, MD
Professor, Departments of Dermatology and
Pathology, Yale University, New Haven,
Connecticut, USA

JENNIFER S. KO, MD, PhD
Staff, Dermatopathology Section, Department
of Pathology, Cleveland Clinic, Cleveland,
Ohio, USA

CECILIA LEZCANO, MD
Department of Pathology, Memorial Sloan
Kettering Cancer Center, New York, New York,
USA

MARIO L. MARQUES-PIUBELLI, MD
Postdoctoral Fellow, Department of
Translational Molecular Pathology, The
University of Texas MD Anderson Cancer
Center, Houston, Texas, USA

JENNIFER M. McNIFF, MD
Director of Dermatopathology, Professor,
Departments of Dermatology and Pathology,
Yale University, New Haven, Connecticut, USA

ROBERTO N. MIRANDA, MD
Professor, Department of Hematopathology,
The University of Texas MD Anderson Cancer
Center, Houston, Texas, USA

PRIYADHARSINI NAGARAJAN, MD, PhD
Assistant Professor, Pathology, The University
of Texas MD Anderson Cancer Center,
Houston, Texas, USA

JEFFREY P. NORTH, MD
Associate Professor, Dermatopathology,
Departments of Dermatology and Pathology,
University of California, San Francisco, School
of Medicine, San Francisco, California, USA

SUSAN PEI, MD
Dermatopathology Fellow, Department of Dermatology, Hospital of the University of Pennsylvania, University of Pennsylvania, Philadelphia, Pennsylvania, USA

ROBERT V. RAWSON, BCom, MBBS, FRCPA
Melanoma Institute Australia, The University of Sydney, North Sydney, New South Wales, Australia; Sydney Medical School, The University of Sydney, Sydney, New South Wales, Australia; Tissue Pathology and Diagnostic Oncology, Royal Prince Alfred Hospital and NSW Health Pathology, New South Wales, Australia

ADAM I. RUBIN, MD
Associate Professor of Dermatology, Pediatrics, and Pathology and Laboratory Medicine, Hospital of the University of Pennsylvania, Children's Hospital of Philadelphia, Perelman School of Medicine at the University of Pennsylvania, University of Pennsylvania, Philadelphia, Pennsylvania, USA

RICHARD A. SCOLYER, BMedSci, MBBS, MD, FRCPA, FRCPath
Professor, Melanoma Institute Australia, The University of Sydney, North Sydney, New South Wales, Australia; Sydney Medical School, The University of Sydney, Sydney, New South Wales, Australia; Tissue Pathology and Diagnostic Oncology, Royal Prince Alfred

Hospital and NSW Health Pathology, New South Wales, Australia

CARLOS A. TORRES-CABALA, MD
Professor, Dermatopathology Section Chief, Departments of Pathology and Dermatology, The University of Texas MD Anderson Cancer Center, Houston, Texas, USA

KATHARINA WIEDEMEYER, MD
Adjunct Assistant Professor, Department of Pathology and Laboratory Medicine, Cumming School of Medicine, University of Calgary, Calgary, Alberta, Canada; Department of Dermatology, University Medical Center, Ruprecht-Karls-University, Heidelberg, Germany

JAMES S. WILMOTT, BSci, PhD
Melanoma Institute Australia, The University of Sydney, North Sydney, New South Wales, Australia; Sydney Medical School, The University of Sydney, Sydney, New South Wales, Australia

BIN ZHANG, MS
Department of Dermatology, Feinberg School of Medicine, Northwestern University, Chicago, Illinois, USA

JEFFREY ZHAO, BA
Department of Dermatology, Feinberg School of Medicine, Northwestern University, Chicago, Illinois, USA

Contents

PRAME (PReferentially expressed Antigen in MElanoma) is a melanoma-associated antigen expressed in cutaneous and ocular melanomas and some other malignant neoplasms, while its expression in normal tissue and benign tumors is limited. Detection of PRAME protein expression by immunohistochemistry in a cohort of 400 melanocytic tumors showed diffuse nuclear immunoreactivity for PRAME in most metastatic and primary melanomas. In contrast, most nevi were negative for PRAME or showed nondiffuse immunoreactivity. The difference in the extent of immunoreactivity for PRAME in unambiguous melanocytic tumors prompted the study of PRAME as an ancillary tool for evaluating melanocytic lesions in more challenging scenarios.

Primary cutaneous T-cell lymphomas pose a diagnostic challenge for dermatopathologists, hematopathologists, and general surgical pathologists. Recognition of gamma/delta phenotype in cutaneous T proliferations has been enhanced by the availability of antibodies against TCRgamma and delta for immunohistochemistry. Thus, reporting gamma/delta phenotype in a cutaneous T-cell lymphoid proliferation may indicate a significant change in therapy and a challenge for dermatologists and oncologists who treat these patients. Herein, we discuss primary cutaneous gamma/delta T-cell lymphoma, its differential diagnosis, and other skin lymphoid proliferations that may show gamma/delta phenotype. Awareness of the occurrence of gamma/delta phenotype in both T-cell lymphomas and benign lymphoid proliferations involving skin is crucial for a better interpretation of histopathologic findings. Integration of clinical presentation, morphology, immunoprofile, and molecular findings is key for a correct diagnosis and appropriate therapy of lesions displaying gamma/delta T-cell phenotype.

This article focuses on various recently described or emerging cutaneous soft tissue neoplasms. These entities encompass a wide range of clinical and histologic characteristics. Emphasis is placed on their distinguishing morphologic and immunophenotypic features compared with entities that enter into their differential diagnosis, as well as novel immunophenotypic and molecular tests that are often necessary for accurate diagnosis of these entities. Entities discussed include EWSR1-SMAD3-rearranged fibroblastic tumor, superficial CD34-positive fibroblastic tumor, epithelioid fibrous histiocytoma, CIC-rearranged sarcomas, and NTRK-rearranged spindle cell tumors.

expression of specific diagnostic markers, such as CDX2 and LEF1 in pilomatrico-mas/pilomatrical carcinomas, and NUT in poromas/porocarcinomas. In these ways, improved understanding of molecular alterations promises to advance diagnostic, prognostic, and therapeutic possibilities for adnexal tumors.

Sebaceous neoplasia primarily includes sebaceous adenoma, sebaceoma, and sebaceous carcinoma (SC). Sebaceous adenoma, sebaceoma, and a subset of cutaneous SC are frequently associated with defective DNA mismatch repair resulting from mutations in MLH1, MSH2, or MSH6. These tumors can be sporadic or associated with Muir-Torre syndrome. SCs without defective DNA mismatch repair have ultraviolet signature mutation or paucimutational patterns. Ocular SCs have low mutation burdens and frequent mutations in ZNF750. Some ocular sebaceous carcinomas have TP53 and RB1 mutations similar to cutaneous SC, whereas others lack such mutations and are associated with human papilloma virus infection.

Pigmented epithelioid melanocytoma (PEM) was originally described based on keen morphologic analysis identifying a group of melanocytic tumors sharing heavily pigmented epithelioid melanocytes. It is defined as heavily pigmented epithelioid, spindled, and dendritic melanocytes with characteristic vesicular nuclei, prominent nucleoli, and melanophages. PEM often involves regional lymph nodes. Recent advances in molecular analysis have allowed for subclassification of PEM into more specific subsets of melanocytic tumors. The most common subsets include PRKCA fusions, which result in pure PEMs with sheets of monomorphic epithelioid melanocytes, and PEMs with combined pattern and mutations in both PRKAR1A and BRAF.

Mucosal melanomas are rare, often aggressive tumors that can arise at any mucosal site but most frequently occur in the head and neck, vulvovaginal, and anorectal regions. They have distinct biological, clinical, and histopathologic features, which have important management implications. Recent whole-genome sequencing studies have led to a greater understanding of the molecular landscape of mucosal melanomas and uncovered oncogenic drivers that could potentially be susceptible to therapeutic manipulation. The authors provide a brief overview of epidemiologic, clinical, and histopathologic features of mucosal melanoma, with particular emphasis on recent advances in understanding, which have arisen from analyzing their molecular landscape.

Although clinicians often put vasculitis and microvascular occlusion in the same differential diagnosis, biopsy findings often are either vasculitis or occlusion. However, both vasculitis and occlusion are present in some cases of levamisole-associated vasculopathy and certain infections. Depth of dermal involvement and vessel size should be reported, because superficial and deep small vessel leukocytoclastic vasculitis and/or involvement of medium-sized vessels may be associated with systemic disease. Microvascular occlusion of vessels in the fat should prompt consideration of calciphylaxis. Clues to ultimate clinical diagnosis can be garnered from depth of involvement, size of vessels affected, and presence of both vasculitis and occlusion.

Nail unit pathology is indispensable to reach an accurate diagnosis of nail tumors as well as inflammatory disorders. This review article provides an update from the most recently published studies on the pathology and management of nail unit tumors and inflammatory disorders. Recent findings of nail clipping histopathology are described first, followed by discussing recent data on the diagnosis and surgical management of several types of nail unit tumors, ending with discussing the recent discoveries in selected nail unit inflammatory disorders.

Dysplastic nevi are distinctive melanocytic lesions in the larger group of atypical nevi. They are often multiple and sporadic with clinical, histopathologic and molecular genetic features intermediate between common acquired nevi and melanoma. Dysplastic nevi may be multiple and familial and may be seen in patients with familial melanoma syndrome. Although their behavior is benign they rarely represent a precursor to melanoma. If clinically suspicious, dysplastic nevi should be removed by excision to allow for adequate histopathologic examination and exclude the possibility of melanoma. It is important to avoid partial sampling as reliable separation from melanoma requires visualization of the entire lesion to allow for examination of important architectural histopathologic features, such as lesional circumscription and symmetry and maturation with depth, and to avoid sampling error.

SURGICAL PATHOLOGY CLINICS

SERIES OF RELATED INTEREST

Clinics in Laboratory Medicine
http://www.labmed.theclinics.com/
Medical Clinics
https://www.medical.theclinics.com/

THE CLINICS ARE AVAILABLE ONLINE!
Access your subscription at:
www.theclinics.com

Preface
Dermatopathology in the Molecular Age

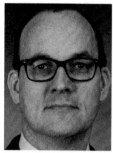

Michael T. Tetzlaff, MD, PhD
Editor

The field of dermatopathology remains one of the most dynamic subspecialties in all of pathology. Accurate diagnoses typically require a systematic integration of histopathologic features together with clinical, immunohistochemical, and molecular findings. As the arsenal of molecular studies applied to skin lesions expands, the complexity of this integration increases. In this issue, we assembled leaders across the spectrum of dermatopathology to provide comprehensive reviews and updates on various topics in the field. Melanocytic lesions are emphasized at multiple points, including a historical overview of dysplastic nevi as well as an update on PRAME immunohistochemistry and applications of this emerging and useful marker. Recent studies on mucosal melanomas identifying histopathologic prognostic biomarkers and molecular drivers are reviewed herein. Finally, there is a comprehensive historical overview and contemporary update on the molecular genetics of pigmented epithelioid melanocytoma. The diagnosis of adnexal tumors similarly remains a formidable challenge, as there can be considerable histopathologic overlap among them. The application of next-generation sequencing studies has changed this field altogether, so a comprehensive update on molecular genetic advances across the spectrum of adnexal tumors is provided. Given their unique biology, an additional article specifically focuses on the molecular genetic features of sebaceous neoplasia. Molecular advances in soft tissue tumors continue to refine their classification, so an article emphasizing new entities in cutaneous soft tissue tumors is provided. There is also a comprehensive update on cutaneous lymphomas as the complexity of these continues to evolve. Similarly, a review of nail pathologic condition contextualizes a rapidly developing area of dermatopathology. Dermatopathology also requires an intricate understanding of inflammatory diseases, and as such, comprehensive overviews of cutaneous vasculitis and connective tissue diseases, including novel biomarkers and molecular studies identifying critical drivers of these processes, are provided. Finally, with the success of immune modulatory agents in the treatment of cancer, the myriad of cutaneous toxicities caused by these agents continues to grow, and a comprehensive update on "oncodermatopathology" is also provided. These updates are written by experts in their respective topic, each of whom is a practicing dermatopathologist who recognizes the salient points that inform and improve the practice of dermatopathology.

Michael T. Tetzlaff, MD, PhD
Dermatopathology and
Oral Pathology Unit
The University of California, San Francisco
1701 Divisadero Street, #280
San Francisco, CA 94115, USA

E-mail address:
michael.tetzlaff@ucsf.edu

Surgical Pathology 14 (2021) xiii
https://doi.org/10.1016/j.path.2021.03.007
1875-9181/21/© 2021 Published by Elsevier Inc.

Michael T. Tetzlaff, MD, PhD
Editor

PRAME Immunohistochemistry as an Ancillary Test for the Assessment of Melanocytic Lesions

Cecilia Lezcano, MD*, Achim A. Jungbluth, MD,
Klaus J. Busam, MD

KEYWORDS

- PReferentially expressed Antigen in MElanoma • Immunohistochemistry • Melanoma • Nevus

Key points

- PRAME (Preferentially expressed Antigen in MElanoma) is a tumor-associated antigen first identified in a melanoma patient and found to be expressed in most melanomas and other malignant neoplasms.
- Detection of PRAME expression in formalin-fixed paraffin-embedded tissue is possible through immunohistochemistry (IHC) with commercially available monoclonal anti-PRAME antibodies.
- PRAME's frequent diffuse pattern of immunoreactivity in in situ and invasive melanoma contrasts with the infrequent and typically focal staining seen in nevi.
- Most metastatic melanomas are positive for PRAME, whereas nodal nevi are not.
- PRAME IHC results showed high concordance with cytogenetic studies in a cohort of melanocytic neoplasms with ambiguous histomorphology; however, these tests are not interchangeable.
- PRAME IHC is a valuable tool in the evaluation of melanocytic lesions; nevertheless, limitations in sensitivity and specificity as well as possible pitfalls need to be kept in mind by practicing pathologists.

ABSTRACT

PRAME (PReferentially expressed Antigen in MElanoma) is a melanoma-associated antigen expressed in cutaneous and ocular melanomas and some other malignant neoplasms, while its expression in normal tissue and benign tumors is limited. Detection of PRAME protein expression by immunohistochemistry in a cohort of 400 melanocytic tumors showed diffuse nuclear immunoreactivity for PRAME in most metastatic and primary melanomas. In contrast, most nevi were negative for PRAME or showed nondiffuse immunoreactivity. The difference in the extent of immunoreactivity for PRAME in unambiguous melanocytic tumors prompted the study of PRAME as an ancillary tool for evaluating melanocytic lesions in more challenging scenarios.

BACKGROUND

PRAME (PReferentially expressed Antigen in MElanoma) is a tumor-associated antigen that was identified by Ikeda and colleagues[1] by autologous T-cell epitope cloning in a patient with metastatic

Department of Pathology, Memorial Sloan Kettering Cancer Center, New York, NY, USA
* Corresponding author. Department of Pathology, Memorial Sloan Kettering Cancer Center, 1275 York Avenue, New York, NY 10065.
E-mail address: lezcanom@mskcc.org

Surgical Pathology 14 (2021) 165–175
https://doi.org/10.1016/j.path.2021.01.001
1875-9181/21/© 2021 Elsevier Inc. All rights reserved.

cutaneous melanoma. The expression of PRAME mRNA was detected by the authors and others not only in cutaneous and ocular melanomas, but also in various nonmelanocytic malignant neoplasms, including carcinomas of pulmonary, renal, and mammary origin, leukemia, synovial sarcoma, and myxoid liposarcoma.[2–10] Conversely, most benign adult tissue showed low or absent PRAME mRNA expression with the exception of the testis, ovary, placenta, adrenals, and endometrium.[1,11] The expression profile of the *PRAME* gene, being expressed in malignant lesions but largely restricted to testis in non-neoplastic tissue, places PRAME in the category of cancer testis antigens (CTAs).[12] This expression profile and its high prevalence in melanoma and other malignant tumors make PRAME particularly attractive for the development of targeted therapies, and clinical trials related to tumor expression of CTAs, including PRAME, are on-going.[7,13–15]

As for most CTAs, *PRAME* gene expression regulation is not yet entirely understood; however, it has been shown to be modulated by epigenetic mechanisms like DNA methylation, being hypermethylated in most normal tissues and hypomethylated in malignant cells.[16–19] Regarding its cellular functions, PRAME has been identified as a repressor of the retinoic acid receptor (RAR) signaling. Retinoic acid through RAR signaling induces proliferation arrest, differentiation, and apoptosis in many cell types. These tumor-suppressive activities are normally mediated by retinoids, and impaired RAR signaling has been implicated in carcinogenesis. PRAME has been shown to interact with RAR in a ligand-dependent manner, repressing the expression of RAR-target genes. Thus, overexpression of PRAME in many malignant neoplasms appears to contribute to cellular mechanisms of growth and tumor survival by antagonizing RAR signaling.[20–22]

PRAME mRNA expression levels have been identified as an important biomarker for metastatic risk stratification of uveal melanomas[23,24] and are part of a 12-gene expression prognostic assay.[23] PRAME is also included in a 23-gene panel assay for cutaneous melanoma diagnosis,[25,26] and in a 2-gene noninvasive molecular assay to assess the need for biopsy of melanocytic lesions.[27]

The availability of commercial monoclonal antibodies for immunohistochemical detection of PRAME protein in formalin-fixed paraffin-embedded tissue has facilitated the in situ evaluation of PRAME expression in histologic sections and allowed for exploration of possible applications in dermatopathology.

PRAME IMMUNOHISTOCHEMISTRY IN PRIMARY CUTANEOUS MELANOMA AND NEVI

In a series of 155 primary cutaneous melanomas, the prevalence and extent of PRAME expression detected by IHC was assessed. These included in situ and invasive melanoma of a wide variety of histologic subtypes, including superficial spreading melanoma, lentigo maligna melanoma, acral melanoma, desmoplastic melanoma, nondesmoplastic nodular melanoma, and a few cases of melanomas less frequently encountered such as nevoid melanoma and melanoma-ex-blue nevus.

In this series, PRAME immunoreactivity was diffuse (ie, present in >75% of tumor cells) in 129 (83.2%) of all primary melanoma cases. Considering a subgroup of only melanoma in situ cases, 45 of 48 (93.8%) cases expressed PRAME in a diffuse pattern (**Fig. 1**). When taking together all histologic subtypes of melanoma with an invasive component, the frequency of diffuse staining for PRAME was 78.5%. However, a marked difference in prevalence of diffuse PRAME expression was seen in desmoplastic versus nondesmoplastic melanoma subtypes. Although diffuse PRAME expression was observed in 88.2% to 90.9% of superficial spreading, acral, nodular, and lentigo maligna melanomas (**Fig. 2**), only 35% of desmoplastic melanomas were diffusely positive for PRAME. In cases of desmoplastic melanoma where only a subset of tumor cells were PRAME positive, these frequently corresponded to the in situ component of the tumor or to the invasive nondesmoplastic component of mixed desmoplastic melanomas (see **Fig. 2**).[28] A similarly high prevalence of PRAME expression in invasive lentigo maligna melanoma has also been reported by others, although the same study found much lower PRAME expression rates in lentigo maligna-type in situ melanoma.[29]

In contrast, of 140 cutaneous nevi, most (86.4%) lacked staining for PRAME. However, a subset of benign nevi showed PRAME immunoreactivity that in most cases was limited to less than 50% of melanocytes (**Fig. 3**). In this initial series, only 1 lesion of a pigmented junctional Spitz nevus from the cheek of a 6-year-old child showed diffuse PRAME staining. In melanomas found to be associated with a melanocytic nevus, only the melanoma tumor cells showed diffuse immunoreactivity for PRAME (**Fig. 4**).

The authors' results have been replicated in a more recent study that reported most malignant melanomas (23/24%; 95.8%) with PRAME immunoreactivity in over 60% of tumor cells, while most nevi,

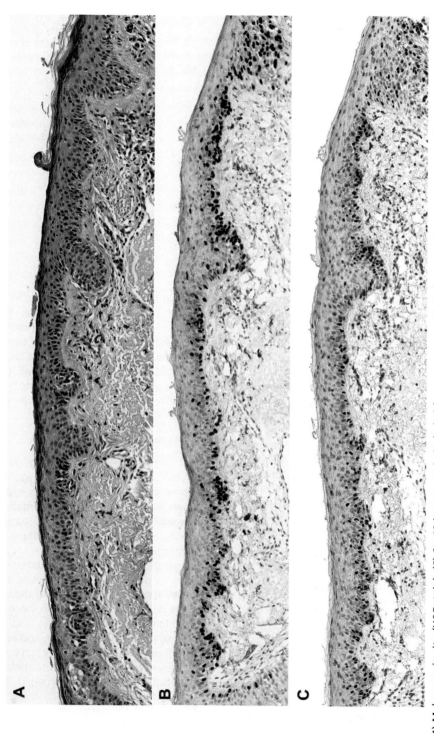

Fig. 1. (A) Melanoma in situ (H&E stain). (B) Sox10 immunostain included for comparison with the extent of staining seen with (C) PRAME, showing nuclear immuno-reactivity diffusely in virtually all tumor cells in this case.

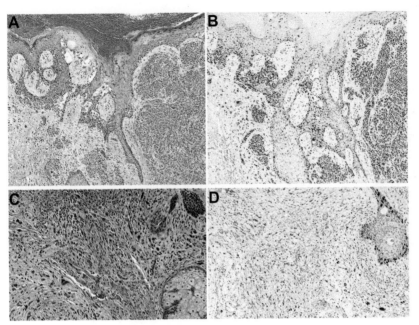

Fig. 2. Primary melanoma. (*A*) H&E stain showing in situ and invasive melanoma. (*B*) Both in situ and invasive melanoma are strongly and diffusely immunoreactive for PRAME in most cases. (*C*) Desmoplastic melanoma, mixed type (H&E). (*D*) PRAME immunoreactivity of the in situ component and subset of the nondesmoplastic invasive tumor cells.

including traumatized, recurrent/persistent, dysplastic, and mitotically active nevi were negative for PRAME (43/45%; 95.6%). This study also reported a single case of a Spitz nevus showing diffuse PRAME expression, although most Spitz nevi (15 of 20) lacked staining for PRAME.[30]

In non-neoplastic skin, nuclear PRAME staining is usually absent, or limited to few scattered melanocytes most frequently encountered in actinically damaged skin.[28,29] The authors have also noted occasional weak nuclear immunoreactivity of stromal cells in scars. Additionally, cytoplasmic PRAME staining is typically seen highlighting the cytoplasm of sebocytes in sebaceous glands. The significance of this finding is unclear. It is consistently observed with the EPR20330 clone, but not with all anti-PRAME antibodies (CL, AAJ, KJB, personal observations, 2017).

Uses include

- Supporting a suspected diagnosis of melanoma or nevus in conjunction with careful morphologic evaluation on hematoxylin and eosin (H&E) stain and correlation with clinical findings and/or additional ancillary tests when applicable
- Assisting in the evaluation of primary tumor staging and Breslow tumor thickness measurement when a dermal melanocytic population with nevoid features is encountered underlying melanoma in situ or when a combination of invasive melanoma and dermal nevic cells is suspected

- Margin assessment of melanoma in situ with broad predominantly lentiginous junctional growth and diffuse immunoreactivity for PRAME; different from other melanocytic markers such as Melan A and Sox10 that highlight all melanocytes, PRAME preferentially highlights melanoma cells and is typically negative in most background non-neoplastic melanocytes

Limitations and pitfalls include:

- Not all melanomas are diffusely positive for PRAME; some are completely negative, while others show only focal or patchy expression.
- Nevi can show PRAME immunoreactivity, but typically in only a subset of tumor cells. Rarely, benign nevi show diffuse PRAME expression.
- Larger series of less frequent tumor subtypes such as melanoma ex-blue nevus and deep penetrating nevi are needed to draw conclusions on the use of PRAME in these melanocytic tumor subsets.
- Intensity of staining can vary, and interpretation of weak immunoreactivity can be difficult.
- Occasional non-neoplastic melanocytes, especially in actinically damaged skin, can be PRAME positive, complicating the use of PRAME IHC for margin assessment, particularly in lower cellularity tumors with irregular borders.
- If a DAB detection system is used, care should be taken to not mistake melanin pigment

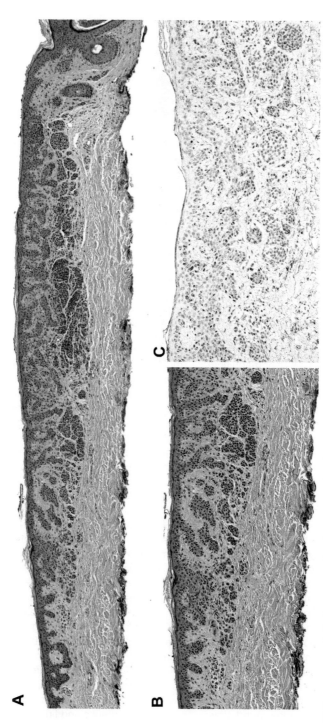

Fig. 3. PRAME immunoreactivity in a nevus. (*A, B*) Compound melanocytic nevus with architectural disorder (H&E stain). (*C*) Subset of PRAME-positive melanocytes at the dermoepidermal junction and in the superficial dermis. Note the melanin pigment within adjacent keratinocytes, which at lower magnification could give a false impression of more extensive PRAME nuclear expression in melanocytes (if using a brown chromogen); examination at medium and high magnification prevents this potential pitfall.

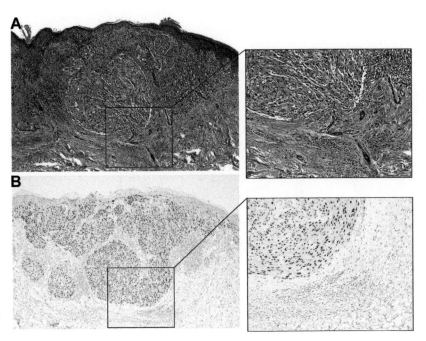

Fig. 4. (*A*) Primary melanoma with associated nevus underlying invasive melanoma cells (H&E). (*B*) IHC for PRAME stains only melanoma cells and is negative in the associated nevus.

within adjacent keratinocytes for PRAME nuclear expression in melanocytes, particularly when examining sections at scanning magnification. A closer look with a higher magnification objective lens should suffice to avoid this pitfall (see **Fig. 3**).

- Tissue sections that underwent decalcification can show a significant decrease in PRAME tumor staining.

PRAME IMMUNOHISTOCHEMISTRY IN CHALLENGING CUTANEOUS MELANOCYTIC TUMORS

Most melanocytic tumors can be readily classified as benign or malignant based on H&E histomorphology and clinical findings. However, ambiguous microscopic features and clinical context occasionally make classification and definitive diagnosis of melanocytic tumors challenging. Cytogenetic tests, including fluorescence in situ hybridization (FISH) for melanoma, genome-wide array comparative genomic hybridization (CGH), and single nucleotide polymorphism (SNP) array have been proven valuable in the assessment of melanocytic tumors.[31–37] Limitations related to these tests include their cost, turnaround time, relatively limited availability, and limitations in their sensitivity and specificity.

In light of the markedly different results of PRAME immunostaining in unequivocally benign versus malignant melanocytic neoplasms,[28] a role for PRAME IHC in the assessment of ambiguous melanocytic tumors was explored. These included melanocytic neoplasms with spitzoid and nevoid features and lesions with dysplastic, combined, or deep-penetrating nevus-like morphology. Given the intrinsic difficulty in confidently classifying the lesions solely on histomorphology and clinical findings,[38,39] evaluation of results concordance with other established ancillary tests (FISH for melanoma and SNP-array) was pursued. A threshold of greater than 75% of tumor cells positive for PRAME was established as in support of a melanoma diagnosis. Absence of PRAME or less than 75% of tumor cells immunoreactive for PRAME was interpreted as insufficient to support melanoma or in favor of an indolent lesion.

There was agreement between PRAME IHC and cytogenetic (FISH and/or SNP-array) results in 90 of 100 cases (90% concordance) and agreement of 92.7% (102 of 110 cases) between PRAME IHC results and final diagnostic interpretation that incorporated all available histomorphologic, clinical, PRAME IHC, and cytogenetic data (**Fig. 5**). Of 10 cases with discordant PRAME IHC and cytogenetic results, 6 corresponded to lesions with nondiffuse PRAME immunoreactivity in which cytogenetic results and final diagnostic interpretation favored melanoma. In 2 cases with diffuse PRAME immunoreactivity and negative cytogenetic results, the final diagnostic interpretation favored malignant melanoma. Conversely, in 2

Fig. 5. PRAME IHC in challenging melanocytic tumors. (*A*, *B*) Atypical compound melanocytic tumor with a junctional component simulating a dysplastic nevus and an unusual dermal component with nevoid features, impaired maturation, and a rare mitotic figure. (*C*) PRAME immunostain diffusely highlights the intraepidermal and dermal tumor cells. (*D*) SNP-array showed several genomic aberrations including gains in chromosome 1q, chromosome 6p, chromosome 9q, and segmental losses in chromosome 11p and 11q. FISH for melanoma confirmed that gains in 6p (RREB1) were present in junctional and dermal components (FISH not shown). Chr, chromosome, seg, segmental.

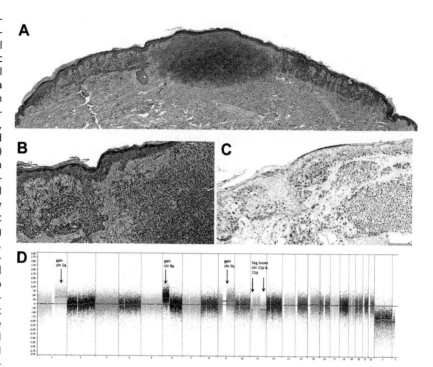

cases with final diagnostic interpretation favoring an indolent Spitz tumor in pediatric patients, PRAME IHC was negative, while cytogenetic studies were suggestive of melanoma. In this cohort of highly challenging melanocytic tumors, the sensitivity of diffuse PRAME immunoreactivity for melanoma was 75%, while its specificity was 98.8%.[40]

Uses and advantages include

- Additional evidence for diagnostic interpretation of difficult cutaneous melanocytic tumors
- Ancillary test that is easy to adopt given technical expertise in immunohistochemistry in most pathology laboratories and commercial availability of reagents including anti-PRAME monoclonal antibody
- Immunohistochemistry offers advantages over molecular tests, including more rapid turn-around time, lower cost, and familiarity of pathologists with test interpretation

Limitations and pitfalls include

- False negative: tumors with absent or focal immunoreactivity for PRAME that in light of other findings are ultimately favored to represent malignant melanoma
- False positive: a few cases with diffuse PRAME immunoreactivity upon review of all combined findings (ie, histomorphology,

clinical, and other ancillary studies such as cytogenetic tests) are indolent tumors (nevi or melanocytomas) with aberrant PRAME expression
- Intermediate extent of PRAME staining (present in >50% but <75% of tumor cells) and/or weak immunoreactivity can be difficult to interpret, limit reproducibility, and ultimately be of little to no value to inform a final diagnosis
- Despite high concordance in results, PRAME IHC is not interchangeable with cytogenetic tests for melanoma
- PRAME IHC cannot replace expert histomorphologic evaluation and correlation with relevant clinical findings.

PRAME IN THE ASSESSMENT OF NODAL MELANOCYTIC DEPOSITS

In the evaluation of 100 lesions of metastatic cutaneous melanoma to lymph nodes, soft tissue, and viscera, the authors found most (92%) were immunoreactive for PRAME, the majority (87%) of which showed diffuse PRAME nuclear staining (ie, present in >75% of tumor cells). When PRAME expression was compared in 14 paired specimens of primary cutaneous and corresponding metastatic melanoma, the extent of PRAME expression was retained or increased in the metastatic lesions.[28]

This prompted the investigation of PRAME as a possible ancillary test for the assessment of nodal melanocytic deposits as metastatic melanoma to lymph nodes can on occasion be difficult to distinguish from nodal nevi. Scenarios where this can pose a challenge include the diagnosis of subcapsular and intraparenchymal nodal nevi, metastatic melanoma confined to the fibrous capsule, and the coexistence of nodal nevi and metastatic melanoma.[41–48]

Thirty lymph nodes with nodal nevi, including 8 cases where nevic melanocytes were present in subcapsular and intraparenchymal location, were negative for PRAME and showed benign cytomorphologic features (ie, small cellular and nuclear size, regular nuclear membranes, inconspicuous or small nucleoli, and absent mitotic activity). Conversely, all 15 melanoma metastases to lymph node examined were diffusely positive for PRAME. These included 10 cases in which metastatic melanoma deposits were seen in perinodal fibrous tissue. The remaining 5 cases showed metastatic melanoma and nodal nevi co-existing in the same lymph node; in these cases, PRAME highlighted only metastatic melanoma cells and was negative in the benign melanocytes of the associated nodal nevus (Fig. 6).

A more recent series comparing the performance of PRAME with p16 IHC in the distinction of nodal melanocytic deposits, found similarly high sensitivity and specificity of PRAME immunostaining for nodal metastatic melanoma, being diffusely positive in 87% of metastatic tumor deposits. Most nodal nevi (43 out of 44) were negative for PRAME; only 1 nodal nevus was reported to show weak focal staining.[49]

Morphologic assessment of nodal melanocytic deposits on H&E routine sections remains paramount. Additionally, correlation of morphologic features between the primary tumor and suspected metastasis and knowledge of the PRAME expression status of the primary melanoma are always important. PRAME IHC may not be informative in the assessment of a nodal melanocytic deposit in the setting of a PRAME-negative primary melanoma.

Uses include:

- PRAME immunostaining of a nodal melanocytic deposit is evidence in support of metastatic melanoma.
- Absence of staining for PRAME in a nodal melanocytic deposit is evidence in support of a morphologically suspected nodal nevus, in particular when the primary melanoma is known to be diffusely positive for PRAME.

Limitations and pitfalls include:

- Not all metastatic melanomas are PRAME positive.
- Lack of PRAME expression in a nodal melanocytic deposit is noninformative in the context of a sentinel lymph node for a PRAME-negative primary melanoma.
- Nonspecific PRAME labeling of scattered hematolymphoid cells in lymph nodes could complicate the use of PRAME IHC as single label in this setting. A PRAME/Melan A double-label immunostain (PRAME nuclear labeling by DAB -brown chromogen- and Melan A cytoplasmic labeling by FastRed -red chromogen) helps circumvent this issue.
- Less frequently encountered variants of nodal nevus, such as blue nevus in lymph nodes, have not yet been evaluated with PRAME IHC.
- Other nonmelanocytic malignant tumors also express PRAME; thus assessment of lymph node metastases of poorly differentiated tumors of unclear primary requires evaluation of other IHC markers to establish tumor lineage.

PRAME IMMUNOHISTOCHEMISTRY IN CONJUNCTIVAL MELANOCYTIC NEVI AND MUCOSAL MELANOMAS

PRAME expression by IHC was found to have value in the distinction of conjunctival nevi from conjunctival melanomas in a study that used a polyclonal rabbit anti-PRAME antibody that showed some cytoplasmic labeling in addition to the expected nuclear immunoreactivity. Using a score that combined staining intensity and extent of immunoreactivity in tumor cells, conjunctival melanomas showed significantly higher levels of PRAME protein expression than conjunctival nevi.[50] A more recent study including mucosal melanomas of sinonasal, gastrointestinal, genitourinary, and oropharyngeal origin also found a high prevalence of PRAME expression.[51]

PRAME IMMUNOHISTOCHEMISTRY IN OTHER MALIGNANT NEOPLASMS

From the initial studies identifying PRAME, it has been known that PRAME mRNA is expressed in a wide variety of malignant neoplasms besides melanoma.[1] Intermediate to occasionally high levels of PRAME protein expression have also been detected by IHC in carcinomas of various origins including the ovary, lung, and breast. In mesenchymal tumors, diffuse PRAME IHC staining is seen in most synovial sarcomas and myxoid liposarcomas.[52] Clear cell sarcomas, which are

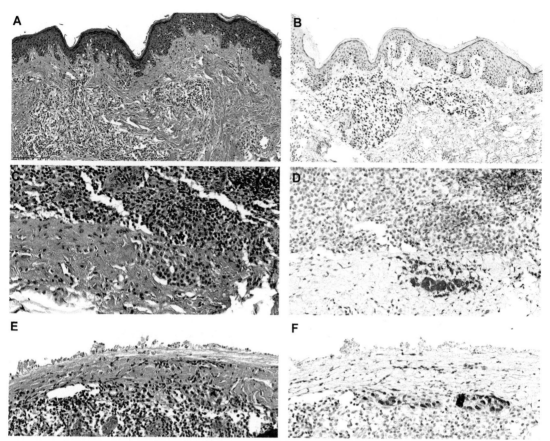

Fig. 6. Melanocytic deposits in a sentinel lymph node for melanoma. (*A*) Excision of a primary melanoma (H&E) that showed (*B*) diffuse immunoreactivity for PRAME. (*C*) The corresponding sentinel lymph node showed capsular and focally subcapsular nevic rests (H&E) (*D*) highlighted only by Melan A with a Melan A/PRAME double immunostain. (*E*) In the same lymph node, an adjacent focus of subcapsular metastatic melanoma is present (*F*) and shows colabeling of red cytoplasmic Melan A and brown nuclear PRAME (Melan A/PRAME double immunostain).

relevant to the differential diagnosis of melanoma because of similarities in histomorphology and expression of most melanocytic differentiation markers, have been found to be negative or show limited PRAME expression.[53]

There are uses and advantages:

- PRAME IHC may become a helpful time- and cost-efficient tool in the selection of best candidates for novel therapies targeting PRAME based on the detected presence and extent of PRAME protein expression across several tumor types.
- High prevalence of diffuse immunoreactivity for PRAME in malignant melanoma versus limited-to-absent expression in clear cell sarcoma shows potential value for diagnosis.

A limitation is that PRAME can be expressed in malignant tumors of various lineages; thus a panel of markers of differentiation, as well as molecular data in certain cases, is required when assessing malignant neoplasms of unknown origin (ie, diffuse PRAME immunostaining does not always equal melanoma).

SUMMARY

Diffuse labeling with PRAME IHC in melanocytic neoplasms is strongly associated with melanoma. Thus, when other findings including histomorphology, clinical context, and when applicable-additional ancillary studies favor melanoma, diffuse immunostaining for PRAME is additional supportive evidence for melanoma. However, it is critical for practicing pathologists to keep in mind that the sensitivity and specificity of PRAME IHC for melanoma are certainly not perfect and do not replace expert histopathologic evaluation.

The potential of PRAME IHC to inform the selection of cases for therapeutic purposes represents an exciting prospect where pathologists may further contribute to patient care.

ACKNOWLEDGMENTS

The authors wish to thank Denise Frosina for excellent technical assistance with the characterization of the antibody. They also thank Yesenia Gonzalez and Maria Sanchez for their assistance with digital images.

DISCLOSURE

The authors have disclosed that they have no significant relationships with, or financial interest in, any commercial companies pertaining to this article.

REFERENCES

1. Ikeda H, Lethe B, Lehmann F, et al. Characterization of an antigen that is recognized on a melanoma showing partial HLA loss by CTL expressing an NK inhibitory receptor. Immunity 1997;6:199–208.
2. Hemminger JA, Toland AE, Scharschmidt TJ, et al. Expression of cancer-testis antigens MAGEA1, MAGEA3, ACRBP, PRAME, SSX2, and CTAG2 in myxoid and round cell liposarcoma. Mod Pathol 2014; 27:1238–45.
3. Iura K, Kohashi K, Hotokebuchi Y, et al. Cancer-testis antigens PRAME and NY-ESO-1 correlate with tumour grade and poor prognosis in myxoid liposarcoma. J Pathol Clin Res 2015;1:144–59.
4. Iura K, Maekawa A, Kohashi K, et al. Cancer-testis antigen expression in synovial sarcoma: NY-ESO-1, PRAME, MAGEA4, and MAGEA1. Hum Pathol 2017;61:130–9.
5. Neumann E, Engelsberg A, Decker J, et al. Heterogeneous expression of the tumor-associated antigens RAGE-1, PRAME, and glycoprotein 75 in human renal cell carcinoma: candidates for T-cell-based immunotherapies? Cancer Res 1998;58:4090–5.
6. Oberthuer A, Hero B, Spitz R, et al. The tumor-associated antigen PRAME is universally expressed in high-stage neuroblastoma and associated with poor outcome. Clin Cancer Res 2004;10:4307–13.
7. Pujol JL, De Pas T, Rittmeyer A, et al. Safety and Immunogenicity of the PRAME cancer immunotherapeutic in patients with resected non-small cell lung cancer: a phase I dose escalation study. J Thorac Oncol 2016;11:2208–17.
8. Roszik J, Wang W-L, Ravi V, et al. Expression and clinical correlations of PRAME in sarcoma subtypes. J Clin Oncol 2016;34:11067.
9. Sanchez MI, Field MG, Kuznetsov JN, et al. The role of PRAME in promoting uveal melanoma metastasis. Abstract in: Proceedings of the AACR Annual Meeting April 1-5, 2017. Cancer Research. Washington, DC: 2017;77.
10. Zhang W, Barger CJ, Eng KH, et al. PRAME expression and promoter hypomethylation in epithelial ovarian cancer. Oncotarget 2016;7: 45352–69.
11. Goodison S, Urquidi V. The cancer testis antigen PRAME as a biomarker for solid tumor cancer management. Biomark Med 2012;6:629–32.
12. Simpson AJ, Caballero OL, Jungbluth A, et al. Cancer/testis antigens, gametogenesis and cancer. Nat Rev Cancer 2005;5:615–25.
13. Gutzmer R, Rivoltini L, Levchenko E, et al. Safety and immunogenicity of the PRAME cancer immunotherapeutic in metastatic melanoma: results of a phase I dose escalation study. ESMO Open 2016;1:e000068.
14. Chang AY, Dao T, Gejman RS, et al. A therapeutic T cell receptor mimic antibody targets tumor-associated PRAME peptide/HLA-I antigens. J Clin Invest 2017;127:2705–18.
15. Gezgin G, Luk SJ, Cao J, et al. PRAME as a potential target for immunotherapy in metastatic uveal melanoma. JAMA Ophthalmol 2017;135:541–9.
16. Schenk T, Stengel S, Goellner S, et al. Hypomethylation of PRAME is responsible for its aberrant overexpression in human malignancies. Genes Chromosomes Cancer 2007;46:796–804.
17. Ortmann CA, Eisele L, Nuckel H, et al. Aberrant hypomethylation of the cancer-testis antigen PRAME correlates with PRAME expression in acute myeloid leukemia. Ann Hematol 2008;87:809–18.
18. Roman-Gomez J, Jimenez-Velasco A, Agirre X, et al. Epigenetic regulation of PRAME gene in chronic myeloid leukemia. Leuk Res 2007;31:1521–8.
19. Luetkens T, Schafhausen P, Uhlich F, et al. Expression, epigenetic regulation, and humoral immunogenicity of cancer-testis antigens in chronic myeloid leukemia. Leuk Res 2010;34:1647–55.
20. Epping MT, Wang L, Edel MJ, et al. The human tumor antigen PRAME is a dominant repressor of retinoic acid receptor signaling. Cell 2005;122:835–47.
21. Salmaninejad A, Zamani MR, Pourvahedi M, et al. Cancer/testis antigens: expression, regulation, tumor invasion, and use in immunotherapy of cancers. Immunol Invest 2016;45:619–40.
22. Wadelin F, Fulton J, McEwan PA, et al. Leucine-rich repeat protein PRAME: expression, potential functions and clinical implications for leukaemia. Mol Cancer 2010;9:226.
23. Field MG, Decatur CL, Kurtenbach S, et al. PRAME as an independent biomarker for metastasis in uveal melanoma. Clin Cancer Res 2016;22:1234–42.
24. Field MG, Durante MA, Decatur CL, et al. Epigenetic reprogramming and aberrant expression of PRAME are associated with increased metastatic risk in Class 1 and Class 2 uveal melanomas. Oncotarget 2016;7:59209–19.

25. Clarke LE, Flake DD 2nd, Busam K, et al. An independent validation of a gene expression signature to differentiate malignant melanoma from benign melanocytic nevi. Cancer 2017;123:617–28.

26. Ko JS, Matharoo-Ball B, Billings SD, et al. Diagnostic distinction of malignant melanoma and benign nevi by a gene expression signature and correlation to clinical outcomes. Cancer Epidemiol Biomarkers Prev 2017;26:1107–13.

27. Ferris LK, Jansen B, Ho J, et al. Utility of a noninvasive 2-gene molecular assay for cutaneous melanoma and effect on the decision to biopsy. JAMA Dermatol 2017;153:675–80.

28. Lezcano C, Jungbluth AA, Nehal KS, et al. PRAME expression in melanocytic tumors. Am J Surg Pathol 2018;42:1456–65.

29. Tio D, Willemsen M, Krebbers G, et al. Differential expression of cancer testis antigens on lentigo maligna and lentigo maligna melanoma. Am J Dermatopathol 2020;42(8):625–7.

30. Raghavan SS, Wang JY, Kwok S, et al. PRAME expression in melanocytic proliferations with intermediate histopathologic or spitzoid features. J Cutan Pathol 2020;47(12):1123–31.

31. Bastian BC, LeBoit PE, Hamm H, et al. Chromosomal gains and losses in primary cutaneous melanomas detected by comparative genomic hybridization. Cancer Res 1998;58:2170–5.

32. Bastian BC, Olshen AB, LeBoit PE, et al. Classifying melanocytic tumors based on DNA copy number changes. Am J Pathol 2003;163:1765–70.

33. Bauer J, Bastian BC. Distinguishing melanocytic nevi from melanoma by DNA copy number changes: comparative genomic hybridization as a research and diagnostic tool. Dermatol Ther 2006;19:40–9.

34. Gerami P, Jewell SS, Morrison LE, et al. Fluorescence in situ hybridization (FISH) as an ancillary diagnostic tool in the diagnosis of melanoma. Am J Surg Pathol 2009;33:1146–56.

35. Gerami P, Li G, Pouryazdanparast P, et al. A highly specific and discriminatory FISH assay for distinguishing between benign and malignant melanocytic neoplasms. Am J Surg Pathol 2012;36:808–17.

36. Gerami P, Zembowicz A. Update on fluorescence in situ hybridization in melanoma: state of the art. Arch Pathol Lab Med 2011;135:830–7.

37. Wang L, Rao M, Fang Y, et al. A genome-wide high-resolution array-CGH analysis of cutaneous melanoma and comparison of array-CGH to FISH in diagnostic evaluation. J Mol Diagn 2013;15:581–91.

38. Gerami P, Busam K, Cochran A, et al. Histomorphologic assessment and interobserver diagnostic reproducibility of atypical spitzoid melanocytic neoplasms with long-term follow-up. Am J Surg Pathol 2014;38:934–40.

39. Barnhill RL, Argenyi ZB, From L, et al. Atypical Spitz nevi/tumors: lack of consensus for diagnosis, discrimination from melanoma, and prediction of outcome. Hum Pathol 1999;30:513–20.

40. Lezcano C, Jungbluth AA, Busam KJ. Comparison of immunohistochemistry for PRAME with cytogenetic test results in the evaluation of challenging melanocytic tumors. Am J Surg Pathol 2020;44:893–900.

41. Holt JB, Sangueza OP, Levine EA, et al. Nodal melanocytic nevi in sentinel lymph nodes. Correlation with melanoma-associated cutaneous nevi. Am J Clin Pathol 2004;121:58–63.

42. Patterson JW. Nevus cell aggregates in lymph nodes. Am J Clin Pathol 2004;121:13–5.

43. Ridolfi RL, Rosen PP, Thaler H. Nevus cell aggregates associated with lymph nodes: estimated frequency and clinical significance. Cancer 1977;39:164–71.

44. Azzopardi JG, Ross CM, Frizzera G. Blue naevi of lymph node capsule. Histopathology 1977;1:451–61.

45. Bautista NC, Cohen S, Anders KH. Benign melanocytic nevus cells in axillary lymph nodes. A prospective incidence and immunohistochemical study with literature review. Am J Clin Pathol 1994;102:102–8.

46. Biddle DA, Evans HL, Kemp BL, et al. Intraparenchymal nevus cell aggregates in lymph nodes: a possible diagnostic pitfall with malignant melanoma and carcinoma. Am J Surg Pathol 2003;27:673–81.

47. Bowen AR, Duffy KL, Clayton FC, et al. Benign melanocytic lymph node deposits in the setting of giant congenital melanocytic nevi: the large congenital nodal nevus. J Cutan Pathol 2015;42:832–9.

48. Carson KF, Wen DR, Li PX, et al. Nodal nevi and cutaneous melanomas. Am J Surg Pathol 1996;20:834–40.

49. See HCS, Finkelman BS, Yeldandi AV. The diagnostic utility of PRAME and p16 in distinguishing nodal nevi from nodal metastatic melanoma. Pathol Res Pract 2020;216(9):153105.

50. Westekemper H, Karimi S, Susskind D, et al. Expression of MCSP and PRAME in conjunctival melanoma. Br J Ophthalmol 2010;94:1322–7.

51. Toyama A, Siegel L, Nelson AC, et al. Analyses of molecular and histopathologic features and expression of PRAME by immunohistochemistry in mucosal melanomas. Mod Pathol 2019;32:1727–33.

52. Jungbluth A, Frosina D, Fayad M, et al. Cancer testis antigen PRAME is abundantly expressed in metastatic melanoma and other malignancies. USCAP 2018 abstracts: pathobiology (1934-1984). Mod Pathol 2018;98:695–711.

53. Raghavan SS, Wang JY, Toland A, et al. Diffuse PRAME expression is highly specific for malignant melanoma in the distinction from clear cell sarcoma. J Cutan Pathol 2020;47(12):1226–8.

Gamma/Delta Phenotype in Primary Cutaneous T-cell Lymphomas and Lymphoid Proliferations
Challenges for Diagnosis and Classification

Carlos A. Torres-Cabala, MD[a,b,*], Auris Huen, MD, PharmD[b],
Swaminathan P. Iyer, MD[c], Roberto N. Miranda, MD[d]

KEYWORDS

- Gamma-delta T-cell lymphoid proliferations of the skin • Primary cutaneous $\gamma\delta$ T-cell lymphoma
- CD30-positive T cell lymphoproliferative disorder • Lymphomatoid papulosis type D
- Hydroa vacciniforme-like lymphoproliferative disorder • Extranodal NK/T-cell lymphoma
- Subcutaneous panniculitis-like T-cell lymphoma
- Primary cutaneous CD8-positive aggressive epidermotropic cytotoxic T-cell lymphoma

Key points

- Gamma/delta phenotype can be detected by immunohistochemistry in a wide range of primary T-cell lymphoid proliferations of the skin.

- Primary cutaneous gamma/delta T-cell lymphoma, the prototype gamma/delta lymphoid proliferation in the skin, is usually clinically aggressive although indolent cases are recognized.

- The predominantly epidermotropic variant of primary cutaneous gamma/delta T-cell lymphoma seems to be distinct—biologically, histopathologically, and clinically—from the dermal/subcutaneous variant.

- The differential diagnosis of primary cutaneous gamma/delta T-cell lymphoma includes other aggressive T-cell lymphomas, mycosis fungoides, and lymphoid proliferations exhibiting the gamma/delta phenotype.

- The diagnosis of primary cutaneous gamma/delta T-cell lymphoma requires clinicopathological correlation and the correct interpretation of histopathologic findings.

ABSTRACT

Primary cutaneous T-cell lymphomas pose a diagnostic challenge for dermatopathologists, hematopathologists, and general surgical pathologists. Recognition of gamma/delta phenotype in cutaneous T proliferations has been enhanced by the availability of antibodies against TCRgamma and delta for immunohistochemistry. Thus, reporting gamma/delta phenotype in a cutaneous T-cell lymphoid proliferation may indicate a significant change in therapy and a challenge for dermatologists and oncologists who treat these patients. Herein, we discuss primary cutaneous gamma/delta T-cell lymphoma, its differential diagnosis, and other skin lymphoid proliferations

[a] Department of Pathology, The University of Texas MD Anderson Cancer Center, 1515 Holcombe Boulevard, Unit 85, Houston, TX 77030, USA; [b] Department of Dermatology, The University of Texas MD Anderson Cancer Center, 1515 Holcombe Boulevard, Unit 1452, Houston, TX 77030, USA; [c] Department of Lymphoma/Myeloma, The University of Texas MD Anderson Cancer Center, 1515 Holcombe Boulevard, Unit 429, Houston, TX 77030, USA; [d] Department of Hematopathology, The University of Texas MD Anderson Cancer Center, 1515 Holcombe Boulevard, Unit 72, Houston, TX 77030, USA
* Corresponding author.
E-mail address: ctcabala@mdanderson.org

Surgical Pathology 14 (2021) 177–194
https://doi.org/10.1016/j.path.2021.03.001
1875-9181/21/© 2021 Elsevier Inc. All rights reserved.

that may show gamma/delta phenotype. Awareness of the occurrence of gamma/delta phenotype in both T-cell lymphomas and benign lymphoid proliferations involving skin is crucial for a better interpretation of histopathologic findings. Integration of clinical presentation, morphology, immunoprofile, and molecular findings is key for a correct diagnosis and appropriate therapy of lesions displaying gamma/delta T-cell phenotype.

OVERVIEW

Primary cutaneous T-cell lymphomas (TCLs) pose a diagnostic challenge for dermatopathologists, hematopathologists, and general surgical pathologists. Recognition of these rare entities is paramount and, as in other types of cutaneous lymphoid infiltrates, correlation with clinical findings is fundamental for appropriate management.[1] In the recent years, recognition of gamma/delta ($\gamma\delta$) phenotype in cutaneous T proliferations has been enhanced by the availability of antibodies against T-cell receptor (TCR)γ and δ for immunohistochemical (IHC) testing on paraffin sections. Thus, reporting $\gamma\delta$ phenotype in a cutaneous T-cell lymphoid proliferation may indicate a significant change in therapy and a challenge for dermatologists and oncologists who treat these patients.

The $\gamma\delta$ T lymphocytes are defined by the expression of $\gamma\delta$ heterodimers in their TCR, as opposed to the more frequent T lymphocytes expressing $\alpha\beta$ TCR. CD4–/CD8– double negative thymic precursors in the bone marrow give rise to $\gamma\delta$ T cells, although some subsets may arise in extrathymic locations.[2] The $\gamma\delta$ T-cell population comprises Vδ1 and Vδ2 subpopulations, based on differences in the variable receptor region. Although Vδ1 are common in the intestine and intraepithelial locations, most $\gamma\delta$ T cells residing in the skin and detected in the blood are Vδ2,[3] where they represent a very small subset (<5%) of the total T lymphocytes. $\gamma\delta$ expression is closely linked to a cytotoxic phenotype. In fact, activated $\gamma\delta$ T cells act as cytotoxic cells and therefore frequently express markers such as T-cell intracellular antigen-1 (TIA-1), granzyme B, and perforin.[4] $\gamma\delta$ T cells also display natural killer (NK)–associated markers such as CD56, supporting their role as killer cells.

It is thought that situations such as chronic immunosuppression or antigenic modulation[5] are involved in the genesis of $\gamma\delta$ T-cell lymphoid proliferations in the skin. Although primary cutaneous $\gamma\delta$ TCL (PC$\delta\gamma$TCL) has been recognized as an aggressive but rare TCL, it is now clear that a $\gamma\delta$ phenotype is not restricted to PC$\gamma\delta$TCL, and it

can be detected in other T-cell lymphoid proliferations with variable clinical behavior. This is in part owing to the increasingly common determination of $\alpha\beta$ or $\gamma\delta$ phenotype in cutaneous lymphoid proliferations by using TCRβ (βF1), TCRγ, and TCRδ antibodies, along with testing for cytotoxic markers.[6]

Our understanding of primary cutaneous lymphoid proliferations has greatly improved in the recent years and is reflected in the revised 2016 World Health Organization classification of cutaneous lymphomas.[7] However, this group of diseases, especially those proliferations with unusual phenotypes, are still in an urgent need for accurate diagnoses and new therapeutic approaches.[8] Elucidation of the clinical significance of the $\gamma\delta$ phenotype in cutaneous T-cell proliferations will improve our understanding of these rare disorders. Herein, we discuss PC$\gamma\delta$TCL, its differential diagnosis, and other skin lymphoid proliferations that may show $\gamma\delta$ phenotype (**Box 1**).

PRIMARY CUTANEOUS $\gamma\delta$ T-CELL LYMPHOMA

PC$\gamma\delta$TCL has long been recognized to harbor a dismal prognosis,[9] although it has been showed that a predominantly epidermotropic presentation of this tumor portends a better prognosis compared with the dermal/subcutaneous-based infiltration.[10,11] Recent genomic analysis of PC$\gamma\delta$TCL suggests that these 2 variants of the disease have different cells of origin (Vδ1 for tumors originating in the upper layers of the skin and Vδ2 for deeper sited proliferations),[12] consistent with the differences in clinical behavior. Furthermore, in contrast with mycosis fungoides, the epidermotropic variant of PC$\gamma\delta$TCL lacks expression of CCR4, a marker of Th2 differentiation, supporting evidence that epidermotropic PC$\gamma\delta$TCL is different from mycosis fungoides (that has been reported to exhibit a $\gamma\delta$ phenotype in rare cases, see Differential diagnosis elsewhere in this article).[13]

CLINICAL PRESENTATION

PC$\gamma\delta$TCL usually presents with multiple rapidly progressive plaques, nodules, or tumors, often ulcerated, on the extremities and trunk (**Fig. 1**). Extracutaneous dissemination, especially mucosal and extranodal sites such as lung, thyroid, breast, or testis is frequent.

Indolent presentations, similar to mycosis fungoides[14] or rheumatologic diseases like lupus erythematous profundus[15,16] have been reported, although it is unclear whether these represent mycosis fungoides with a $\gamma\delta$ phenotype or truly indolent PC$\gamma\delta$TCL (see Differential diagnosis elsewhere in this article). Rapid progression after protracted course is rarely noted.[17] Nonaggressive cases with subcutaneous involvement have also been described.[18]

MICROSCOPIC FEATURES

The infiltrate is composed of medium to large size cytologically atypical lymphocytes with protean distribution in the epidermis, dermis, and often subcutis. Some cases may present with a strikingly paucicellular and predominantly epidermotropic infiltrate by atypical lymphocytes[19] (Fig. 2). Interface changes and hemorrhage are common.

ANCILLARY STUDIES

By immunohistochemistry (IHC), the tumor cells are typically CD3+, CD7+, and commonly double negative for both CD4 and CD8. Some cases are CD8+, and CD5 is commonly lost. The atypical lymphocytes express TIA-1, granzyme B, and perforin (Fig. 3). CD30 may be expressed. It seems that more cases of dermal or subcutaneous PC$\gamma\delta$TCL are CD56+ in contrast to the predominantly epidermotropic variant.[10,20] EBER (Epstein–Barr virus-encoded small RNA) by in situ hybridization (ISH) is negative.

By definition, the tumor cells display a γ/δ phenotype. The recently developed antibody against TCRδ has been validated and reported to be specific and comparable with the previous TCRγ.[21] Rarely, cases may show lack of expression of both TCRβ (βF1) and δ or γ, indicating a TCR silent phenotype.[22] Immunophenotypic 'shift' that consists in the gain or loss of markers such as CD4, CD5, CD7, CD8, CD30, or CD56 with disease progression is not uncommon and suggests antigenic modulation.[5] It should be emphasized that $\gamma\delta$ phenotype can be detected in other conditions, tumoral and inflammatory, and thus by itself it should not be taken as an indicator of aggressive behavior.[23]

MOLECULAR PATHOLOGY FEATURES

TCR γ and β gene rearrangements studies usually detect monoclonality. Highly complex cytogenetic abnormalities were detected in a single case.[24] Mutations in the JAK/STAT, MAPK, MYC, and chromatin pathways have been recently reported.[12]

DIFFERENTIAL DIAGNOSIS

The clinicopathologic differential diagnosis includes other cytotoxic lymphomas and lymphoproliferative disorders such as primary cutaneous CD8-positive aggressive epidermotropic cytotoxic TCL (PCAECTCL), extranodal NK/TCL (ENKTCL), nasal type,[25] subcutaneous panniculitis-like TCL (SPTCL),[26] and CD30-positive T-cell lymphoproliferative disorders such as lymphomatoid papulosis (LyP) type D (Table 1).[27]

There is still debate about the existence of mycosis fungoides with $\gamma\delta$ phenotype. We postulate that predominantly epidermotropic $\gamma\delta$ TCLs and mycosis fungoides with $\gamma\delta$ phenotype probably belong to the same group of diseases,[10] but are perhaps different from classic $\alpha\beta$ mycosis

---

Box 1

Facts to consider in the evaluation of $\gamma\delta$ and cytotoxic TCLs and lymphoproliferative disorders

- Both malignant a benign T-lymphoid proliferations may show a $\gamma\delta$ phenotype

- The $\gamma\delta$ phenotype usually correlates with cytotoxicity; this does not necessarily indicate a malignant behavior of the lesion

- Increased, likely reactive, $\gamma\delta$ T cells can be seen in:

  ○ Some B-cell lymphomas

  ○ Subcutaneous panniculitis-like TCL

  ○ Reactive and inflammatory conditions

- TIA-1, granzyme B, and perforin are cytotoxic molecules detected by immunohistochemistry

- Nonactivated cytotoxic phenotype is suggested by expression of TIA-1 but lack of expression of granzyme B and perforin

- $\gamma\delta$ T-cell proliferations usually display a double CD4/CD8 negative phenotype but can be CD8+

- Cytotoxic T-cell proliferations are commonly CD8+; CD4/CD8 double negative and CD4+ phenotypes can also be seen

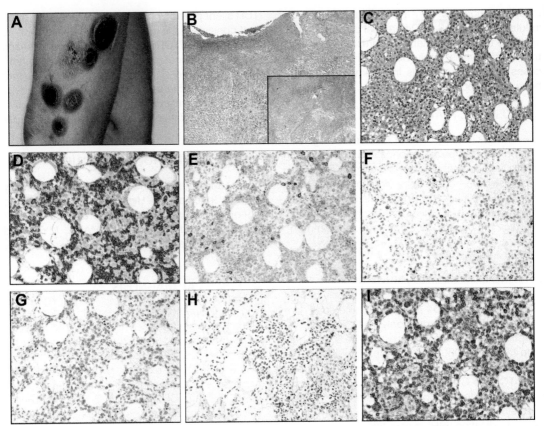

Fig. 1. PCδγTCL, dermal/subcutaneous pattern. (*A*) Ulcerated, rapidly progressive dermal and subcutaneous nodules are seen. Some lesions are necrotic and show eschar appearance. (*B*) The lymphoid infiltrate occupies the whole dermis and overlying ulceration is noted. There is involvement of the subcutaneous adipose tissue (*inset*) (stain: hematoxylin and eosin; original magnification ×40). (*C*) The atypical lymphocytes range from small to medium size. Focal rimming of adipocytes is seen (stain: hematoxylin and eosin; original magnification ×200). (*D*) The atypical lymphocytes are positive for CD3 (stain: immunohistochemistry; original magnification ×200). (*E*) Scattered CD4-positive T cells are present. Histiocytes are weakly positive for CD4 (stain: immunohistochemistry; original magnification ×200). (*F*) A double negative CD4/CD8 phenotype is confirmed by CD8 (stain: immunohistochemistry; original magnification ×200). (*G*) CD56 is weakly expressed in most of the tumor cells (stain: immunohistochemistry; original magnification ×200). (*H*) The tumor cells are negative for TCRβ that highlights scattered reactive small lymphocytes (stain: immunohistochemistry; original magnification ×200). (*I*) TCRδ labels the lymphoma cells, demonstrating the γδ phenotype of this lymphoma (stain: immunohistochemistry; original magnification ×200).

fungoides. In a recent molecular study, 38% of mycosis fungoides cases with γδ phenotype were clinically, genetically, and transcriptionally indistinguishable from PCγδTCL,[12] supporting this contention.

Rare presentations of other lymphomas with γδ phenotype in the skin, such as γδ hepatosplenic TCL,[28] may represent a pitfall in the diagnosis. Last, primary cutaneous peripheral TCL, not otherwise specified, may show similar IHC phenotype, including double negativity for CD4 and CD8 and cytotoxic profile, but, by definition, it should not display γδ phenotype.[29] Numerous γδ T cells can be detected in B-cell lymphomas.[30]

THERAPY AND PROGNOSIS

The standard treatment is a combination of chemotherapy with or without radiation therapy. Brentuximab vedotin, an anti-CD30 directed antibody–drug conjugate (anti–CD30-ADC) has been used in these patients with good efficacy and tolerance.[31] Of 7 patients who underwent allogeneic stem cell transplant, at 5 years follow-up, 4 were alive and 3 were disease free.[32] A single case with complete response to bendamustine has been reported.[33] Radiation therapy, in particular intensity modulated approach,[34] has been reported as effective in selected cases.

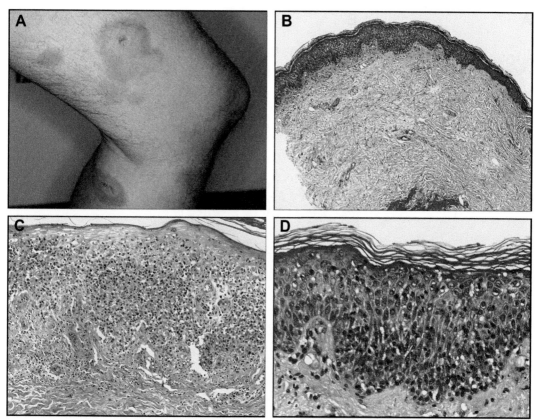

Fig. 2. PCδγTCL, predominantly epidermotropic. (*A*) At initial examination, this patient presented with eczematous patches, similar to mycosis fungoides. (*B*) The process is predominantly epidermotropic without involvement of the dermis or subcutis (stain: hematoxylin and eosin; original magnification ×40). (*C*) Some areas show epidermal acanthosis with dyskeratotic keratinocytes and underlying vascular congestion with hemorrhage (stain: hematoxylin and eosin; original magnification ×200). (*D*) The tumor lymphocytes show cytologic atypia and hyperchromasia, with prominent upward migration (stain: hematoxylin and eosin; original magnification ×400).

PRIMARY CUTANEOUS CD8-POSITIVE AGGRESSIVE EPIDERMOTROPIC CYTOTOXIC T-CELL LYMPHOMA

This nomenclature was first used by Berti and associates[35] to describe a very rare and rapidly progressive lymphoma, currently considered a provisional category in the 2016 revision of the World Health Organization classification of cutaneous lymphomas.

CLINICAL PRESENTATION

PCAECTCL presents with extensive rapidly progressive necrotic tumors or plaques. Mucous membrane involvement is frequent.[36] A more protracted clinical course with patches or plaques preceding an aggressive phase has also been reported[36] and observed by the authors (**Fig. 4**).

MICROSCOPIC FEATURES

Atypical medium to large size lymphocytes are concentrated in the superficial dermis and show epidermotropism that tends to be marked, with pagetoid pattern of infiltration and Pautrier microabscesses in cases showing extreme epidermal involvement. Adnexotropism is common.[36] Dermal and subcutaneous infiltration can be seen.

ANCILLARY STUDIES

The tumor cells are positive for CD3 and CD8 with variable loss of expression of pan T-cell markers (CD2, CD5, and CD7). In a large series, a subset of cases with CD4–/CD8– double negative phenotype was included in the PCAECTCL category.[36] Cytotoxic markers are usually expressed and CD57 may be positive. CD30 is usually negative although rare cases may be partially positive.[36]

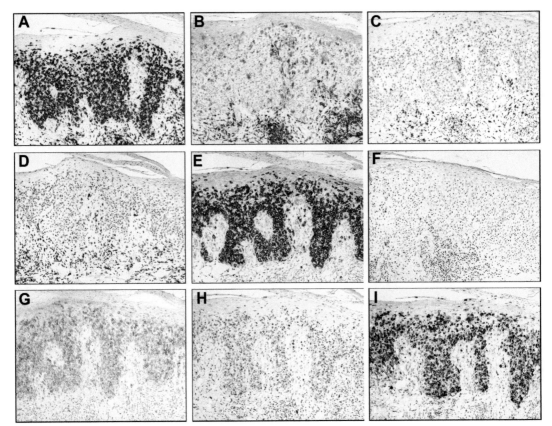

Fig. 3. PCδγTCL, predominantly epidermotropic. (*A*) The epidermotropic tumor cells are positive for CD3 (stain: immunohistochemistry; original magnification ×200). (*B*) CD4 is negative in the tumor cells and highlights intra-epidermal Langerhans and dermal lymphocytes (stain: immunohistochemistry; original magnification ×200). (*C*) The tumor cells are mostly negative for CD8, with only weak labeling in some of the cells (stain: immunohisto-chemistry; original magnification ×200). (*D*) Loss of CD5 is noted in the tumor lymphocytes (stain: immunohisto-chemistry; original magnification ×200). (*E*) Strong positivity for TCRδ is noted in the tumor cells (stain: immunohistochemistry; original magnification ×200). (*F*) TCRb (bF1) labels dermal lymphocytes only, supporting the γδ phenotype of the tumor (stain: immunohistochemistry; original magnification ×200). (*G*) The tumor cells are positive for CD56 (stain: immunohistochemistry; original magnification ×200). (*H*) TIA-1 labels the tumor cells (stain: immunohistochemistry; original magnification ×200). (*I*) The cells are strongly positive for granzyme B, in keeping with the activated cytotoxic nature of the tumor (stain: immunohistochemistry; original magnification ×200).

Tumors usually express TCRβ by IHC; however, in the aforementioned series,[36] double negative (TCR silent) or double positive αβ/γδ phenotype was noted in a few cases. EBER ISH is negative.

MOLECULAR PATHOLOGY FEATURES

Monoclonal TCR gene rearrangements are commonly detected. Through array comparative genomic hybridization, numerous aberrations such as gains in 7q, 8q24.3, and 17q, along with loss of 9p21.3 have been found.[37] However, these genetic abnormalities did not correlate with clinical outcomes and were not specific, suggesting a secondary event.[37]

DIFFERENTIAL DIAGNOSIS

Clinically, this tumor may mimic inflammatory conditions like pytiriasis lichenoides et varioliformis acute, pyoderma gangrenosum,[38] erythema multiforme[39] and infectious processes. LyP type D may closely simulate PCAECTCL histopathologically.[40] Clinical presentation, and in the case of LyP, expression of CD30 should help in the differential diagnosis. Distinction from other cytotoxic primary cutaneous lymphomas requires demonstration of αβ phenotype (to distinguish this tumor from PCγδTCL) and negativity for EBER (to distinguish it from EBV-positive cytotoxic lymphomas and lymphoproliferative disorders).

Table 1
PCδγTCL and its differential diagnosis

	Clinical Features	Histopathologic Findings	Immunophenotype	γδ Expression	Molecular Findings
PCδγTCL	Nodules or tumor that rapidly progress. Indolent and protracted presentations with progression to aggressive presentations are rarely seen	Atypical lymphocytes involving subcutis, dermis and epidermis. Epidermotropic variant. Interface changes, hemorrhage	CD3+, CD7+, CD5−, CD4−, CD8− It can be CD8+ TIA-1+, granzyme B+, perforin+ CD56+/−, CD30−/+ Immunophenotypic shift may be frequent EBER ISH negative	TCRδ+, TCRγ+, TCRβ (βF1)− Rarely TCR silent	Monoclonal TCR gene rearrangements Complex cytogenetics Mutations in JAK/STAT, MAPK, MYC, and chromatin pathways
PCAECTCL	Rapidly progressive necrotic tumors. Mucosal involvement. Rare protracted course Poor prognosis	Atypical lymphocytes involving epidermis and superficial dermis with marked epidermotropism. Subcutaneous involvement may be seen	CD3+, CD8+, CD4−, CD2+/−, CD5+/−, CD7+/− It can be CD4−/CD8− according to one series TIA-1+, granzyme B+, perforin+ CD56+/−, CD30− (usually) EBER ISH negative	TCRβ (βF1)+ TCRδ−, TCRγ− Rarely TCR silent and TCR αβ/γδ double positive	Monoclonal TCR gene rearrangements Gains in 7q, 8q24.3, and 17q Loss of 9p21.3
Hydroa vacciniforme-like lymphopro-liferative disorder	Children and adolescents with recurrent papules and vesicles leaving scars Benign to malignant behavior	Spongiosis, edema Polymorphous lymphocytic infiltrate with variable atypia	CD3+, CD8+, CD4−/+ CD2+/−, CD5+/−, CD7+/− It can be CD4−/CD8− It can have NK phenotype (CD56+, CD2+, CD3ε−, CD4−, CD8−) TIA-1+, granzyme B+, perforin+ EBER ISH positive	TCRβ (βF1)+ TCRδ−, TCRγ− Frequent TCRδ+, TCRγ+, TCRβ, (βF1)− TCR silent (NK)	Monoclonal TCR gene rearrangements (T-cell) Genetically heterogeneous
Extranodal (cutaneous) NK/TCL, nasal type	Adults with ulcerated and necrotic tumors Malignant, poor prognosis	Small to large atypical lymphocytes with angioinvasion and necrosis	CD56+, CD2+, CD3ε−, CD4−, CD8−, CD5− It can be T-cell: CD3+, CD5+, CD8+, CD4− TIA-1+, granzyme B+, perforin+ EBER ISH positive	TCR silent (NK) TCRβ (βF1)+ TCRδ−, TCRγ− Some TCRδ+, TCRγ+, TCRβ, (βF1)−	Monoclonal TCR gene rearrangements Complex cytogenetics Somatic mutations in *DDX3X, JAK-STAT, TP53, RAS, MYC, CDKN2A*

(continued on next page)

Table 1
(continued)

	Clinical Features	Histopathologic Findings	Immunophenotype	γδ Expression	Molecular Findings
SPTCL	Young women with subcutaneous nodules in lower extremities and trunk Usually good prognosis	Subcutaneous infiltrate by atypical lymphocytes rimming adipocytes, with necrosis, karyorrhexis, and hematophagocytosis It should be distinguished from PCδγTCL	CD3+, CD8+, CD4– CD2+/–, CD5+/–, CD7+/– Ki67 high CD56–, CD30– TIA-1+, granzyme B+, perforin+ EBER ISH negative	TCRβ (βF1)+ TCRδ–, TCRγ–	Monoclonal TCR gene rearrangements Germline mutations of *HAVCR2* (TIM-3), in cases presenting with hemophagocytic lymphohistiocytosis
CD30+ T-cell lymphoproliferative disorders (LyP type D)	Multiple papules that wax and wane, indolent behavior	Monomorphous lymphoid infiltrate with epidermotropism Neutrophils and eosinophils scant to absent	CD3+, CD8+, CD4–, CD30+ CD2+/–, CD5+/–, CD7+/– TIA-1+/–, granzyme B+/–, perforin+/– EBER ISH negative	TCRβ (βF1)+ TCRδ–, TCRγ– Some cases are TCRδ+, TCRγ+, TCRβ (βF1)–	Frequent monoclonal TCR gene rearrangements
Inflammatory T-cell lymphoid proliferations	Infections, chronic dermatitis, trauma	Lymphoid infiltrates with variable atypia and involvement of epidermis and dermis	CD3+, CD8+/–, CD4–/+	Can be TCRδ+, TCRγ+, TCRβ (βF1)–	Not applicable

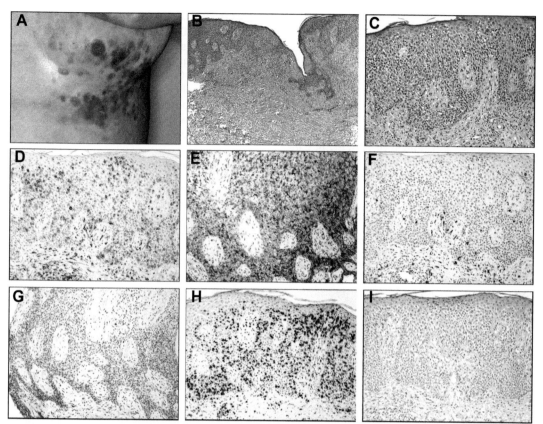

Fig. 4. PCAECTCL. (*A*) This patient presented with a history of patches and plaques that after a few months displayed the typical aggressive behavior of this tumor. (*B*) The skin biopsy reveals an almost exclusively epidermotropic infiltrate (stain: hematoxylin and eosin; original magnification ×40). (*C*) Single atypical lymphocytes involve the epidermis without formation of microabscesses (stain: hematoxylin and eosin; original magnification ×200). (*D*) The atypical lymphocytes are CD3-positive (stain: immunohistochemistry; original magnification ×200). (*E*) The tumor lymphocytes were diffusely positive for CD8 in the initial biopsy, and negative for CD4 (not shown) (stain: immunohistochemistry; original magnification ×200). (*F*) After a few months of therapy the tumor switched to double CD8/CD4-negative, a phenotype that may be seen in this lymphoma (stain: CD8 immunohistochemistry; original magnification ×200). (*G*) The tumor cells are essentially negative for CD30 (stain: immunohistochemistry; original magnification ×200). (*H*) TCRβ (βF1) highlights the epidermotropic tumor cells (stain: immunohistochemistry; original magnification ×200). (*I*) The tumor cells are negative for TCRδ (stain: immunohistochemistry; original magnification ×200).

THERAPY AND PROGNOSIS

Chemotherapy is used in these cases. Isolated reports on successful therapies include brentuximab vedotin[41] and stem cell transplantation. The prognosis is usually poor.

EPSTEIN–BARR VIRUS–POSITIVE T/NATURAL KILLER CELL LYMPHOMAS AND LYMPHOID PROLIFERATIONS

These are NK/T lymphomas and lymphoproliferative disorders that are associated with Epstein–Barr virus (EBV) infection. These diseases are more commonly seen in Latin America and East Asia, where EBV infection is prevalent. In the skin, 2 main categories of tumors are considered: hydroa vacciniforme-like lymphoproliferative disorder (HV-LPD) and extranodal (cutaneous) NK/TCL, nasal type. Whereas HV-LPD is considered a manifestation of chronic active EBV infection and comprises a spectrum of benign and malignant disorders such as classic HV, intermediate forms, and HV-like TCL,[42] ENKTCL is invariably an aggressive lymphoma with high mortality rate.

CLINICAL PRESENTATION

HV-LPD is more common in children and adolescents and is characterized by recurrent papules and vesicles on sun-exposed skin that heal leaving varioliform scars[43] (**Fig. 5**). Central facial edema is common. Severe cases may present with systemic symptoms and progression to lymphoma.[44]

ENKTCL usually occurs in adults as cutaneous ulcerated and necrotic tumors.

MICROSCOPIC FEATURES

The microscopic appearance of HV-LPD is variable. Spongiosis and vesicle formation, dermal edema, and a polymorphous lymphoid infiltrate in a perivascular, periadnexal, or diffuse distribution are noted. Involvement of the subcutis may be present.

ENKTCL is often associated with extensive necrosis and ulceration. The tumor lymphocytes range from small to large and pleomorphic and usually show angioinvasion.

ANCILLARY STUDIES

HV-LPD is usually a CD8+, EBER+ T-cell process, with frequent expression of TIA-1, granzyme B, and perforin by IHC.[45] Loss of pan T-cell markers is variable. Rarely, the lesion cells are CD4/CD8 double negative, CD4+ or CD56+, the latter indicating a NK phenotype.[46] CD30 may be expressed by a subset of lymphocytes. The T lymphocytes commonly express βF1 indicating an α/β phenotype, but a γ/δ phenotype seems to be frequent.[23]

ENKTCL is more often an NK proliferation, positive for CD2, CD56, and CD3ε by IHC (**Fig. 6**). Pan T-cell markers such as CD3, CD4, CD8, and CD5 are usually negative. The TCLs are a minority of cases and are CD3+, CD8+, and CD5+.[46] Both NK and T lymphomas express cytotoxic markers. EBER ISH is positive. As in HV-LPD, the TCLs frequently show α/β phenotype; however, cases of γ/δ phenotype are well-recognized.[47]

MOLECULAR PATHOLOGY FEATURES

Monoclonal TCR gene rearrangements can be detected in cases of HV-LPD and ENKTCL of T-cell lineage. HV-LPD is a genetically heterogeneous disease that may be more associated with epigenetic or environmental changes.[47] In contrast, ENKTCL has been found to harbor complex genomic abnormalities, the most frequent being 6q21 deletion, 1q21 gain, and 17p11 deletion.[46] Several somatic mutations involving genes such as *DDX3X*, *JAK-STAT*, *TP53*, *RAS*, *MYC*, and *CDKN2A*, among others, have been identified.[46]

DIFFERENTIAL DIAGNOSIS

The clinical presentation and geographic occurrence of most cases of HV-LPD should help in the differential diagnosis between this and other EBV-positive cytotoxic lymphomas. Conversely,

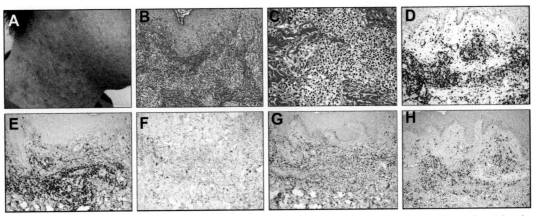

Fig. 5. HV-LPD. (*A*) Some cases may present in young adults, like this patient from Peru. Papules and vesicles that heal leaving scars are characteristic of this entity. (*B*) A superficial perivascular lymphoid infiltrate occupying the superficial and mid-dermis is present (stain: hematoxylin and eosin; original magnification ×40). (*C*) The infiltrate is polymorphous and composed of small to medium size lymphocytes with variable cytologic atypia (stain: hematoxylin and eosin; original magnification ×100). (*D*) CD3 demonstrates the T nature of the infiltrate (stain: immunohistochemistry; original magnification ×100). (*E*) The infiltrate is CD8-positive (stain: immunohistochemistry; original magnification ×100). (*F*) Scattered CD30-positive cells are seen (stain: immunohistochemistry; original magnification ×100). (*G*) TIA-1 is expressed by the lesion cells, supporting a cytotoxic phenotype (stain: immunohistochemistry; original magnification ×100). (*H*) EBER demonstrates diffuse positivity in the lesion (ISH, ×100). (Clinical photograph *Courtesy of* Francisco Bravo MD, Lima, Peru.)

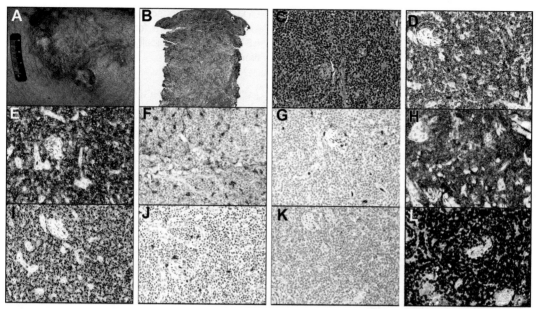

Fig. 6. Extranodal (cutaneous) NK/TCL, nasal type. (*A*) Indurated lesions with hemorrhagic and necrotic appearance are seen in this case. (*B*) A punch biopsy reveals diffuse pandermal infiltrate by lymphoid cells (stain: hematoxylin and eosin; original magnification ×20). (*C*) The cells are monomorphic, medium size cells that tend to distribute around blood vessels (stain: hematoxylin and eosin; original magnification ×200). (*D*) CD3 is diffusely positive in this case, and mostly cytoplasmic (stain: immunohistochemistry; original magnification ×200). (*E*) The tumor cells were also diffusely positive for CD7 (stain: immunohistochemistry; original magnification ×200). (*F*) CD4 was negative in the tumor cells (stain: immunohistochemistry; original magnification ×200). (*G*) CD8 highlights rare lymphocytes while the tumor cells are negative (stain: immunohistochemistry; original magnification ×200). (*H*) CD56 is strongly expressed by the tumor cells (stain: immunohistochemistry; original magnification ×200). (*I*) The cytotoxic nature of these NK cells is demonstrated by expression of TIA-1 (stain: immunohistochemistry; original magnification ×200). (*J*) TCRβ highlights scattered TCRαβ lymphocytes (stain: immunohistochemistry; original magnification ×200). (*K*) TCRδ is negative in the infiltrate (stain: immunohistochemistry; original magnification ×200). (*L*) EBER is diffusely expressed by the tumor cells (ISH, ×200).

although HV-LPD may be clinically similar to LyP, positivity for EBER favors HV-LPD.

The wide range of histopathologic appearances of ENKTCL makes its diagnosis at many times challenging. Inflammatory conditions may be entertained in early lesions, although obvious lymphomatous proliferations need to be distinguished from other cutaneous cytotoxic lymphomas. The clinical presentation should help in the distinction between ENKTCL and HV-LPD. LyP type E, PCγδTCL, SPTCL, and peripheral TCL not otherwise specified are all negative for EBER ISH.

THERAPY AND PROGNOSIS

Because HV-LPD comprises a spectrum of benign and malignant presentations, therapy depends on the extent of the disease. It seems that HV-LPD with EBV-infected γδ T cells may show a better prognosis.[47] Localized ENKTCL is treated with high-dose radiotherapy, and allogeneic hematopoietic cell transplantation is recommended for most cases.[48] The prognosis is poor.

SUBCUTANEOUS PANNICULITIS-LIKE T-CELL LYMPHOMA

SPTCL is a cytotoxic lymphoma that almost exclusively involves subcutaneous adipose tissue. It is an intriguing disease associated with autoimmune disorders and generally exhibits a good prognosis.

CLINICAL PRESENTATION

SPTCL mainly affects young women and presents as multiple subcutaneous nodules or plaques with predilection for the lower extremities and trunk.[48] Patients may present with systemic symptoms and hemophagocytic lymphohistiocytosis. An association with lupus erythematous is well-documented.

MICROSCOPIC FEATURES

SPTCL typically affects the subcutis without involvement of dermis and epidermis. The infiltrate consists of atypical lymphocytes with conspicuous rimming adipocytes. An associated reactive infiltrate, sometimes dense and/or granulomatous, can be present. Karyorrhexis and fat necrosis are frequent, and hematophagocytosis may be seen.

ANCILLARY STUDIES

By IHC, the tumor cells are positive for CD3, CD8, and βF1 and show an activated cytotoxic phenotype (Fig. 7). A loss of pan T-cell markers (CD2, CD5, and CD7) is sometimes detected. The cells are usually negative for CD4, CD56, CD30, and EBER ISH. Ki67 typically demonstrates a high proliferation index.[49]

MOLECULAR PATHOLOGY FEATURES

Monoclonal rearrangements of TCR are detected in most cases. Germline mutations of *HAVCR2*, a gene that encodes T-cell immunoglobulin mucin 3 (TIM-3), have been linked to SPTCL presenting with hemophagocytic lymphohistiocytosis[50] and detected in tumors not associated with autoimmune disease.[51]

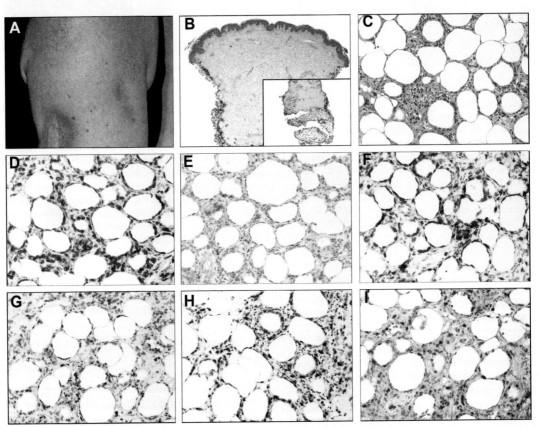

Fig. 7. SPTCL. (A) This patient presented with subcutaneous nodules associated with areas of lipoatrophy. (B) A skin biopsy shows unremarkable epidermis and deep dermis. Only the subcutaneous adipose tissue (inset) is involved by a lobular infiltrate (stain: hematoxylin and eosin; original magnification ×40). (C) The subcutaneous infiltrate is composed of small and medium sized atypical lymphocytes, admixed with some histiocytes. Focal rimming of adipocytes is seen (stain: hematoxylin and eosin; original magnification ×200). (D) CD3 better demonstrates the arrangement of the atypical lymphocytes around adipocytes (stain: immunohistochemistry; original magnification ×200). (E) The tumor cells are negative for CD4 that weakly labels scattered histiocytes (stain: immunohistochemistry; original magnification ×200). (F) In contrast, the lymphocytes are positive for CD8 (stain: immunohistochemistry; original magnification ×200). (G) TIA-1 is positive in most of the lymphocytes, supporting a cytotoxic type of lymphoma (stain: immunohistochemistry; original magnification ×200). (H) The tumor lymphocytes express βF1 (stain: immunohistochemistry; original magnification ×200). (I) TCRγ highlights numerous small lymphocytes, interpreted as reactive γδ T cells, not infrequently found in this lymphoma (stain: immunohistochemistry; original magnification ×200).

DIFFERENTIAL DIAGNOSIS

Lupus erythematous profundus may precede or overlap with SPTCL and, therefore, distinguishing these 2 diseases may be very difficult. Lymphoid aggregates with germinal center formation, hyaline degeneration of the fat, and a low Ki67 proliferation index[49] are more common in lupus erythematous profundus than in SPTCL. Plasma cells and aggregates of plasmacytoid dendritic cells (detected with CD123) also favor lupus erythematous profundus. Atypical lobular lymphocytic panniculitis is a term sometimes used for lymphoid panniculitis that showed TCR clonality, but do not completely fulfill the diagnostic criteria for SPTCL.[52] Other cytotoxic lymphomas such as ENKTCL and PCγδTCL are distinguished from SPTCL by their positivity for EBER and γδ phenotype, respectively.

THERAPY AND PROGNOSIS

SPTCL is often an indolent lymphoma with more than 80% survival at 5 years.[48] Immunosuppression with systemic steroids, cyclosporine A, bexarotene, or methotrexate is the first line of therapy. Patients with hemophagocytic lymphohistiocytosis require more aggressive treatments, such as chemotherapy and hematopoietic stem cell transplantation.[53]

CD30-POSITIVE T-CELL LYMPHOPROLIFERATIVE DISORDERS THAT MAY SHOW γδ AND CYTOTOXIC PHENOTYPE

Primary cutaneous CD30-positive T-cell lymphoproliferative disorders comprise LyP and primary cutaneous anaplastic large cell lymphoma (PC-ALCL). These lymphoid processes can be CD8 positive and frequently express cytotoxic markers.[54] In the absence of critical clinical information, the histopathologic and immunophenotypic findings seen in indolent entities can be easily misinterpreted as those of aggressive lymphomas, as demonstrated in reports of CD8-positive LyP with cytotoxic phenotype[55] that most likely represent cases of the recently accepted variants of LyP, named types D[56] and E.[57]

CLINICAL PRESENTATION

In the largest series of CD8+ LyP and PC ALCL to date,[40] these tumors did not differ clinically from other phenotypic variants. In general, crops of multiple papules followed by spontaneous remission characterize LyP, while solitary or localized grouped tumors and papules constitute the common clinical presentation of PC-ALCL. LyP type E tends to present with few or solitary lesions that show extensive ulceration and necrosis (eschar-like appearance), making the clinical distinction between LyP and other processes more challenging.

MICROSCOPIC FEATURES

In contrast with the more common types of LyP (like type A), type D reveals a more homogeneous perivascular, nodular, or diffuse lymphoid infiltrate composed of lymphocytes varying in size and associated with only scattered, if any, neutrophils or eosinophils.[40] Epidermotropism may be marked in LyP type D, and folliculotropism can be seen. LyP type E is characterized by angiocentric infiltrates associated with extensive necrosis and often thrombosis. Clusters of eosinophils are commonly seen and focal epidermotropism may be detected.[57]

Cytotoxic phenotype can be detected in a large proportion of PC-ALCL. Among the several histopathologic variants of PC-ALCL,[58] no definite microscopic findings have been reported to be linked to cytotoxic phenotype in PC-ALCL.

ANCILLARY STUDIES

By IHC, these processes can be characterized as T-cell proliferations by positivity for CD3, CD2, CD5, or CD7, although the loss of expression of 1 or more of these markers is fairly common. LyP type D is, by definition, a CD8+ proliferation, CD4-negative, with variable labeling for CD30. These processes generally express at least one cytotoxic marker,[56] usually TIA-1 or granzyme B.[59] Some cases are of γδ phenotype, revealed by positivity for TCRδ or TCRγ and lack of βF1 (Fig. 8).

Most cases of LyP type E are CD8+, although CD4+ cells can be seen composing the angioinvasive infiltrates.[57] CD30 is usually present and TIA-1 detected in most of the cases. In the original series by Kempf and colleagues,[57] no cases showing γδ phenotype were reported. EBER by ISH is negative in all cases.

Cytotoxic markers can be detected by IHC in up to 62% of cases of PC-ALCL.[60] The expression of CD8 is rather uncommon (18% according to Massone and colleagues[60]) and is usually concomitant to cytotoxic phenotype. γδ phenotype in PC-ALCL seems to be extremely rare, with no cases reported in a large series of cutaneous lymphomas.[23] As in CD4+ PC-ALCL, the expression of Epithelial membrane antigen (EMA) seems to

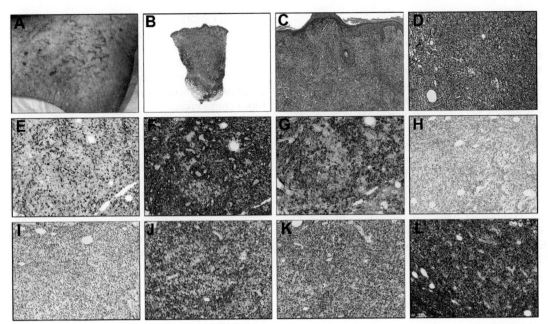

Fig. 8. LyP type D with γδ phenotype. (A) The most common clinical presentation is that of multiple papules, sometimes ulcerated, that self-regress and recur. (B) This skin punch shows a pandermal infiltrate with extension into the underlying subcutaneous adipose tissue (stain: hematoxylin and eosin; original magnification ×20). (C) Epidermotropism and even folliculotropism can be seen in CD30-positive T-cell lymphoproliferative disorders (stain: hematoxylin and eosin; original magnification ×40). (D) The infiltrate in LyP, in contrast with other types of LyP is rather monotonous, composed of small and large lymphocytes. Other cells such as neutrophils and eosinophils are rarely present (stain: hematoxylin and eosin; original magnification ×100). (E) Loss of expression of CD3 in at least a subset of the lesion cells is frequently detected (stain: immunohistochemistry; original magnification ×100). (F) The infiltrate is strongly and diffusely positive for CD8 (stain: immunohistochemistry; original magnification ×100). (G) CD30 is expressed by most of the cells in the infiltrate (stain: immunohistochemistry; original magnification ×100). (H) The lesion cells are negative for CD56 (stain: immunohistochemistry; original magnification ×100). (I) The lesion cells are negative for βF1 that highlights rare small reactive lymphocytes (stain: immunohistochemistry; original magnification ×100). (J) TCRδ labels the lesion cells, supporting the γδ phenotype of this LyP (stain: immunohistochemistry; original magnification ×100). (K) A cytotoxic phenotype is supported by granular cytoplasmic expression of TIA-1 and granzyme B (L) (stain: immunohistochemistry; original magnification ×100).

be rare. MUM-1 (IRF4) has been reported to be at least focally expressed in both CD8+ LyP and PC-ALCL.[59]

MOLECULAR PATHOLOGY FEATURES

Clonal TCR gene rearrangements are frequently demonstrated in these disorders. LyP with 6p25.3 rearrangements can be CD8+ and express cytotoxic markers.[61] 6p25.3 rearrangements, involving *DUSP22/IRF4* and detected by FISH, were present in at least 1 case of CD8+ PC-ALCL.[62] Similarly, the rare PC-ALCL with *ALK* translocations can have CD8+ phenotype and frequently express TIA-1.[63]

DIFFERENTIAL DIAGNOSIS

The main differential diagnosis of LyP type D is PCAECTCL,[40] from which it is distinguished based

on clinical presentation and CD30 expression. PCδγTCL may be considered in select cases and, in such instances, clinical correlation is crucial. LyP type E may mimic angioinvasive lymphomas such as NK/TCL, nasal type; however, EBER is consistently negative in LyP, and their respective clinical courses are different. CD8+ PC-ALCL should be distinguished from mycosis fungoides with large cell transformation, a task usually made according to clinical history. Loss of pan T-cell markers other than CD7 may suggest PC-ALCL over mycosis fungoides with large cell transformation, and expression of GATA-3 may indicate mycosis fungoides with large cell transformation rather than ALCL.[64]

THERAPY AND PROGNOSIS

LyP is usually a self-limited process for which therapy is seldom required, harboring an excellent prognosis. PC-ALCL is treated with surgery and local radiation therapy, and its prognosis is in general good. Brentuximab vedotin has demonstrated efficacy in both PC-ALCL and LyP.[65]

INFLAMMATORY CONDITIONS THAT MAY DISPLAY γδ T LYMPHOCYTIC INFILTRATES

Cutaneous γδ T lymphocytes are activated by trauma (like burns), malignancy, and/or infection.[66] It is known that, once activated, γδ T cells change morphology from dendritic (hence their designation as dendritic epidermal T cells) to round and induce wound healing, leukocyte recruitment, chronic inflammation, and keratinocyte proliferation.[66] Also, a subset of γδ T cells (γδ 17 cells) produce IL-17, in addition to T helper 17 CD4+ T cells (Th17).[67]

High numbers of IL-17–producing γδ T cells have been identified in psoriasis[68] and increased IL-4 producing γδ T lymphocytes have been detected in the skin of patients with allergic contact dermatitis caused by corticosteroids.[69] The lymphoid infiltrates of pytiriasis lichenoides et varioliformis acute can show γδ phenotype and may mimic PCδγTCL.[70] T-cell proliferations with γδ phenotype have been observed in S maltophilia[71] and herpesvirus infections,[72] and in association with a tick bite.[73]

SUMMARY

Although the γδ phenotype of the TCR was originally associated with an aggressive cutaneous lymphoma known as PCδγTCL, the availability of antibodies for use in formalin fixed, paraffin-embedded tissues has expanded the spectrum of benign and malignant lymphoproliferative disorders associated with TCR γδ expression. An awareness of the occurrence of γδ phenotype in both TCLs and benign lymphoid proliferations involving skin is crucial for a better interpretation of the histopathologic findings. Integration of clinical presentation, morphology, immunoprofile, and molecular findings is key for a correct diagnosis and appropriate therapy of lesions displaying a γδ T-cell phenotype.

CLINICS CARE POINTS

- Primary cutaneous TCLs are rare and represent a diagnostic and therapeutic challenge for pathologists and clinicians.

- The γδ phenotype can be detected in a wide range of T-cell lymphoid proliferations of the skin, both benign and malignant.

- Adequate interpretation of γδ phenotype in a cutaneous T-cell lymphoid proliferation needs careful correlation with other histopathologic and clinical findings, because it does not necessarily imply malignant or more aggressive behavior.

- PCδγTCL, the prototype of these diseases, needs to be distinguished from other processes by adequate evaluation of histopathologic findings and clinical presentation.

- It seems that the predominantly epidermotropic variant of PCδγTCL portends a better prognosis than the classic dermal/subcutaneous presentation and that these 2 variants originate from different γδ T cells.

DISCLOSURE

S.P. Iyer reports research grants from Merck, Seattle Genetics, Rhizen, Affimed, Spectrum, Trillium, CrisprRx, Novartis; Speaking: Target Oncology, Curio Biosciences outside the submitted work.

REFERENCES

1. Torres-Cabala CA. Diagnosis of T-cell lymphoid proliferations of the skin: putting all the pieces together. Mod Pathol 2020;33(Suppl 1):83–95.

2. Tripodo C, Iannitto E, Florena AM, et al. Gamma-delta T-cell lymphomas. Nat Rev Clin Oncol 2009; 6(12):707–17.

3. Foppoli M, Ferreri AJ. Gamma-delta t-cell lymphomas. Eur J Haematol 2015;94(3):206–18.

4. Swerdlow SH, Jaffe ES, Brousset P, et al. Cytotoxic T-cell and NK-cell lymphomas: current questions and controversies. Am J Surg Pathol 2014;38(10): e60–71.

5. Agbay RL, Torres-Cabala CA, Patel KP, et al. Immunophenotypic shifts in primary cutaneous gamma-delta T-Cell lymphoma suggest antigenic modulation: a study of sequential biopsy specimens. Am J Surg Pathol 2017;41(4):431–45.

6. Santucci M, Pimpinelli N, Massi D, et al. Cytotoxic/natural killer cell cutaneous lymphomas. Report of EORTC Cutaneous Lymphoma Task Force Workshop. Cancer 2003;97(3):610–27.

7. Berti EWR, Guitart J, Jaffe ES, et al. Primary cutaneous peripheral T-cell lymphomas, rare subtypes. In: Elder DE, Scolyer RA, Willemze R, editors. WHO classification of skin tumours. 4th edition. Lyon: International Agency for Research on Cancer; 2018. p. 248–53.

8. van der Weyden C, McCormack C, Lade S, et al. Rare T-Cell subtypes. Cancer Treat Res 2019;176: 195–224.

9. Toro JR, Beaty M, Sorbara L, et al. gamma delta T-cell lymphoma of the skin: a clinical, microscopic, and molecular study. Arch Dermatol 2000;136(8): 1024–32.

10. Merrill ED, Agbay R, Miranda RN, et al. Primary cutaneous T-Cell lymphomas showing gamma-delta (gammadelta) phenotype and predominantly epidermotropic pattern are clinicopathologically distinct from classic primary cutaneous gammadelta T-cell lymphomas. Am J Surg Pathol 2017;41(2): 204–15.

11. Guitart J, Weisenburger DD, Subtil A, et al. Cutaneous gammadelta T-cell lymphomas: a spectrum of presentations with overlap with other cytotoxic lymphomas. Am J Surg Pathol 2012;36(11):1656–65.

12. Daniels J, Doukas PG, Escala MEM, et al. Cellular origins and genetic landscape of cutaneous gamma delta T cell lymphomas. Nat Commun 2020;11(1): 1806.

13. Jour G, Aung PP, Merrill ED, et al. Differential expression of CCR4 in primary cutaneous gamma/delta (gammadelta) T cell lymphomas and mycosis fungoides: significance for diagnosis and therapy. J Dermatol Sci 2018;89(1):88–91.

14. Kempf W, Kazakov DV, Scheidegger PE, et al. Two cases of primary cutaneous lymphoma with a gamma/delta+ phenotype and an indolent course: further evidence of heterogeneity of cutaneous gamma/delta+ T-cell lymphomas. Am J Dermatopathol 2014;36(7):570–7.

15. von Ducker L, Fleischer M, Stutz N, et al. Primary cutaneous gamma-delta T-Cell lymphoma with long-term indolent clinical course initially mimicking lupus erythematosus profundus. Front Oncol 2020; 10:133.

16. Yi L, Qun S, Wenjie Z, et al. The presenting manifestations of subcutaneous panniculitis-like T-cell lymphoma and T-cell lymphoma and cutaneous gammadelta T-cell lymphoma may mimic those of rheumatic diseases: a report of 11 cases. Clin Rheumatol 2013;32(8):1169–75.

17. Alexander RE, Webb AR, Abuel-Haija M, et al. Rapid progression of primary cutaneous gamma-delta T-cell lymphoma with an initial indolent clinical presentation. Am J Dermatopathol 2014;36(10):839–42.

18. Khallaayoune M, Grange F, Condamina M, et al. Primary cutaneous gamma-delta T-cell lymphoma: not an aggressive disease in all cases. Acta Derm Venereol 2020;100(1):adv00035.

19. Ramani NS, Curry JL, Merrill ED, et al. Primary cutaneous gamma-delta (gamma/delta) T-cell lymphoma: an unusual case with very subtle histopathological findings. Am J Dermatopathol 2016;38(10):e147–9.

20. Cocks M, Porcu P, Wick MR, et al. Recent advances in cutaneous t-cell lymphoma: diagnostic and prognostic considerations. Surg Pathol Clin 2019;12(3): 783–803.

21. Pulitzer M, Geller S, Kumar E, et al. T-cell receptor-delta expression and gammadelta+ T-cell infiltrates in primary cutaneous gammadelta T-cell lymphoma and other cutaneous T-cell lymphoproliferative disorders. Histopathology 2018;73(4):653–62.

22. Junkins-Hopkins JM. Aggressive cutaneous T-cell lymphomas. Semin Diagn Pathol 2017;34(1):44–59.

23. Rodriguez-Pinilla SM, Ortiz-Romero PL, Monsalvez V, et al. TCR-gamma expression in primary cutaneous T-cell lymphomas. Am J Surg Pathol 2013;37(3):375–84.

24. Yamamoto-Sugitani M, Kuroda J, Shimura Y, et al. Comprehensive cytogenetic study of primary cutaneous gamma-delta T-cell lymphoma by means of spectral karyotyping and genome-wide single nucleotide polymorphism array. Cancer Genet 2012;205(9):459–64.

25. Geller S, Myskowski PL, Pulitzer M. NK/T-cell lymphoma, nasal type, gammadelta T-cell lymphoma, and CD8-positive epidermotropic T-cell lymphoma-clinical and histopathologic features, differential diagnosis, and treatment. Semin Cutan Med Surg 2018;37(1):30–8.

26. Willemze R. Cutaneous lymphomas with a panniculitic presentation. Semin Diagn Pathol 2017;34(1): 36–43.

27. Badje ED, Tejasvi T, Hristov A. gammadelta lymphomatoid papulosis type D: a histologic mimic of primary cutaneous gammadelta T-cell lymphoma. JAAD Case Rep 2019;5(3):264–6.

28. Santonja C, Carrasco L, Perez-Saenz MLA, et al. A skin plaque preceding systemic relapse of gamma-delta hepatosplenic T-Cell Lymphoma. Am J Dermatopathol 2020;42(5):364–7.

29. Wang C, Reusser N, Shelton M, et al. An unusual case of cytotoxic peripheral T-cell lymphoma. JAAD Case Rep 2015;1(5):257–60.

30. Ishida M, Iwai M, Yoshida K, et al. Primary cutaneous B-cell lymphoma with abundant reactive gamma/delta T-cells within the skin lesion and peripheral blood. Int J Clin Exp Pathol 2014;7(3): 1193–9.

31. Talpur R, Chockalingam R, Wang C, et al. A single-center experience with brentuximab vedotin in gamma delta T-Cell Lymphoma. Clin Lymphoma Myeloma Leuk 2016;16(2):e15–9.

32. Isufi I, Seropian S, Gowda L, et al. Outcomes for allogeneic stem cell transplantation in refractory mycosis fungoides and primary cutaneous gamma Delta T cell lymphomas. Leuk Lymphoma 2020;1–7.

33. Kreuter A, Koushk-Jalali B, Mitrakos G, et al. Bendamustine Monotherapy for Primary Cutaneous Gamma-Delta T-Cell Lymphoma. JAMA Dermatol

2020. https://doi.org/10.1001/jamadermatol.2020. 1231. Epub ahead of print. PMID: 32584930.

34. Obeid JP, Gutkin PM, Lewis J, et al. Volumetric modulated arc therapy and 3-dimensional printed bolus in the treatment of refractory primary cutaneous gamma delta lymphoma of the bilateral legs. Pract Radiat Oncol 2019;9(4):220–5.

35. Berti E, Tomasini D, Vermeer MH, et al. Primary cutaneous CD8-positive epidermotropic cytotoxic T cell lymphomas. A distinct clinicopathological entity with an aggressive clinical behavior. Am J Pathol 1999;155(2):483–92.

36. Guitart J, Martinez-Escala ME, Subtil A, et al. Primary cutaneous aggressive epidermotropic cytotoxic T-cell lymphomas: reappraisal of a provisional entity in the 2016 WHO classification of cutaneous lymphomas. Mod Pathol 2017;30(5):761–72.

37. Fanoni D, Corti L, Alberti-Violetti S, et al. Array-based CGH of primary cutaneous CD8+ aggressive EPIDERMO-tropic cytotoxic T-cell lymphoma. Genes Chromosomes Cancer 2018;57(12):622–9.

38. Deenen NJ, Koens L, Jaspars EH, et al. Pitfalls in diagnosing primary cutaneous aggressive epidermotropic CD8(+) T-cell lymphoma. Br J Dermatol 2019;180(2):411–2.

39. Tomasini C, Novelli M, Fanoni D, et al. Erythema multiforme-like lesions in primary cutaneous aggressive cytotoxic epidermotropic CD8+ T-cell lymphoma: a diagnostic and therapeutic challenge. J Cutan Pathol 2017;44(10):867–73.

40. McQuitty E, Curry JL, Tetzlaff MT, et al. The differential diagnosis of CD8-positive ("type D") lymphomatoid papulosis. J Cutan Pathol 2014;41(2):88–100.

41. Cyrenne BM, Subtil A, Girardi M, et al. Primary cutaneous aggressive epidermotropic cytotoxic CD8(+) T-cell lymphoma: long-term remission after brentuximab vedotin. Int J Dermatol 2017;56(12):1448–50.

42. Quintanilla-Martinez L, Ridaura C, Nagl F, et al. Hydroa vacciniforme-like lymphoma: a chronic EBV+ lymphoproliferative disorder with risk to develop a systemic lymphoma. Blood 2013;122(18):3101–10.

43. Magana M, Sangueza P, Gil-Beristain J, et al. Angiocentric cutaneous T-cell lymphoma of childhood (hydroa-like lymphoma): a distinctive type of cutaneous T-cell lymphoma. J Am Acad Dermatol 1998;38(4): 574–9.

44. Iwatsuki K, Xu Z, Ohtsuka M, et al. Cutaneous lymphoproliferative disorders associated with Epstein-Barr virus infection: a clinical overview. J Dermatol Sci 2000;22(3):181–95.

45. Barrionuevo C, Anderson VM, Zevallos-Giampietri E, et al. Hydroa-like cutaneous T-cell lymphoma: a clinicopathologic and molecular genetic study of 16 pediatric cases from Peru. Appl Immunohistochem Mol Morphol 2002;10(1):7–14.

46. Montes-Mojarro IA, Kim WY, Fend F, et al. Epstein - Barr virus positive T and NK-cell lymphoproliferations:

47. morphological features and differential diagnosis. Semin Diagn Pathol 2020;37(1):32–46.

47. Cohen JI, Iwatsuki K, Ko YH, et al. Epstein-Barr virus NK and T cell lymphoproliferative disease: report of a 2018 international meeting. Leuk Lymphoma 2020;61(4):808–19.

48. Damasco F, Akilov OE. Rare Cutaneous T-Cell Lymphomas. Hematol Oncol Clin North Am 2019;33(1): 135–48.

49. Sitthinamsuwan P, Pattanaprichakul P, Treetipsatit J, et al. Subcutaneous panniculitis-like T-Cell lymphoma versus lupus erythematosus panniculitis: distinction by means of the periadipocytic cell proliferation index. Am J Dermatopathol 2018;40(8):567–74.

50. Gayden T, Sepulveda FE, Khuong-Quang DA, et al. Germline HAVCR2 mutations altering TIM-3 characterize subcutaneous panniculitis-like T cell lymphomas with hemophagocytic lymphohistiocytic syndrome. Nat Genet 2018;50(12):1650–7.

51. Polprasert C, Takeuchi Y, Kakiuchi N, et al. Frequent germline mutations of HAVCR2 in sporadic subcutaneous panniculitis-like T-cell lymphoma. Blood Adv 2019;3(4):588–95.

52. Magro CM, Schaefer JT, Morrison C, et al. Atypical lymphocytic lobular panniculitis: a clonal subcutaneous T-cell dyscrasia. J Cutan Pathol 2008;35(10): 947–54.

53. Geller S, Myskowski PL, Pulitzer M, et al. Cutaneous T-cell lymphoma (CTCL), rare subtypes: five case presentations and review of the literature. Chin Clin Oncol 2019;8(1):5.

54. Boulland ML, Wechsler J, Bagot M, et al. Primary CD30-positive cutaneous T-cell lymphomas and lymphomatoid papulosis frequently express cytotoxic proteins. Histopathology 2000;36(2):136–44.

55. Wu WM, Tsai HJ. Lymphomatoid papulosis histopathologically simulating angiocentric and cytotoxic T-cell lymphoma: a case report. Am J Dermatopathol 2004;26(2):133–5.

56. Saggini A, Gulia A, Argenyi Z, et al. A variant of lymphomatoid papulosis simulating primary cutaneous aggressive epidermotropic CD8+ cytotoxic T-cell lymphoma. Description of 9 cases. Am J Surg Pathol 2010;34(8):1168–75.

57. Kempf W, Kazakov DV, Scharer L, et al. Angioinvasive lymphomatoid papulosis: a new variant simulating aggressive lymphomas. Am J Surg Pathol 2013;37(1):1–13.

58. Massone C, El-Shabrawi-Caelen L, Kerl H, et al. The morphologic spectrum of primary cutaneous anaplastic large T-cell lymphoma: a histopathologic study on 66 biopsy specimens from 47 patients with report of rare variants. J Cutan Pathol 2008; 35(1):46–53.

59. Martires KJ, Ra S, Abdulla F, et al. Characterization of primary cutaneous CD8+/CD30+ lymphoproliferative disorders. Am J Dermatopathol 2015;37(11):822–33.

60. Massone C, Cerroni L. Phenotypic variability in primary cutaneous anaplastic large T-cell lymphoma: a study on 35 patients. Am J Dermatopathol 2014;36(2):153–7.

61. Karai LJ, Kadin ME, Hsi ED, et al. Chromosomal rearrangements of 6p25.3 define a new subtype of lymphomatoid papulosis. Am J Surg Pathol 2013;37(8):1173–81.

62. Onaindia A, Montes-Moreno S, Rodriguez-Pinilla SM, et al. Primary cutaneous anaplastic large cell lymphomas with 6p25.3 rearrangement exhibit particular histological features. Histopathology 2015;66(6):846–55.

63. Melchers RC, Willemze R, van de Loo M, et al. Clinical, histologic, and molecular characteristics of anaplastic lymphoma kinase-positive primary cutaneous anaplastic large cell lymphoma. Am J Surg Pathol 2020;44(6):776–81.

64. Hsi AC, Lee SJ, Rosman IS, et al. Expression of helper T cell master regulators in inflammatory dermatoses and primary cutaneous T-cell lymphomas: diagnostic implications. J Am Acad Dermatol 2015; 72(1):159–67.

65. Duvic M, Tetzlaff MT, Gangar P, et al. Results of a Phase II Trial of Brentuximab Vedotin for CD30+ Cutaneous T-Cell Lymphoma and Lymphomatoid Papulosis. J Clin Oncol 2015;33(32):3759–65.

66. Fay NS, Larson EC, Jameson JM. Chronic Inflammation and gammadelta T Cells. Front Immunol 2016;7: 210.

67. Akitsu A, Iwakura Y. Interleukin-17-producing gammadelta T (gammadelta17) cells in inflammatory diseases. Immunology 2018;155(4):418–26.

68. Laggner U, Di Meglio P, Perera GK, et al. Identification of a novel proinflammatory human skin-homing Vgamma9Vdelta2 T cell subset with a potential role in psoriasis. J Immunol 2011;187(5):2783–93.

69. Baeck M, Soria A, Marot L, et al. Characterization of the T cell response in allergic contact dermatitis caused by corticosteroids. Contact Dermatitis 2013;68(6):357–68.

70. King RL, Yan AC, Sekiguchi DR, et al. Atypical cutaneous gammadelta T cell proliferation with morphologic features of lymphoma but with clinical features and course of PLEVA or lymphomatoid papulosis. J Cutan Pathol 2015;42(12):1012–7.

71. Kash N, Vin H, Danialan R, et al. Stenotrophomonas maltophilia with histopathological features mimicking cutaneous gamma/delta T-cell lymphoma. Int J Infect Dis 2015;30:7–9.

72. Crowson AN, Saab J, Magro CM. Folliculocentric herpes: a clinicopathological study of 28 patients. Am J Dermatopathol 2017;39(2):89–94.

73. Martin SM, Flowers R, Saavedra AP, et al. A reactive peripheral gamma-delta T-cell lymphoid proliferation after a tick bite. Am J Dermatopathol 2019;41(7): e73–5.

Update on Cutaneous Soft Tissue Tumors

Josephine K. Dermawan, MD, PhD[a], Jennifer S. Ko, MD, PhD[b], Steven D. Billings, MD[b],*

KEYWORDS

- *EWSR1-SMAD3*-rearranged fibroblastic tumor • Superficial CD34-positive fibroblastic tumor
- Epithelioid fibrous histiocytoma • *CIC*-rearranged sarcoma
- *NTRK*-rearranged spindle cell neoplasm

Key points

- *EWSR1-SMAD3*-positive fibroblastic tumor is a recently described, benign superficial acral fibroblastic tumor positive for ERG by immunohistochemistry and harbors a recurrent *EWSR1-SMAD3* gene fusion.

- Superficial CD34-positive fibroblastic tumor is a low-grade spindle cell neoplasm with striking nuclear pleomorphism, low mitotic activity, and diffuse CD34 immunoreactivity.

- Epithelioid fibrous histiocytoma is a benign, polypoid, epithelioid neoplasm distinct from benign fibrous histiocytoma and harbors *ALK* gene rearrangements and overexpresses ALK by immunohistochemistry.

- *CIC* rearranged sarcomas are high-grade, undifferentiated round cell sarcomas that most commonly harbor *CIC-DUX4* gene fusions and show greater morphologic heterogeneity and worse prognosis compared with Ewing sarcoma.

- *NTRK*-rearranged spindle cell tumors are a heterogenous, emerging group of soft tissue tumors with S100 and CD34 coexpression that range from benign, low-grade tumors including lipofibromatosis-like neural tumors to high-grade spindle cell tumors with aggressive clinical behaviors, and are amenable to TRK-targeted therapies.

ABSTRACT

This article focuses on various recently described or emerging cutaneous soft tissue neoplasms. These entities encompass a wide range of clinical and histologic characteristics. Emphasis is placed on their distinguishing morphologic and immunophenotypic features compared with entities that enter into their differential diagnosis, as well as novel immunophenotypic and molecular tests that are often necessary for accurate diagnosis of these entities. Entities discussed include *EWSR1-SMAD3*-rearranged fibroblastic tumor, superficial CD34-positive fibroblastic tumor, epithelioid fibrous histiocytoma, *CIC*-rearranged sarcomas, and *NTRK*-rearranged spindle cell tumors.

EWSR1-SMAD3-REARRANGED FIBROBLASTIC TUMOR

INTRODUCTION

EWSR1-SMAD3-rearranged fibroblastic tumors (ESFT) is a recently characterized benign

[a] Soft Tissue and Bone Pathology Section, Department of Pathology, Cleveland Clinic, 9500 Euclid Avenue, L25, Cleveland, OH 44195, USA; [b] Dermatopathology Section, Department of Pathology, Cleveland Clinic, 9500 Euclid Avenue, L25, Cleveland, OH 44195, USA
* Corresponding author.
E-mail address: billins@ccf.org

Surgical Pathology 14 (2021) 195–207
https://doi.org/10.1016/j.path.2021.03.002

surgpath.theclinics.com

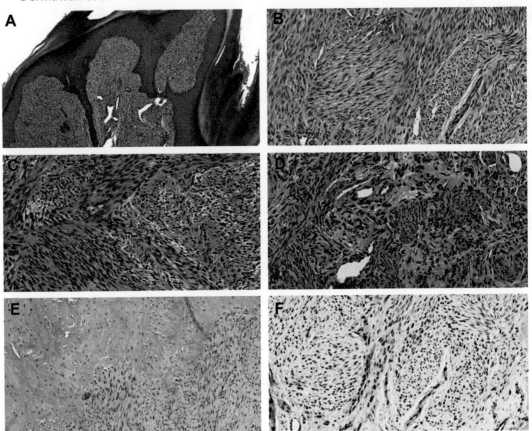

Fig. 1. *EWSR1-SMAD3*-positive fibroblastic tumor in acral skin (*A*) (hematoxylin and eosin [H&E], original magnification ×70) composed of cellular intersecting fascicles of bland spindle cells in a collagenous stroma (*B–D*) (H&E, original magnification ×200) in the peripheral zone and a central hypocellular, hyalinized area (*E*) (H&E, original magnification ×200). (*F*) Tumor cells are positive for ERG by immunohistochemistry (original magnification ×200).

superficial acral fibroblastic spindle cell tumor.[1,2] It is classified as an emerging entity in the fifth edition of the World Health Organization Classification of Tumors for Soft Tissue and Bone Tumors.[3]

CLINICAL FEATURES

ESFT occurs in patients with broad age range (1–68 years old; mean, 36 years old) with a female predilection. Typically presenting as small, painless, superficial nodular tumors, most of these tumors are located in the dermis or subcutaneous tissue of acral skin (feet more than hands) (**Fig. 1**A). Tumor size ranges between 1 and 2 cm in greatest dimension.[1–3]

MICROSCOPIC FEATURES

Tumors may present in the subcutis or dermis. Tumors involving the superficial dermis often abut the epidermis. The tumors have a nodular or vaguely lobular growth pattern. Dermal tumors often have subcutaneous fat infiltration. In many cases, the tumors show two components: a more cellular peripheral zone and an acellular center: the peripheral zone consists of intersecting cellular fascicles of bland fibroblastic spindle cells against a collagenous to myxoid stroma without cytologic atypia or increased mitotic activity (**Fig. 1**B–D), whereas the center appears hypocellular or acellular and shows prominent hyalinization (**Fig. 1**E), reminiscent of collagen rosettes, with some cases showing stippled calcifications focally. In other cases, the cellular, fascicular zones intermingle with the hyalinized areas without distinct zonation.[1,2,4]

IMMUNOHISTOCHEMISTRY

The fibroblastic spindle cells consistently show strong and diffuse nuclear expression for ERG (**Fig. 1**F), and are negative for SMA, CD34, CD31, and S100 protein.[1,2]

Molecular Testing

This tumor is characterized by a gene fusion between exon 7 of *EWSR1* and exon 5 or exon 6 of *SMAD3*. SMAD3 is a signal transducer in the TGF-β/Smad signaling pathway, which is involved in extracellular matrix synthesis by fibroblasts.[5]

DIFFERENTIAL DIAGNOSIS

Superficial acral fibromyxomas (or digital fibromyxomas) show a strong predilection for the subungual regions of the digits, and consists of bland spindled to stellate cells arranged in storiform to loose fascicles in myxoid to collagenous stroma with variably prominent vasculature, and lacks the distinct cellular intersecting fascicles and hyalinized areas in ESFT. Half of all cases contain multinucleated cells. CD34 is positive in 70% to 90% of tumors, and RB1 expression is often lost.[6,7] Myopericytomas, including myofibromas, are benign, well-circumscribed, nodular lesions of variable cellularity composed of bland, ovoid to short spindled cells arranged in a multilayered, concentric growth pattern around numerous small vessels, and are consistently positive for SMA.[8] Dermatofibrosarcoma protuberans (DFSP) is a locally aggressive fibroblastic neoplasm that is more infiltrative and classically shows "honeycombing" of fat. It is composed of uniform, elongated spindled cells arranged in tight cartwheel or storiform growth patterns. DFSP expresses CD34 by immunohistochemistry and is characterized by *COL1A1-PDGFB* gene fusions.[9] Acral DFSP is rare, but usually has conventional features of DFSP.[9] Low-grade fibromyxoid sarcomas may present as superficial tumors,[10] but acral presentation is exceptional.[11] Low-grade fibromyxoid sarcomas are composed of bland spindled cells and alternating fibrous and myxoid stroma. Low-grade fibromyxoid sarcomas can also show collagen rosettes, but they are consistently positive for MUC4 and harbors a gene fusion for *FUS-CREB3L2* or *YAP1-KMT2A*.[12] Soft tissue perineuriomas are benign peripheral nerve sheath tumors that typically show elongated, slender spindle cells arranged in a whorled growth pattern. They consistently express focal to diffuse EMA, are often CD34-positive, and positive for GLUT-1 and claudin-1 in a subset.[13]

PROGNOSIS

ESFT are benign neoplasms that rarely recur after incomplete surgical excision.

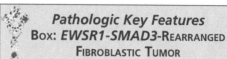

Pathologic Key Features
Box: *EWSR1-SMAD3*-REARRANGED FIBROBLASTIC TUMOR

1. Benign, small, superficial acral fibroblastic tumor occurring over a broad age range

2. Peripheral zone of cellular, intersecting fascicles and central, acellular, hyalinized zone

3. Diffuse nuclear ERG immunoreactivity; negative for CD34 and SMA

4. Recurrent *EWSR1-SMAD3* gene fusion

SUPERFICIAL CD34-POSITIVE FIBROBLASTIC TUMOR

INTRODUCTION

Superficial CD34-positive fibroblastic tumor is a low-grade cutaneous neoplasm characterized by cellular proliferation of CD34-positive spindled cells with marked nuclear pleomorphism.[14,15]

CLINICAL FEATURES

Most cases occur in middle-aged adults (median age, 37 years) as slow-growing, painless, superficial soft tissue masses in the lower extremities, ranging from 1 to 10 cm. The most common locations are thighs, arms, buttocks, and shoulders.[14–17]

MICROSCOPIC FEATURES

Relatively circumscribed to partially infiltrative and largely confined to the superficial subcutis (**Fig. 2**A), this tumor is composed of large spindled to epithelioid cells arranged in cellular fascicles and solid sheets. The tumor cells are characterized by abundant, granular to glassy, eosinophilic cytoplasm and moderate to striking nuclear pleomorphism, including bizarre, hyperchromatic nuclei, variably prominent nucleoli, and intranuclear pseudoinclusions (**Fig. 2**B–D). Some tumors can have areas with ectatic blood vessels (**Fig. 2**E) and admixture of chronic inflammatory cell infiltrate. Despite the significant cytologic atypia, mitotic activity is disproportionately low (<1/50 high-powered fields) to the degree of cytologic atypia, and tumor necrosis is only rarely identified. Often, there is a background of chronic inflammation with lymphocytes and mast cells.[14,15]

IMMUNOHISTOCHEMISTRY

Superficial CD34-positive fibroblastic tumor consistently expresses CD34 (**Fig. 2**F) and is

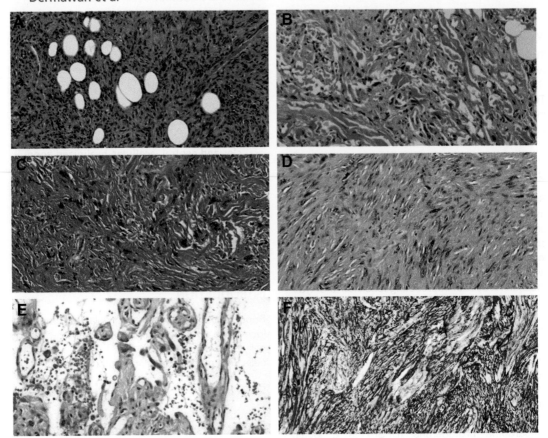

Fig. 2. Superficial CD34-positive fibroblastic tumor infiltrating superficial subcutis (*A*) (H&E, original magnification ×100), composed of large, pleomorphic, spindled to epithelioid cells with abundant eosinophilic cytoplasm arranged in cellular fascicles and solid sheets (*B–D*) (H&E, original magnification ×200). (*E*) Areas with ectatic blood vessels are sometimes present (H&E, original magnification ×200). (*F*) Tumor cells are diffusely positive for CD34 by immunohistochemistry (original magnification ×200).

frequently immunoreactive, at least focally, for cytokeratins, particularly AE1/AE3. Expression of INI-1 is retained.

Molecular Testing

PRDM10 gene rearrangements have been reported in a few cases of superficial CD34-positive fibroblastic tumors, but it is unknown if this is a consistent feature.[18]

DIFFERENTIAL DIAGNOSIS

Other pleomorphic soft tissue neoplasms, myxofibrosarcomas, atypical fibroxanthomas, and undifferentiated pleomorphic sarcomas show a much higher mitotic rate that is usually proportionate to the degree of nuclear pleomorphism.[19] Myxoinflammatory fibroblastic sarcomas share some morphologic features, including bizarre nuclear atypia with a low mitotic rate and prominent chronic inflammatory cell infiltrate.[20] However, myxoinflammatory fibroblastic sarcoma has a predilection for acral locations and shows more prominent myxoid areas with pseudolipoblasts, lacks diffuse CD34

expression, and is characterized by gene rearrangements involving *TGFBR3* and *MGEA5* in a subset of cases.[21] DFSP is usually centered in the dermis, as opposed to the subcutis, and despite also showing CD34 immunoreactivity, is composed of spindle cells with monomorphic cytology.[9] Epithelioid sarcomas, which can also show coexpression of CD34 and cytokeratins, typically show tumor cell palisading around central necrosis or hyalinized areas in the classical (distal) type, and prominent rhabdoid cytology in the proximal type. Tumor cells consistently show loss of INI-1.[22–24] Pleomorphic hyalinizing angiectatic tumor also shows CD34-positive pleomorphic cells with low mitotic rate, but the ectatic, hyalinized blood vessels in pleomorphic hyalinizing angiectatic tumor are significantly more striking, and pleomorphic hyalinizing angiectatic tumor contains areas with hemosiderin-rich bland spindle cell proliferation.[25,26]

PROGNOSIS

Most tumors behave in an indolent fashion with excellent prognosis and low risk of recurrence.

Only one case with lymph node metastasis has been reported to date.[14,15]

> ### Pathologic Key Features
> ### : SUPERFICIAL CD34-POSITIVE FIBROBLASTIC TUMOR
>
> 1. Superficial, low-grade cellular spindle cell neoplasm
>
> 2. Large eosinophilic cells with abundant granular to glassy cytoplasm
>
> 3. Marked nuclear pleomorphism but low mitotic count
>
> 4. Diffuse CD34 and frequent cytokeratin immunoreactivity

EPITHELIOID FIBROUS HISTIOCYTOMA

INTRODUCTION

Epithelioid fibrous histiocytoma (EFH) is a benign, polypoid, cutaneous neoplasm composed of ALK-positive epithelioid cells.[27,28]

CLINICAL FEATURES

EFH most commonly arises in young to middle-aged adults with a female predominance and usually occurs in the lower extremities, followed by the upper extremities, trunk, and head and neck. EFH usually presents as an exophytic, red to red-brown nodule, and could be mistaken for Spitz nevus or hemangioma clinically.

MICROSCOPIC FEATURES

Tumors usually present as exophytic, polypoid and well-circumscribed skin nodules with an epidermal collarette (**Fig. 3**A). Tumor cells are

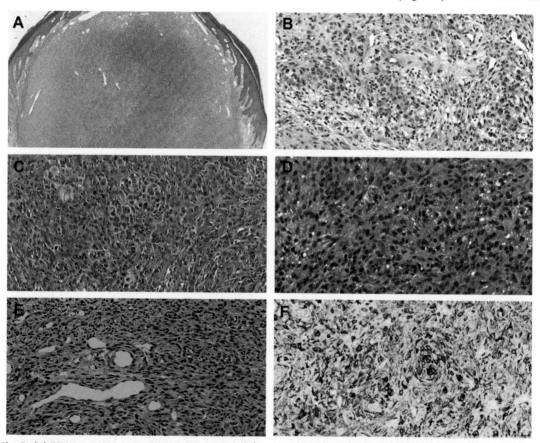

Fig. 3. (*A*) EFH presenting as a polypoid dermal nodule with an epidermal collarette (H&E, original magnification ×10). (*B–D*) EFH is composed of uniformly plump, epithelioid to polygonal tumor cells with abundant cytoplasm with bland cytology (H&E, original magnification ×200). (*E*) Tumor periphery often contains ectatic, thin-walled blood vessels (H&E, original magnification ×200). (*F*) Tumor cells are characteristically diffusely and strongly positive for ALK, especially the DF53 antibody clone, by immunohistochemistry (original magnification ×200).

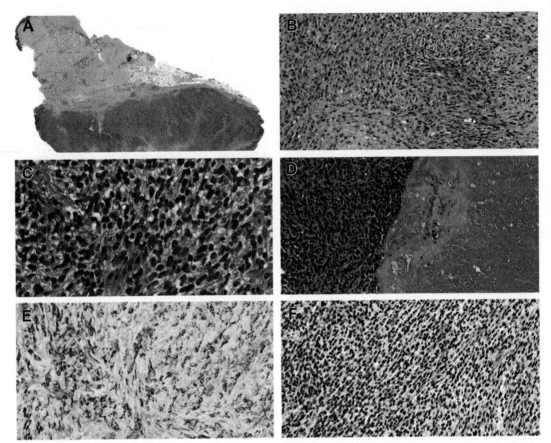

Fig. 4. (*A*) *CIC*-rearranged sarcoma can sometimes present as a cutaneous tumor (H&E, original magnification ×10) and is composed of undifferentiated round cells arranged in solid sheets. (*B*, *C*) Tumor cells show at least mild nuclear pleomorphism with prominent nucleoli and are variably epithelioid, spindled, or even plasmacytoid in morphology (H&E, original magnification ×200). (*D*) Geographic tumor necrosis is often present (H&E, original magnification ×200). (*E*) CD99 immunoreactivity is almost always present but patchy (original magnification ×200). (*F*) Tumor cells with *CIC-DUX4* rearrangements show strong and diffuse nuclear DUX4 positivity (original magnification ×200).

uniform, plump, epithelioid to polygonal, and frequently binucleate cells with abundant pale pink to amphophilic cytoplasm, vesicular nuclei, and small nucleoli (**Fig. 3**B–D). Ectatic, thin-walled blood vessels at the periphery are frequently present (**Fig. 3**E). Unlike conventional benign fibrous histiocytomas (dermatofibromas), EFH typically shows only limited to no peripheral collagen trapping.[27,28]

IMMUNOHISTOCHEMISTRY

ALK expression by immunohistochemistry (particularly the ALK D5F3 antibody clone) is highly specific and seen in about 90% of cases (**Fig. 3**F).[28] EMA is frequently positive (about 65% of cases).[29] SMA and desmin are largely negative.

Molecular Testing

Approximately 90% of EFH harbors gene rearrangements for *ALK*, most commonly partnered with *SQSTM1* and *VCL*.[30,31] Because *ALK* rearrangements have not been described in conventional benign fibrous histiocytomas, many authors believe that, rather than being a rare morphologic variant, EFH is a biologically distinct entity.

DIFFERENTIAL DIAGNOSIS

Epithelioid sarcomas also show variably epithelioid to spindled cells with abundant pink cytoplasm and frequently express EMA and frequently involve the superficial dermis. However, they show a greater degree of nuclear atypia and loss if INI-1 expression.[22–24] Spitz nevus contains nests of large epithelioid cells extending from the epidermis into the reticular dermis in a wedge-shaped configuration. It may have a junctional component and is positive for S100 protein and melanocytic markers.[32] Cutaneous syncytial myoepithelioma also arises in the superficial dermis and is composed of uniform, ovoid to spindled cells with pale eosinophilic cytoplasm with frequent EMA expression. However, they are less polypoid; lack ectatic vasculature; and also express variable S100 protein and other myoepithelial markers, such as GFAP, SMA, and p63.[33] Cellular neurothekeoma is a lobulated neoplasm with a predilection for the face, shoulders, and upper limbs. Although also composed of epithelioid to slightly spindled cells with moderate to abundant pale eosinophilic cytoplasm and vesicular nuclei, the cells in cellular neurothekeomas are characteristically arranged in a distinctive nested pattern and consistently express NKI/C3 (CD63), and are negative for EMA and ALK.[34]

PROGNOSIS

EFH is a benign neoplasm and only rarely shows local recurrence.

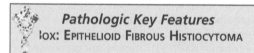

Pathologic Key Features
Box: Epithelioid Fibrous Histiocytoma

1. Benign exophytic and well-circumscribed cutaneous neoplasm with epidermal collarette

2. Composed of uniform, plump epithelioid cells with abundant pink to amphophilic cytoplasm

3. ALK is overexpressed by immunohistochemistry in most cases

4. Characterized by ALK gene rearrangements

CIC-rearranged sarcoma

INTRODUCTION

CIC-rearranged sarcomas are high-grade, undifferentiated, round cell sarcomas that harbor CIC-related gene fusions, most commonly CIC-DUX4.[35,36]

CLINICAL FEATURES

Most CIC-rearranged sarcomas present as a mass, with or without pain, in deep soft tissues of the limbs or trunk, but can present in the skin (Fig. 4A).[37] Although this tumor has been reported in a wide age range of patients, from children to elderly adults, there is a strong predilection for young adults (25–35 years old).

MICROSCOPIC FEATURES

The tumors are composed of predominantly undifferentiated round cells arranged in sheets and lobules. Many tumors also variably have epithelioid, spindled, rhabdoid, and plasmacytoid cells. Although uniform, at least a mild degree of nuclear pleomorphism is invariably present. Tumor cells are small to medium-sized with pale eosinophilic to clear cytoplasm, round to ovoid nuclei, vesicular chromatin, and variably prominent nucleoli (Fig. 4B, C). Usually embedded in a fibrotic stroma, some tumors show prominent myxoid areas. Geographic tumor necrosis is often a prominent feature (Fig. 4D), and mitotic activity is brisk.[35–37]

IMMUNOHISTOCHEMISTRY

CIC-rearranged sarcomas frequently express CD99, but usually in a patchy, heterogenous fashion rather than a diffuse and membranous pattern (Fig. 4E). They also frequently express nuclear WT1 and ETV4,[38] and are negative for NKX2-2. Nuclear expression of DUX4 has been reported as a highly sensitive and specific marker for CIC-rearranged sarcomas with CIC-DUX4 fusions (Fig. 4F).[39] Other authors have found immunohistochemical stains for ETV4 to be superior.[40]

Molecular Testing

The CIC-DUX4 fusion is detected in 95% of cases. Rarely, non-DUX4 partners including FOXO4, LEUTX, NUTM1, and NUTM2A have been reported.[41–43] In some studies ETV transcriptional upregulation has been shown to be more reliable than RNA sequencing or fluorescent in situ hybridization to confirm the diagnosis.[40]

DIFFERENTIAL DIAGNOSIS

Ewing sarcoma is characterized by uniform small round cells with round nuclei, fine chromatin, and indistinct nucleoli. It lacks the more prominent nuclear pleomorphism, morphologic heterogeneity, myxoid stroma, and geographic tumor necrosis seen in CIC-rearranged sarcomas. Ewing sarcoma also typically shows strong and diffuse membranous CD99 expression and stains with NKX2-2. Most Ewing sarcomas harbor gene fusion involving EWSR1 and occasionally FUS, fused with genes in the ETS family of transcription factors, including *FLI1*, *ERG*, and *FEV*.[44] Other cutaneous entities that can also show a small round cell morphology, including lymphoma, Merkel cell carcinoma, melanoma, and rhabdomyosarcoma, are readily differentiated by immunohistochemical stains.

PROGNOSIS

CIC-rearranged sarcomas are highly aggressive tumors with frequent metastases and a dismal response to Ewing sarcoma chemotherapeutic regimens. It has an estimated 5-year overall survival rate of 17% to 43%, which is significantly worse than that of Ewing sarcoma. Cutaneous *CIC*-rearranged sarcoma also seems to behave in an aggressive fashion, unlike cutaneous Ewing sarcoma.[37]

Pathologic Key Features
Box: CIC-Rearranged Sarcomas

1. Highly aggressive, undifferentiated round cell sarcomas with *CIC* gene rearrangement

2. Diffuse sheets of undifferentiated round cells with frequent tumor necrosis

3. Greater degree of nuclear pleomorphism and morphologic heterogeneity than Ewing sarcoma

4. Variable CD99 reactivity and express WT1, ETV4, and DUX4 by immunohistochemistry

5. Inferior response to chemotherapy and survival compared with Ewing sarcoma

---

NTRK-REARRANGED SPINDLE CELL NEOPLASM

INTRODUCTION

This is an emerging group of rare soft tissue tumors defined by *NTRK* gene rearrangements with a wide morphologic spectrum and frequent coexpression of S100 protein and CD34.[45] It is classified as a provisional entity in the fifth edition of the World Health Organization Classification of Tumors for Soft Tissue and Bone Tumors, and includes lipofibromatosis-like neural tumors (LPF-NT) and spindle cell tumors that closely resemble peripheral nerve sheath tumors.[3] The canonical infantile fibrosarcoma (IFS) with *ETV6-NTRK3* fusions is regarded as a separate category and is not discussed here.[46]

CLINICAL FEATURES

Most of these tumors occur in the first two decades of life. LPF-NT predominantly occurs in children. Most LPF-NT present as a palpable, painless mass in superficial and deep soft tissues in the extremities or trunk.[47,48] Spindle cell tumors that closely resemble peripheral nerve sheath tumors predominate in children and young adults, and occur in various sites including soft tissue, bone, and visceral organs.[49,50]

MICROSCOPIC FEATURES

NTRK-rearranged spindle cell neoplasms display a wide range of morphologic spectrum. One distinct morphologic pattern is the so-called LPF-NT, a distinct soft tissue tumor that primarily occurs in the extremities and trunk of children. LPF-NT is a hypocellular neoplasm that is highly infiltrative in the superficial subcutis and resembles lipofibromatosis. However, LPF-NT displays a more pronounced spindle cell component, which is composed of monomorphic, delicate, bland spindle cells with tapering nuclei and indistinct cytoplasm arranged in short fascicles within a fibrous stroma.[47,48] LPF-NT typically shows a low mitotic count and lacks tumor necrosis.

Another morphologically distinct group encompasses spindle cell tumors that resemble low- to intermediate-grade malignant peripheral nerve sheath tumor (MPNST). Tumors are composed of moderately cellular proliferation of uniform spindle cells with ovoid-to-spindled, hyperchromatic nuclei with scant cytoplasm arranged in streaming short fascicles or haphazardly in solid sheets. These tumors are characteristically associated with stromal or perivascular bandlike hyalinization and keloidal collagen. Some display a zoned appearance with hypercellular areas merging with paucicellular areas, similar to MPNST. Although most tumors are low grade, some could display high-grade histologic features including hypercellularity with herringbone-like intersecting fascicles, high mitotic count, and tumor necrosis, thus resembling high-grade MPNSTs or adult-type fibrosarcomas (**Fig. 5**A–E).[49–54]

Finally, one single study to date has reported spindle cell sarcomas with *NTRK1*-associated gene fusions displaying myopericytoma- or hemangiopericytoma-like architectures. They are characterized by numerous thick-walled vessels with nodular, myxohyaline proliferation of SMA-positive cells. These tumors resemble infantile hemangiopericytoma and myopericytoma and show mitotic activity greater than 10/10 high power fields.[55]

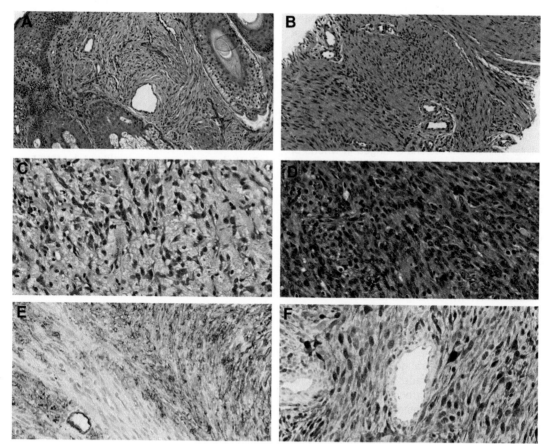

Fig. 5. NTRK-rearranged spindle cell neoplasm has a predilection for superficial soft tissue (*A*) (H&E, original magnification ×200) and show a wide morphologic spectrum, from low-grade lipofibromatosis-like neural tumor (*B*) (H&E, original magnification ×200), moderately cellular patternless pattern (*C*) (H&E, original magnification ×400), to high-grade MPNST-like hypercellular, intersecting fascicles (*D*) (H&E, original magnification ×400). Tumor cells show variable coexpression of CD34 (*E*) and S100 (*F*) (original magnification ×400).

IMMUNOHISTOCHEMISTRY

Most tumors show variable coexpression of S100 protein (**Fig. 5**F) and CD34, and are negative for SOX10. H3K27me3 expression is retained. Tumors with *NTRK* fusions are also reactive to pan-TRK monoclonal antibodies, which are not completely specific.[56,57] Molecular testing is necessary to confirm the presence of *NTRK* fusions.

Molecular Testing

Most tumors harbor gene fusions involving *NTRK1*, and rarely *NTRK2* and *NTRK3*, including *LMNA-NTRK1* (interstitial deletions), or *TPR-* and *TPM3-NTRK1* (unbalanced insertions).[49–54] *NTRK3*-fusion-positive soft tissue tumors reportedly show higher grade morphology and behave in a more clinically aggressive manner.[49–54] Alternative fusions involving *RAF1*, *BRAF*, and *RET* have also been reported.[49,58–61] Detection of

NTRK fusions is necessary for determination of targeted therapy (see later).

DIFFERENTIAL DIAGNOSIS

MPNST also shows monomorphic, hyperchromatic spindle cells arranged in fascicles and solid sheets. However, MPNST often expresses at least focal SOX10 and S100, shows loss of H3K27me3 (more frequent in high-grade MPNST), does not harbor kinase fusions, and could occur in association with neurofibromatosis 1 or arise in a preexisting neurofibroma.[62] Cutaneous MPNST is exceptionally rare. IFS typically occurs at birth or in the first 2 years of life, with a predilection for the extremities. IFS typically shows monomorphic spindled to ovoid cells arranged in a fascicular/ herringbone pattern with staghorn vasculature and mixed inflammation. They stain variably with SMA, CD34, S100, and desmin; reacts with the pan-TRK antibody; and harbors the *ETV6-NTRK3* fusion. IFS has a favorable outcome and is treated with conservative surgical resection in most cases.[46] Lipofibromatosis also shows bland, uniform spindle cells in fascicles that infiltrate into adipose tissue. Lipofibromatosis, however, characteristically shows pseudolipoblast-like cells and are variably positive for CD34 and SMA, whereas stains for S100 protein are negative.[63] Myopericytomas or myofibromas are superficial, cellular spindle cell lesions arranged in whorls or nodules, and are consistently positive for SMA.[8] Solitary fibrous tumors are also characterized by a haphazard or "patternless" spindle cell arrangement with hyalinized stromal and perivascular collagen. However, solitary fibrous tumors are usually well-demarcated and harbor a NAB2-STAT6 fusion, which is readily detected by STAT6 immunoreactivity. Molecular testing remains the mainstay of diagnosis for definitive classification of NTRK-rearranged tumors.[64]

PROGNOSIS

Prognosis of NTRK-rearranged tumors largely correlates with histologic grade. LPF-NTs have a propensity for local recurrence with incomplete excision, but do not metastasize.[47,48] NTRK-rearranged tumors with higher histologic grade were shown to have metastatic potential.[49–54] Importantly, because NTRK1, NTRK2, and NTRK3 encode for the tropomyosin receptor tyrosine kinases TRKA, TRKB, and TRKC, respectively, NTRK fusions led to activation of oncogenic signaling pathways that could be targeted by TRK inhibitors.[65–67]

Pathologic Key Features
Box: NTRK-Rearranged
Spindle Cell Neoplasm

1. Emerging soft tissue entity that includes wide morphologic spectrum: LPF-NT and spindle cell tumors resembling peripheral nerve sheath tumors, and defined by kinase fusions involving NTRK1, NTRK2, NTRK3, BRAF, RAF1, RET, and so forth

2. Mostly involves children and young adults in superficial soft tissues of the extremities and trunk, but could involve visceral organs

3. LPF-NT are highly infiltrative within subcutaneous fat with haphazardly arranged monomorphic spindle cells with low mitotic count

4. Spindle cell tumors resembling peripheral nerve sheath tumors comprise moderately to highly cellular proliferation of spindle cells associated with keloid-like, hyalinized collagen, and display low- to high-grade phenotypes

5. Most tumors show variable coexpression of S100 protein and CD34 but lack SOX10 immunoreactivity

6. LPF-NT are locally aggressive but follow a benign clinical course

7. High-grade tumors resemble high MPNST or adult-type fibrosarcomas show aggressive clinical behavior

8. Tumors with NTRK fusions can be targeted with TRK tyrosine kinase inhibitors

CLINICS CARE POINTS

- EWSR1-SMAD3-positive fibroblastic tumor are benign neoplasms that rarely recur after incomplete surgical excision.

- Superficial CD34-positive fibroblastic tumors behave in an indolent fashion with excellent prognosis and low risk of recurrences.

- Epithelioid fibrous histiocytoma is a benign neoplasm and only rarely shows local recurrence.

- CIC-rearranged sarcomas, included the cutaneous one, are highly aggressive tumors with frequent metastases and a dismal response to Ewing sarcoma chemotherapeutic regimens. It has an estimated 5-year overall survival rate of 17% to 43.

- Prognosis of NTRK-rearranged tumors largely correlates with histologic grade. Lipofibromatosis-like neural tumors have a propensity for local recurrence with incomplete excision, but do not metastasize. NTRK-rearranged tumors with higher histologic grade were shown to have metastatic potential. Importantly, these tumors harbor NTRK fusions, which are targetable by tyrosine kinase inhibitors.

DISCLOSURE

The authors have nothing to disclose.

REFERENCES

1. Kao YC, Flucke U, Eijkelenboom A, et al. Novel EWSR1-SMAD3 gene fusions in a group of acral fibroblastic spindle cell neoplasms. Am J Surg Pathol 2018;42:522–8.

2. Michal M, Berry RS, Rubin BP, et al. EWSR1-SMAD3-rearranged fibroblastic tumor: an emerging entity in an increasingly more complex group of fibroblastic/myofibroblastic neoplasms. Am J Surg Pathol 2018;42:1325–33.

3. Antonescu CR, Suurmeijer AJH. WHO Classification of Tumours Editorial Board. EWSR1-SMAD3-positive fibroblastic tumour (emerging). WHO Classification of Tumours Soft tissue and Bone Tumours, 5th edition. Lyon: IARC Press; 2020:76-77.

4. Zhao L, Sun M, Lao IW, et al. EWSR1-SMAD3 positive fibroblastic tumor. Exp Mol Pathol 2019;110:104291.

5. Verreccha F, Chu ML, Mauviel A. Identification of novel TGF-beta/Smad gene targets in dermal fibroblasts using a combined cDNA microarray/promoter transactivation approach. J Biol Chem 2001;276:17058–62.

6. Fetsch JF, Laskin WB, Miettinen M. Superficial acral fibromyxoma: a clinicopathologic and immunohistochemical analysis of 37 cases of a distinctive soft tissue tumor with a predilection for the fingers and toes. Hum Pathol 2001;32:704–14.

7. Hollmann TJ, Bovée JV, Fletcher CD. Digital fibromyxoma (superficial acral fibromyxoma): a detailed characterization of 124 cases. Am J Surg Pathol 2012;36:789–98.

8. Mentzel T, Dei Tos AP, Sapi Z, et al. Myopericytoma of skin and soft tissues: clinicopathologic and immunohistochemical study of 54 cases. Am J Surg Pathol 2006;30:104–13.

9. Shah KK, McHugh JB, Folpe AL, et al. Dermatofibrosarcoma protuberans of distal extremities and acral sites: a clinicopathologic analysis of 27 cases. Am J Surg Pathol 2018;42:413–9.

10. Billings SD, Giblen G, Fanburg-Smith JC. Superficial low-grade fibromyxoid sarcoma (Evans tumor): a clinicopathologic analysis of 19 cases with a unique observation in the pediatric population. Am J Surg Pathol 2005;29:204–10.

11. Saab-Chalhoub MW, Al-Rohil RN. Low-grade fibromyxoid sarcoma of acral sites: case report and literature review. J Cutan Pathol 2019;46:271–6.

12. Doyle LA, Möller E, Dal Cin P, et al. MUC4 is a highly sensitive and specific marker for low-grade fibromyxoid sarcoma. Am J Surg Pathol 2011;35:733–41.

13. Hornick JL, Fletcher CD. Soft tissue perineurioma: clinicopathologic analysis of 81 cases including those with atypical histologic features. Am J Surg Pathol 2005;29:845–58.

14. Carter JM, Weiss SW, Linos K, et al. Superficial CD34-positive fibroblastic tumor: report of 18 cases of a distinctive low-grade mesenchymal neoplasm of intermediate (Borderline) Malignancy. Mod Pathol 2014;27:294–302.

15. Lao IW, Yu L, Wang J. Superficial CD34-positive fibroblastic tumour: a clinicopathological and immunohistochemical study of an additional series. Histopathology 2017;70:394–401.

16. Hendry SA, Wong DD, Papadimitriou J, et al. Superficial CD34-positive fibroblastic tumour: report of two new cases. Pathology (Phila) 2015;47:479–82.

17. Batur S, Ozcan K, Ozcan G, et al. Superficial CD34 positive fibroblastic tumor: report of three cases and review of the literature. Int J Dermatol 2019;58:416–22.

18. Puls F, Pillay N, Fagman H, et al. PRDM10-rearranged soft tissue tumor: a clinicopathologic study of 9 cases. Am J Surg Pathol 2019;43:504–13.

19. Yang H, Yu L. Cutaneous and superficial soft tissue CD34 spindle cell proliferation. Arch Pathol Lab Med 2017;141:1092–100.

20. Montgomery EA, Devaney KO, Giordano TJ, et al. Inflammatory myxohyaline tumor of distal extremities with virocyte or Reed-Sternberg-like cells: a distinctive lesion with features simulating inflammatory conditions, Hodgkin's disease, and various sarcomas. Mod Pathol 1998;11:384–91.

21. Antonescu CR, Zhang L, Nielsen GP, et al. Consistent t(1;10) with rearrangements of TGFBR3 and MGEA5 in both myxoinflammatory fibroblastic sarcoma and hemosiderotic fibrolipomatous tumor. Genes Chrom Cancer 2011;50:757–64.

22. Enzinger FM. Epithelioid sarcoma: a sarcoma simulating a granuloma or a carcinoma. Cancer 1970;26:1029–41.

23. Miettinen M, Fanburg-Smith JC, Virolainen M, et al. Epithelioid sarcoma: an immunohistochemical analysis of 112 classical and variant cases and a discussion of the differential diagnosis. Hum Pathol 1999;30:934–42.

24. Guillou L, Wadden C, Coindre JM, et al. Proximal-type" epithelioid sarcoma, a distinctive aggressive neoplasm showing rhabdoid features. Clinicopathologic, immunohistochemical, and ultrastructural study of a series. Am J Surg Pathol 1997;21:130–46.

25. Smith ME, Fisher C, Weiss SW. Pleomorphic hyalinizing angiectatic tumor of soft parts. A low-grade neoplasm resembling neurilemoma. Am J Surg Pathol 1996;20:21–9.

26. Folpe AL, Weiss SW. Pleomorphic hyalinizing angiectatic tumor: analysis of 41 cases supporting evolution from a distinctive precursor lesion. Am J Surg Pathol 2004;28:1417–25.

27. Singh Gomez C, Calonje E, Fletcher CD. Epithelioid benign fibrous histiocytoma of skin: clinicopathological analysis of 20 cases of a poorly known variant. Histopathology 1994;24:123–9.

28. Doyle LA, Mariño-Enriquez A, Fletcher CD, et al. ALK rearrangement and overexpression in epithelioid fibrous histiocytoma. Mod Pathol 2015;28:904–12.

29. Doyle LA, Fletcher CD. EMA positivity in epithelioid fibrous histiocytoma: a potential diagnostic pitfall. J Cutan Pathol 2011;38:697–703.

30. Jedrych J, Nikiforova M, Kennedy TF, et al. Epithelioid cell histiocytoma of the skin with clonal ALK gene rearrangement resulting in VCL-ALK and SQSTM1-ALK gene fusions. Br J Dermatol 2015; 172:1427–9.

31. Dickson BC, Swanson D, Charames GS, et al. Epithelioid fibrous histiocytoma: molecular characterization of ALK fusion partners in 23 cases. Mod Pathol 2018;31:753–62.

32. Paniago-Pereira C, Maize JC, Ackerman AB. Nevus of large spindle and/or epithelioid cells (Spitz's nevus). Arch Dermatol 1978;114:1811–23.

33. Jo VY, Antonescu CR, Zhang L, et al. Cutaneous syncytial myoepithelioma: clinicopathologic characterization in a series of 38 cases. Am J Surg Pathol 2013;37:710–8.

34. Hornick JL, Fletcher CD. Cellular neurothekeoma: detailed characterization in a series of 133 cases. Am J Surg Pathol 2007;31:329–40.

35. Yoshimoto T, Tanaka M, Homme M, et al. CIC-DUX4 induces small round cell sarcomas distinct from Ewing sarcoma. Cancer Res 2017;77:2927–37.

36. Antonescu CR, Owosho AA, Zhang L, et al. Sarcomas with CIC-rearrangements are a distinct pathologic entity with aggressive outcome: a clinicopathologic and molecular study of 115 cases. Am J Surg Pathol 2017;41:941–9.

37. Ko JS, Marusic Z, Azzato EM, et al. Superficial sarcomas with CIC rearrangement are aggressive neoplasms: a series of eight cases. J Cutan Pathol 2020;47:509–16.

38. Hung YP, Fletcher CD, Hornick JL. Evaluation of ETV4 and WT1 expression in CIC-rearranged sarcomas and histologic mimics. Mod Pathol 2016; 29(11):1324-1334.

39. Siegele B, Roberts J, Black JO, et al. DUX4 immunohistochemistry is a highly sensitive and specific marker for CIC-DUX4 fusion-positive round cell tumor. Am J Surg Pathol 2017;41(3):423-429.

40. Kao YC, Sung YS, Chen CL, et al. ETV transcriptional upregulation is more reliable than RNA sequencing algorithms and FISH in diagnosing round cell sarcomas with CIC gene rearrangements. Genes Chromosomes Cancer 2017;56:501–10.

41. Loarer FL, Pissalous D, Watson S, et al. Clinicopathologic features of CIC-NUTM1 sarcomas, a new molecular variant of the family of CIC-fused sarcomas. Am J Surg Pathol 2019;43:268–76.

42. Sugita S, Arai Y, Aoyama T, et al. NUTM2A-CIC fusion small round cell sarcoma: a genetically distinct variant of CIC-rearranged sarcoma. Hum Pathol 2017;65:225–30.

43. Sugita S, Arai Y, Tonooka A, et al. A novel CIC-FOXO4 gene fusion in undifferentiated small round cell sarcoma: a genetically distinct variant of Ewing-like sarcoma. Am J Surg Pathol 2014;38:1571–6.

44. Yoshida A, Goto K, Kodaira M, et al. CIC-rearranged sarcomas: a study of 20 cases and comparisons with Ewing sarcomas. Am J Surg Pathol 2016;40:313–23.

45. Antonescu CR. Emerging soft tissue tumors with kinase fusions: an overview of the recent literature with an emphasis on diagnostic criteria. Genes Chromosomes Cancer 2020;59:437–44.

46. Davis JL, Lockwood CM, Albert CM, et al. Infantile NTRK-associated mesenchymal tumors. Pediatr Dev Pathol 2018;21:68–78.

47. Agaram NP, Zhang L, Sung YS, et al. Recurrent NTRK1 gene fusions define a novel subset of locally aggressive lipofibromatosis-like neural tumors. Am J Surg Pathol 2016;40:1407–16.

48. Panse G, Reisenbichler E, Snuderl M, et al. LMNA-NTRK1 rearranged mesenchymal tumor (lipofibromatosis-like neural tumor) mimicking pigmented dermatofibrosarcoma protuberans. J Cutan Pathol 2021;48:290–4.

49. Suurmeijer AJH, Dickson BC, Swanson D, et al. A novel group of spindle cell tumors defined by S100 and CD34 co-expression shows recurrent fusions involving RAF1, BRAF, and NTRK1/2 genes. Genes Chromosomes Cancer 2018;57:611–21.

50. Yamazaki F, Nakatani F, Asano N, et al. Novel NTRK3 fusions in fibrosarcomas of adults. Am J Surg Pathol 2019;43:523–30.

51. Suurmeijer AJ, Dickson BC, Swanson D, et al. The histologic spectrum of soft tissue spindle cell tumors with NTRK3 gene rearrangements. Genes Chromosomes Cancer 2019;58:739-46.

52. Chiang S, Cotzia P, Hyman DM, et al. NTRK fusions define a novel uterine sarcoma subtype with features of fibrosarcoma. Am J Surg Pathol 2018;42:791–8.

53. Croce S, Hostein I, Longacre TA, et al. Uterine and vaginal sarcomas resembling fibrosarcoma: a clinicopathological and molecular analysis of 13 cases showing common NTRK-rearrangements and the description of a COL1A1-PDGFB fusion novel to uterine neoplasms. Mod Pathol 2019;32:1008-22.

54. Olson N, Rouhi O, Zhang L, et al. A novel case of an aggressive superficial spindle cell sarcoma in an adult resembling fibrosarcomatous dermatofibrosarcoma protuberans and harboring an EML4-NTRK3 fusion. J Cutan Pathol 2018;45:933-9.

55. Haller F, Knopf J, Ackermann A, et al. Pediatric and adult soft tissue sarcomas with NTRK1 gene fusions: a subset of spindle cell sarcomas unified by a prominent myopericytic/haemangiopericytic pattern. J Pathol 2016;238:700–10.

56. Hechtman JF, Benayed R, Hyman DM, et al. Pan-Trk immunohistochemistry is an efficient and reliable

screen for the detection of NTRK fusions. Am J Surg Pathol 2017;41:1547–51.

57. Hung YP, Fletcher CD, Hornick JL. Evaluation of pan-TRK Immunohistochemistry in infantile fibrosarcoma, lipofibromatosis-like neural tumour and histological mimics. Histopathology 2018;73:634–44.

58. Kao YC, Fletcher CDM, Alaggio R, et al. Recurrent BRAF gene fusions in a subset of pediatric spindle cell sarcomas: expanding the genetic spectrum of tumors with overlapping features with infantile fibrosarcoma. Am J Surg Pathol 2018;42:28–38.

59. Antonescu CR, Dickson BC, Swanson D, et al. Spindle cell tumors with RET gene fusions exhibit a morphologic spectrum akin to tumors with NTRK gene fusions. Am J Surg Pathol 2019;43:1384–91.

60. Davis JL, Vargas SO, Rudzinski ER, et al. Recurrent RET gene fusions in paediatric spindle mesenchymal neoplasms. Histopathology 2020;76:1032–41.

61. Michal M, Ptakova N, Martinek P, et al. S100 and CD34 positive spindle cell tumor with prominent perivascular hyalinization and a novel NCOA4-RET fusion. Genes Chromosomes Cancer 2019;58:680-5.

62. Miettinen MM, Antonescu CR, Fletcher CD, et al. Histopathologic evaluation of atypical neurofibromatous tumors and their transformation into malignant peripheral nerve sheath tumor in patients with neurofibromatosis 1-a consensus overview. Hum Pathol 2017;67:1–10.

63. Fetsch JF, Miettinen M, Laskin WB, et al. A clinicopathologic study of 45 pediatric soft tissue tumors with an admixture of adipose tissue and fibroblastic elements, and a proposal for classification as lipofibromatosis. Am J Surg Pathol 2000;24: 1491–500.

64. Chmielecki J, Crago AM, Rosenberg M, et al. Whole-exome sequencing identifies a recurrent NAB2-STAT6 fusion in solitary fibrous tumors. Nat Genet 2013;45:131–2.

65. Laetsch TW, DuBois SG, Mascarenhas L, et al. Larotrectinib for paediatric solid tumours harbouring NTRK gene fusions: phase 1 results from a multicentre, open-label, phase 1/2 study. Lancet Oncol 2018;19:705–14.

66. Hsiao SJ, Zehir A, Sireci AN, et al. Detection of tumor NTRK gene fusions to identify patients who may benefit from tyrosine kinase (trk) inhibitor therapy. J Mol Diagn 2019;21:553–71.

67. Cocco E, Scaltriti M, Drilon A. NTRK fusion-positive cancers and TRK inhibitor therapy. Nat Rev Clin Oncol 2018;15:731–47.

Cutaneous Toxicities in the Setting of Immune Checkpoint Blockade:
The Era of Oncodermatopathology

Jonathan L. Curry, MD[a,b,c],*, Susan Y. Chon, MD[c],
Mario L. Marques-Piubelli, MD[b], Emily Y. Chu, MD, PhD[d]

KEYWORDS

- Cutaneous toxicities • Immune checkpoint inhibitor • Oncodermatopathology

Key points

- In the era of oncodermatopathology, the diagnosis of cutaneous immune-related adverse events (irAEs) from immune checkpoint inhibitor (ICI) therapy is critical for patient care.
- The diagnosis of cutaneous irAEs from ICI therapy poses challenges because skin toxicities show diverse clinical and histopathologic features.
- A multidisciplinary approach with the clinical oncology team, dermatologists, and dermatopathologists is necessary to diagnose and manage cutaneous irAEs.

ABSTRACT

Advancements in cancer therapy with monoclonal immune checkpoint antibody blockade have impacted the practice of all medical specialties. Cutaneous immune-related adverse events (irAEs) are a frequent, unintended, off-target consequence of immune checkpoint inhibitor (ICI) therapy that have ushered in the era of oncodermatopathology. Knowledge of the diverse morphologic types of cutaneous irAEs from ICI therapy allows further classification of cutaneous irAEs according to major histopathologic reaction patterns. Early studies suggest that immune mechanisms of lichenoid dermatitis irAE, psoriasiform dermatitis irAE, and bullous pemphigoid irAE show some similarities and differences from their histopathologic counterparts not associated with ICI therapy.

OVERVIEW

The discovery of cytotoxic T-lymphocyte-associated protein 4 (CTLA-4) and programmed cell death protein 1 (PD-1)/programmed death-ligand 1 (PD-L1) immune checkpoint signaling and the development of monoclonal antibodies that block these receptor-ligand interactions on T cells and/or tumor cells to enhance and sustain immune function have revolutionized the field of oncology.[1] This paradigm shift in cancer therapy has brought great excitement because a large subset of patients treated with immune checkpoint inhibitors (ICIs) have shown durable antitumor responses and survival benefits comparable with those achieved with conventional chemotherapy.[2–4]

An unintended consequence of ICI therapy is the development of immune-related adverse events (irAEs), which may occur in any organ system.[5] The skin is a frequent site of irAEs, which

[a] Department of Pathology, The University of Texas MD Anderson Cancer Center, Houston, TX 77030, USA;
[b] Department of Translational Molecular Pathology, The University of Texas MD Anderson Cancer Center, Houston, TX 77030, USA; [c] Department of Dermatology, The University of Texas MD Anderson Cancer Center, Houston, TX 77030, USA; [d] Department of Dermatology, The University of Pennsylvania, Philadelphia, PA 19104, USA
* Corresponding author. Department of Pathology, The University of Texas MD Anderson Cancer Center, Houston, TX 77030.
E-mail address: jlcurry@mdanderson.org

Surgical Pathology 14 (2021) 209–224
https://doi.org/10.1016/j.path.2021.01.002

may occur in 15% to 35% of patients receiving ICI therapy.[6–8] In ~2% of patients, cutaneous irAEs can be life threatening.[5,9] Management of cutaneous irAEs remains a challenge, and more effective therapy to combat irAEs while still preserving antitumor immunity is needed. A contributing factor to the challenges of cutaneous irAEs is the diverse spectrum of morphologies that may develop in the skin.[10] The era of oncodermatopathology has begun, which means cutaneous irAEs must now be considered in the clinical and histopathologic differential diagnosis in patients receiving ICI therapy. Dermatologists and dermatopathologists need to be familiar with cutaneous irAEs in order to make diagnoses and manage skin toxicities without compromising the antitumor response from ICI therapy. Furthermore, identifying immunologic pathways driving cutaneous irAEs may expose targetable immune mediators and lead to the development of more efficacious antitoxicity therapies.

sites.[19,20] Targetoid, annular erythematous macules of erythema multiforme (EM)–like lesions may occur on the extremities (**Fig. 3**). Lichenoid, erythematous papules and plaques with more eczematous features (**Fig. 4**) may also be encountered as well as lesions that may show recognizable features of psoriasis and Grover-like reactions.[8,21] In addition, ICI therapy may induce pigmentary alteration, and patients may manifest hypopigmented patches of vitiligo (**Fig. 5**) and regressed melanocytic nevi and melanoma.[22,23] Dermal and subcutaneous nodules of sarcoid-like granulomas or panniculitis (**Fig. 6**) and cutaneous bullae of bullous pemphigoid (**Fig. 7**) are infrequent but known complications of ICI therapy.[24–27] Exceedingly rare is the development of lipoatrophy, fat necrosis, and Stevens-Johnson syndrome (SJS)/toxic epidermal necrolysis (TEN).[28–30] The clinical morphologic features of cutaneous irAEs are diverse and require astute dermatologists and dermatopathologists for specific clinical and histopathologic diagnoses.

CLINICAL FEATURES

Cutaneous irAEs from ICI therapy are visible and often occur earlier on the skin than in other organs.[11] Cutaneous irAEs may occur 2 to 3 weeks after initiating therapy; however, lesions may be seen within days of treatment and even several months after cessation of ICI therapy.[11–13] The clinical features of cutaneous irAEs from ICI therapy are diverse, but associated pruritus is a frequent complication.[14] A morbilliform, maculopapular cutaneous reaction (**Fig. 1**) is a commonly encountered cutaneous irAE with ICI therapy.[15,16] Lesions generally are low grade and predominantly involve the trunk.[17,18] However, connective tissue disease–like reactions with discoid lesions of lupus and erythema and papules of dermatomyositis (**Fig. 2**) may occur on the face and sun-exposed

MICROSCOPIC FEATURES AND DIAGNOSIS

The histopathologic features of cutaneous irAEs are diverse and may generally be categorized as (1) inflammatory adverse skin reactions, (2) cutaneous epithelial neoplasm–associated adverse skin reactions, and (3) melanocyte-specific adverse skin reactions.[14,31] Of these 3 categories, the inflammatory reactions account for most cutaneous irAEs and include a vast array of lesions that may be further subclassified according to the following histopathologic features: (1) squamoinflammatory, (2) vesiculobullous and vesiculopustular, (3) connective tissue disease–like, (4) vasculitide, and (5) granulomatous/sarcoid-like (**Table 1**).[8–11,19,21,24–27,31–42] Of the inflammatory reaction subclassifications, the squamoinflammatory

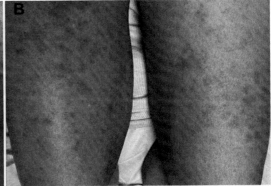

Fig. 1. Clinical features of morbilliform immune-related adverse event secondary to immune checkpoint inhibitor therapy. Erythematous, pruritic macules located on the (*A*) trunk and (*B*) extremities.

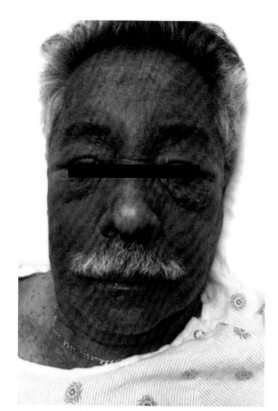

Fig. 2. Clinical features of connective tissue disease–like immune-related adverse event secondary to immune checkpoint inhibitor therapy. Patient with heliotrope rash of dermatomyositis-like irAE.

and the vesiculobullous and vesiculopustular are the most diverse.

INFLAMMATORY ADVERSE SKIN REACTIONS

Squamoinflammatory Immune-Related Adverse Events

The histopathologic features of the squamoinflammatory cutaneous irAEs from ICI therapy include superficial perivascular dermatitis with eosinophils and a dermal hypersensitivity reaction (DHR) (**Fig. 8**). Overlying scale and spongiosis are not prominent histopathologic features of the DHR. Most DHRs are readily recognized by dermatologists as mild erythema and are typically not biopsied because they are low-grade cutaneous irAEs that can be managed with topical therapies. In contrast, the lichenoid dermatitis (LD) irAE is the most frequently encountered cutaneous reaction from ICI therapy submitted for histopathologic examination. More than 50% of biopsies typically show an LD-irAE reaction pattern.[5–8,24,25,31,32,34] LD-irAE may show histopathologic features that are identical to those of lichen planus (LP), with hyperkeratosis, hypergranulosis, and irregular

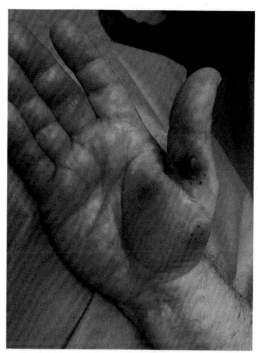

Fig. 3. Clinical features of erythema multiforme-like immune-related adverse event secondary to immune checkpoint inhibitor therapy. Targetoid, erythematous macules on acral skin.

acanthosis with a band-like dense inflammatory infiltrate along the dermal-epidermal junction (DEJ) (**Fig. 9**). Associated dyskeratosis and colloid bodies may be observed. The inflammatory infiltrate is composed predominantly of lymphocytes and histiocytes. Eosinophils and plasma cells are not prominent; however, multiple biopsies at various anatomic sites from a single patient may show variability in histopathologic features, with

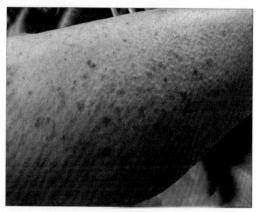

Fig. 4. Clinical features of lichenoid dermatitis immune-related adverse event secondary to immune checkpoint inhibitor therapy. Multiple erythematous papules are distributed on the trunk and on the extremities.

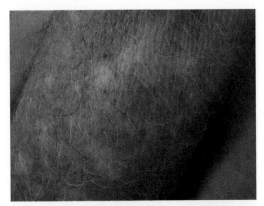

Fig. 5. Clinical features of vitiligo-like immune-related adverse event secondary to immune checkpoint inhibitor therapy. There are irregular, hypopigmented patches scattered on the extremities.

more prominent spongiosis, parakeratosis, and eosinophilic inflammation in some lesions.[32] The variability of histopathologic morphologies is a clue to the diagnosis of LD-irAE from LP in the setting of ICI therapy.

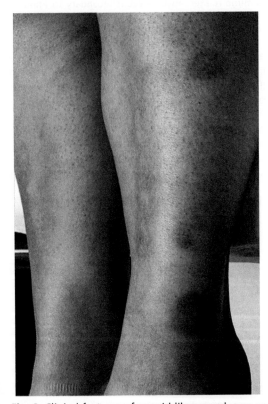

Fig. 6. Clinical features of sarcoid-like granulomas or panniculitis immune-related adverse event secondary to immune checkpoint inhibitor therapy. Indurated nodules with bruise-like features are present on the lower extremity.

A variant of LD-irAE is the hypertrophic pattern. Histopathologically, there is exuberant epidermal hyperplasia with some cytologic atypia of keratinocytes and associated lichenoid inflammation. Single lesions may show features that mimic a superficially well-differentiated squamous cell carcinoma (SCC). Clinical information of ICI therapy and presentation of multiple plaques and nodules are critical for distinguishing hyperplastic LD-irAE from superficially invasive well-differentiated SCC. Histopathologic clues of hypertrophic LD-irAE include epidermal hypermaturation, lichenoid inflammation concentrated at the base of broadened rete ridges, and lichenoid inflammation at the periphery of the biopsy separate from the area of exuberant epidermal hyperplasia and keratinocyte atypia.[43] Lichen nitidus (LN) irAE is another variant of LD-irAE that may be encountered in the setting of ICI therapy.[44] LN-irAEs show focal lichenoid inflammation with a collaret of elongated rete ridges or a ball-and-claw pattern. LN-irAE can be diagnosed when combined with clinical features of micropapules in patients receiving ICI therapy.[44]

The lymphocytic infiltrate in cutaneous irAE may show cytologic atypia and notable epidermal and follicular involvement that may be concerning histopathologically for mycosis fungoides. LD-irAE may additionally show immunohistochemical features of mycosis fungoides with predominance of cluster of differentiation (CD) 4+ cells over CD8+ cells in the epidermis, follicular epithelium, and dermis.[45] Furthermore, lesions may show monoclonal T-cell receptor gene rearrangement in multiple biopsies from a single patient at different time points.[45] Clinical correlation is essential to avoid a diagnosis of mycosis fungoides in a patient treated with ICI therapy.

Psoriasiform dermatitis (PD) irAE is an emerging cutaneous irAE reaction pattern.[8] Lesions may show features of psoriasis vulgaris with broad areas of hyperkeratosis and parakeratosis, hypogranulosis, and uniform epidermal hyperplasia. Lesions may show extravasation of neutrophils in the papillary dermis and exocytosis into the epidermis. Histopathologic features not typical of psoriasis vulgaris, such as spongiosis, irregular epidermal hyperplasia, and eosinophilic inflammation, may also be seen in PD-irAE.[46] Diagnosis of PD-irAE by a dermatopathologist is important because biologic therapy intended for psoriasis vulgaris (eg, interleukin [IL]-17A inhibitor) may be used in a subset of patients to treat this form of cutaneous irAE. In our experience, IL-17A blockade showed dramatic improvement in a patient with PD-irAE

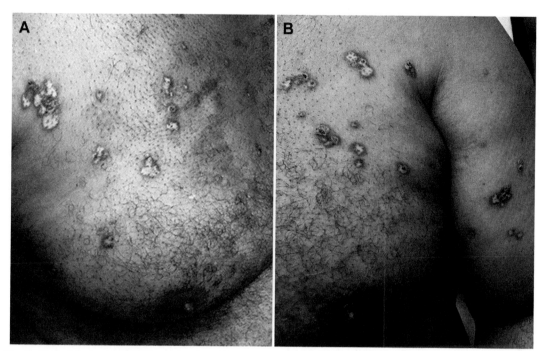

Fig. 7. Clinical features of bullous pemphigoid immune-related adverse event secondary to immune checkpoint inhibitor therapy. (*A*) Multiple ruptured, eroded blisters are present on the chest, and (*B*) a tense blister is evident adjacent to a ruptured blister.

without compromising the ICI anticancer therapy.[46]

Pityriasiform dermatitis (**Fig. 10**) and folliculitis may also be encountered with ICI therapy.[31] Pityriasiform dermatitis irAE may show features of either guttate psoriasis or pityriasis lichenoides–like reactions.[31,46]

Vesiculobullous and Vesiculopustular Immune-Related Adverse Events

Vesiculobullous and vesiculopustular reaction patterns from ICI therapy include autoimmune bullous and nonautoimmune cutaneous irAEs. Bullous pemphigoid (BP) irAE is the most frequently encountered autoimmune bullous disorder that develops in the context of ICI therapy.[8,25,31,47] Clinically, histologically, and immunologically, BP-irAE is identical to de novo BP not associated with ICI therapy. BP-irAE shows a subepidermal blister with associated lymphocytic inflammation with eosinophils in the dermis and within the blister cavity (**Fig. 11**). Periodic acid–Schiff (PAS) stain or anti–type IV collagen highlights the basement membrane zone at the floor of the blister. Direct immunofluorescence (DIF) studies reveal linear immunoglobulin (Ig) G and C3 along the basement membrane zone.[25] A subset of BP-irAE may show predominance of neutrophils in the inflammatory infiltrate.[48] Paraneoplastic pemphigus (PNP) may

show a DIF reaction pattern of BP as well as pemphigus vulgaris.[49] Histologic features of PNP are variable, and PNP-like irAE may show a similar array of morphologies, including interface changes with dyskeratosis, suprabasal blister, acantholysis, and lymphocytic inflammation with eosinophils.[27] Clinical suspicion, DIF and/or serologic studies, and histopathologic features are necessary to identify PNP-like irAE in the era of oncodermatopathology. Other autoimmune bullous irAEs infrequently encountered include dermatitis herpetiformis and linear IgA reactions.[10,40]

Nonautoimmune vesiculobullous and vesiculopustular irAEs include spongiotic dermatitis (**Fig. 12**), acute generalized exanthematous pustulosis (AGEP)–like reactions, acantholytic dyskeratosis (Grover-like), interface dermatitis (EM-like) (**Fig. 13**), and SJS/TEN. The histopathologic features of these nonautoimmune vesiculobullous and vesiculopustular irAEs are identical to their respective dermatitides not associated with ICI therapy; thus, in the era of oncodermatopathology, there should be a high index of suspicion that a variety of inflammatory dermatitides may be related to ICI therapy, and clinical information is critical for diagnosis.

Grover-like irAE may be recognized by focal suprabasal acantholysis of keratinocytes, corp ronds, and corp grains. Lesions may show a dermal lymphocytic inflammation with notable

Table 1
Histopathologic categories of inflammatory adverse skin reactions from immune checkpoint inhibition

Histopathologic Category	Diagnosis of Cutaneous irAEs
Squamoinflammatory	Dermal hypersensitivity reaction Lichenoid dermatitis[a] Psoriasiform dermatitis Pityriasiform dermatitis[b] Folliculitis
Vesiculobullous and vesiculopustular	Spongiotic dermatitis Interface dermatitis (EM-like)[c] AGEP-like SJS/TEN Bullous pemphigoid Dermatitis herpetiformis Paraneoplastic pemphigus-like Linear IgA Grover-like
Connective tissue disease–like	Lupus[d] Dermatomyositis
Vasculitide	Leukocytoclastic vasculitis Pyoderma gangrenosum Sweet syndrome
Granulomatous/ sarcoid-like	Sarcoid-like Erythema nodosum–like Mixed lobular and septal panniculitis Granuloma annulare–like Lipoatrophy-fat necrosis

Abbreviations: AGEP, acute generalized exanthematous pustulosis; IgA, immunoglobulin A.
[a] Variants: hypertrophic, acantholytic, mycosis fungoides–like.
[b] Pityriasis lichenoides–like
[c] Variant: bullous EM–like
[d] Variant: subacute, discoid.

eosinophils.[27] Bullous EM–like irAE is a variant of EM-like irAE that may occur and shows histopathologic features of an interface dermatitis with dyskeratosis and an associated blister cavity.[32] Infrequently, life-threatening dermatologic irAEs with features of SJS/TEN may occur.[29] Biopsies show full-thickness necrosis of the epidermis and, as with SJS/TEN not associated with ICI therapy, there may be variability in the quantity of the inflammatory infiltrate within the lesion.[30]

Connective Tissue Disease–Like Immune-Related Adverse Events

Connective tissue disease-like irAEs include lupus erythematosus–like and dermatomyositis-like lesions.[11,19,20] ICI therapy may exacerbate symptoms in patients with a known history of connective tissue disorder. Lupus-like lesions may show interface changes with associated perivascular and periadnexal lymphocytic inflammation. Discoid lesions show hyperkeratosis, follicular plugging, and a brisk periadnexal and superficial and deep perivascular lymphocytic inflammation. Similar to dermatomyositis unrelated to ICI, dermatomyositis-like irAE shows interface changes and less inflammatory infiltrate. Visualization of increased dermal mucin in connective tissue disease–like irAEs may be appreciated with colloidal iron or Alcian blue stains.

Vasculitide Immune-Related Adverse Events

Vasculitide irAEs are an increasing complication in ICI therapy.[48,50] Leukocytoclastic vasculitis irAE shows histopathologic features of dermal small vessel vascular damage with fibrinoid necrosis of the vessel wall and associated neutrophilic inflammation.[51] Neutrophilic dermatosis irAEs may show dense dermal inflammation with neutrophils and associated papillary dermal edema, similar to histopathologic features shown in Sweet syndrome.[39]

Granulomatous/Sarcoid-like Immune-Related Adverse Events

Granulomatous/sarcoid–like irAEs encompass panniculitides associated with ICI therapy. The histomorphology may involve sarcoid-like granulomas in the skin and/or subcutis with or without associated lymphocytic inflammatory infiltrate (**Fig. 14**). Sarcoid-like granulomas may be confined to the skin or present with skin and lymph node involvement in a subset of patients.[24] Panniculitides (**Fig. 15**) may be predominantly septal with erythema nodosum (EN)–like histomorphology or mixed septal and lobular with mixed inflammatory infiltrate of lymphocytes, histiocytes, neutrophils, and eosinophils.[34] Granulomatous/ sarcoid-like irAEs may be deeply situated in the soft tissue, and patients may have lymphadenopathy. Lesions are PET–computed tomography fluorodeoxyglucose F 18 avid and may thus clinically and radiographically mimic disease recurrence, but may also represent markers of therapy

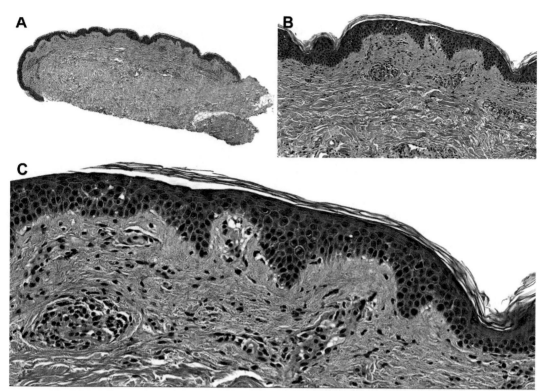

Fig. 8. Histopathologic features of a dermal hypersensitivity reaction immune-related adverse event secondary to immune checkpoint inhibitor therapy. (*A*) Low-magnification section shows skin with a mild, superficial, perivascular inflammatory infiltrate (hematoxylin-eosin [H&E], original magnification ×40). (*B*) The epidermis shows minimal histopathologic changes (H&E, original magnification ×80). (*C*) The perivascular infiltrate is composed of lymphocytes and scattered eosinophils (H&E, original magnification ×200).

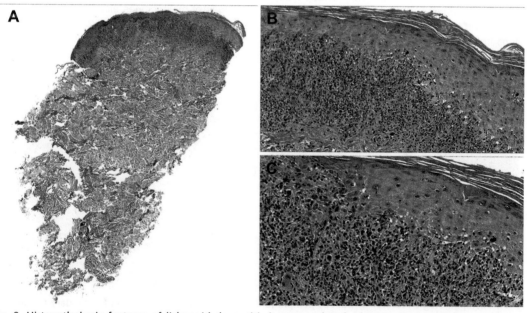

Fig. 9. Histopathologic features of lichenoid dermatitis immune-related adverse event secondary to immune checkpoint inhibitor therapy. (*A*) Low-magnification section shows skin with a dense, band-like inflammatory infiltrate in superficial dermis (H&E, original magnification ×40). (*B*) Epidermis with hyperkeratosis, wedge-shaped hypergranulosis, and dyskeratosis (H&E, original magnification ×100). (*C*) Lichenoid infiltrate composed of lymphocytes, pigmented macrophages, and colloid bodies (H&E, original magnification ×150).

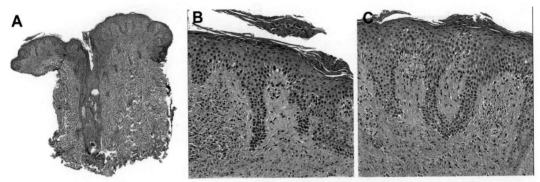

Fig. 10. Histopathologic features of pityriasiform dermatitis immune-related adverse event secondary to immune checkpoint inhibitor therapy. (*A*) Low-magnification section shows skin with focal mounds of parakeratosis and superficial and deep perivascular dermal infiltrate (H&E, original magnification ×40). (*B, C*) Epidermis shows mild spongiosis with focal mounds of parakeratosis (H&E, original magnification ×150).

response in a subset of patients. Awareness of this pattern of irAEs in the era of oncodermatopathology is important for appropriate cancer management by the oncology team.[24]

CUTANEOUS EPITHELIAL NEOPLASM–ASSOCIATED ADVERSE SKIN REACTIONS

Cutaneous epithelial neoplasms are an infrequent complication in ICI therapy; in contrast, these types of cutaneous toxicities are commonly associated with targeted therapy (eg, vemurafenib).[31,52] Keratoacanthomas with endophytic, cup-shaped squamous proliferation with well-differentiated keratinocytes and prurigo nodularis lesions from ICI therapy may occur.[31,53]

MELANOCYTE-SPECIFIC ADVERSE SKIN REACTIONS

irAEs from ICI therapy that targets melanocytes and melanoma show characteristic histopathologic features in the skin.[23] These features include a completely regressed melanocytic lesion (eg, nevi or melanoma) with histopathologic features of pigmentary alteration and melanophages in the dermis and the absence of viable neoplastic cells; melanocytic nevi with regression changes noted by attenuated normal rete ridge pattern, dermal fibrosis, vascular proliferation, and partial absence of melanocytes; and vitiligo changes with loss of melanocytes along the DEJ (**Fig. 16**). Biopsy of the skin of vitiligo-like irAEs may histopathologically appear normal; however, a Sox10

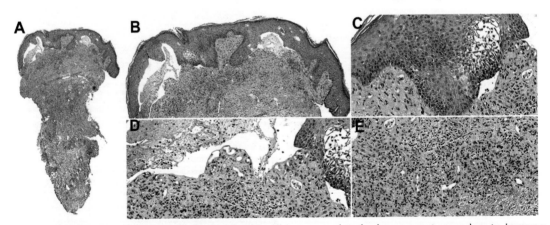

Fig. 11. Histopathologic features of bullous pemphigoid immune-related adverse event secondary to immune checkpoint inhibitor therapy. (*A*) Low magnification shows skin with subepidermal blister (H&E, original magnification ×40). (*B*) Subepidermal blister and associated dermal inflammation (H&E, original magnification ×80). (*C*) Epidermis with eosinophilic spongiosis (H&E, original magnification ×100). (*D, E*) Blister cavity and dermis with inflammatory infiltrate and numerous eosinophils ([*D*] H&E, original magnification ×100 and [*E*] H&E, original magnification ×200).

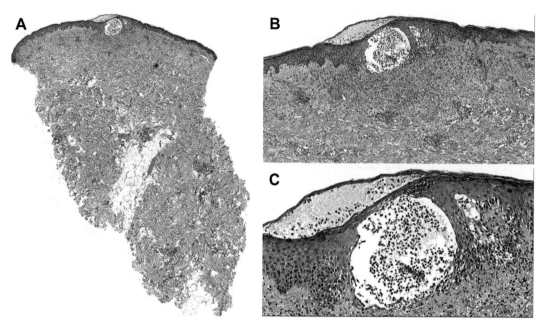

Fig. 12. Histopathologic features of spongiotic dermatitis immune-related adverse event secondary to ICI therapy. (*A*) Low-magnification section shows skin with spongiotic vesicle formation and inflammatory infiltrate in superficial dermis (H&E, original magnification ×40). (*B*) Epidermis shows intraepithelial vesicle with spongiosis, dyskeratosis, and superficial dermal inflammation with eosinophils (H&E, original magnification ×100). (*C*) Spongiotic vesicle with dyskeratosis and eosinophils in epidermis and superficial dermis (H&E, original magnification ×150).

or melanocytic marker (eg, HMB45) may confirm the detection of reduced numbers of normal melanocytes along the DEJ and a diagnosis of vitiligo-like irAE from ICI therapy.

DIFFERENTIAL DIAGNOSIS

In the era of oncodermatopathology, ICI therapy–associated cutaneous irAEs need to be excluded

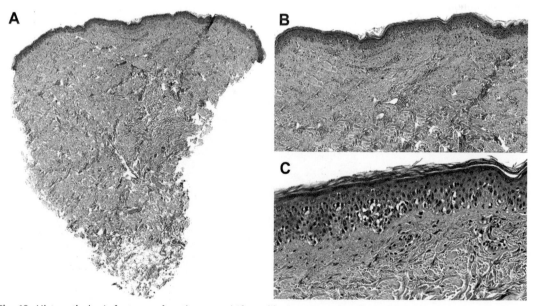

Fig. 13. Histopathologic features of erythema multiform–like immune-related adverse event secondary to immune checkpoint inhibitor therapy. (*A*) Low-magnification section of skin shows pauci-inflammatory interface infiltrate (H&E, original magnification ×40). (*B*) DEJ with vacuolar changes and sparse lymphocytic infiltrate (H&E, original magnification ×100). (*C*) Epidermis with rare dyskeratotic cells (H&E, original magnification ×200).

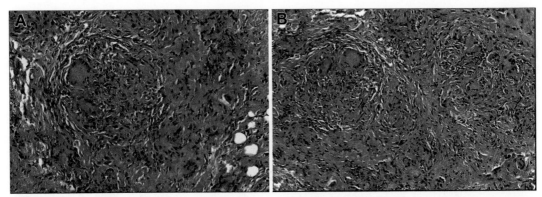

Fig. 14. Histopathologic features of granulomatous dermatitis/sarcoid–like immune-related adverse event secondary to immune checkpoint inhibitor therapy. (*A, B*) Granulomatous inflammation of deep dermis composed of well-formed granulomas and numerous multinucleated giant cells and absence of necrosis (H&E, original magnification ×200).

in any patients with cancer who develop cutaneous lesions during therapy. Because of the diverse morphologies of cutaneous irAEs, the differential diagnosis is vast and poses challenges. Cutaneous irAEs may be categorized as (1) inflammatory adverse skin reactions, (2) cutaneous epithelial neoplasm–associated adverse skin reactions, and (3) melanocyte-specific adverse skin reactions. Inflammatory reactions, which have been further subcategorized according to histopathologic reaction pattern (see **Table 1**), may aid dermatologists and dermatopathologists in classifying the diverse cutaneous irAEs.[14,31] The histomorphologic features of cutaneous irAEs mimic skin conditions unrelated to ICI therapy in

patients without cancer; thus, knowledge of clinical history together with the major tissue inflammatory reactions and patterns of inflammation aids in the diagnosis of inflammatory cutaneous irAEs.[14]

The most common biopsied inflammatory adverse skin reactions from ICI therapy is LD-irAE. LP is the main histopathologic differential diagnosis of LD-irAE, and both conditions may show identical histomorphologic features.[32] However, LD-irAE may show histopathologic variability with greater spongiosis and eosinophilic inflammation among multiple biopsies from a patient that may aid in distinguishing it from LP. A lichenoid drug reaction not associated with ICI therapy is

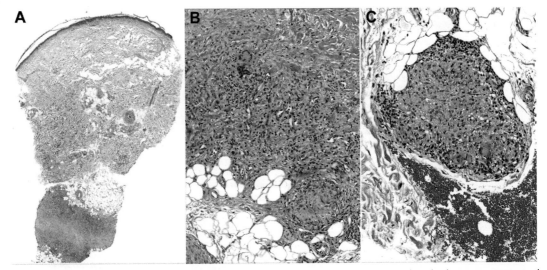

Fig. 15. Histopathologic features of erythema nodosum–like panniculitis immune-related adverse event secondary to immune checkpoint inhibitor therapy. (*A*) Low-magnification section shows septal panniculitis, widening of the septa, and fibrosis (H&E, original magnification ×40). (*B*) Lobular septa with lymphocytic inflammation, giant cells, and granulomas (H&E, original magnification ×100); (*C*) Involvement of noncaseating granulomas into lobules adjacent to the septa (H&E, original magnification ×200).

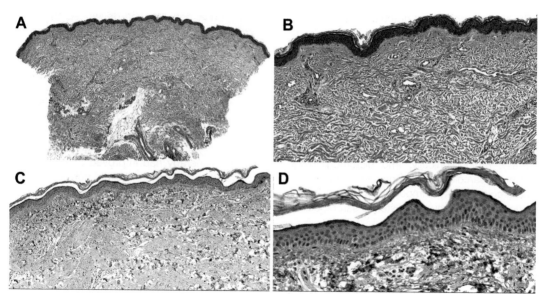

Fig. 16. Histopathologic features of vitiligo-like immune-related adverse event secondary to immune checkpoint inhibitor therapy. (*A*) Low-magnification section shows unremarkable normal-appearing skin (H&E, original magnification ×40). (*B*) Normal-appearing epidermis and absence of significant inflammatory infiltrate (H&E, original magnification ×100). (*C, D*) Panmelanocytic cocktail (HMB45 and antityrosinase) shows markedly reduced density of melanocytes along the DEJ (immunohistochemistry, antipanmelanocytic cocktail, original magnification ×100 and ×400, respectively).

also in the differential diagnosis. Obtaining clinical information and history of ICI therapy is critical, and, at times, distinguishing lichenoid drug reactions not associated with ICI therapy from LD-irAE cannot be done with absolute certainty. Variants of LD-irAE include the hypertrophic form and lesions that resemble mycosis fungoides.[43,45] Hypertrophic LD-irAE may mimic a well-differentiated, superficially invasive SCC. Clinical information about recent onset of multiple nodules and the histomorphology of the lichenoid infiltrate concentrated at broadened rete ridges are needed to avoid a diagnosis of SCC. LD-irAEs may show histopathologic and molecular features of mycosis fungoides and clinical presentation of sudden onset of patches and/or plaques in contrast with a long history of patches evolving to plaques; this information is crucial in distinguishing LD-irAE from mycosis fungoides.

Distinguishing cutaneous graft-versus-host disease (GVHD) from lichenoid/interface irAE in patients who undergo allogenic stem cell transplant who also have received ICI therapy may not be feasible.[54] Histopathologically, an acute pattern of GVHD may show identical features to those of EM-like irAE. Furthermore, histopathologically, chronic lichenoid GVHD may appear similar to LD-irAE. Further investigations into the immunopathogenesis of these dermatoses may provide insight into immune mediators that drive these reactions.

PD-irAE may show some histopathologic features of psoriasis vulgaris.[8] PD-irAE has a more acute onset than does psoriasis vulgaris; therefore, psoriatic plaque of psoriasis vulgaris may be more prominent. Thus, histopathologically, the scale and acanthosis of PD-irAE may be thinner compared with the plaque of psoriasis vulgaris. Furthermore, spongiosis and eosinophilic inflammation may be more prominent in PD-irAE than in psoriasis vulgaris.[46]

BP-irAE is the most commonly encountered autoimmune bullous disorder from ICI therapy. BP-irAE shows identical clinical, histopathologic, and immunologic features to de novo BP not associated with ICI therapy. A clinical history of ICI therapy is necessary for distinguishing BP-irAE from de novo BP. PNP-like irAE may show features similar to those of PNP.[27] Furthermore, PNP-like irAE may show immunologic overlap from BP-irAE and de novo BP; thus, the histopathologic features of interface changes and blister cavity with acantholysis and dyskeratosis may aid in distinguishing PNP-like irAEs from BP-irAE and de novo BP. Grover-like irAE may also show suprabasal acantholysis and dyskeratosis; however, the presence of papules rather than of tense bullae aids in distinguishing Grover-like irAE from PNP-like irAE. Grover disease without associated ICI therapy may have identical histopathologic features to Grover-like irAE; thus, clinical information is necessary.

The histomorphology of granulomatous/sarcoid-like irAE includes septal panniculitis, and the histopathologic differential includes EN.[34] Distinguishing EN not associated with ICI therapy from granulomatous/sarcoid-like irAE that shows EN-like features requires clinical information of ICI therapy. Collection of epithelioid histiocytes without necrosis-forming sarcoidal granulomas may occur in the dermis, subcutis, lymph nodes, and visceral sites during ICI therapy.[24] Sarcoid-like irAE may clinically, radiographically, and histomorphologically mimic sarcoidosis. Recognition of granulomatous/sarcoid-like irAE is important in avoiding a new diagnosis of cutaneous or systemic sarcoidosis in patients receiving ICI therapy.[24]

The differential diagnosis for cutaneous epithelial neoplasms associated adverse skin reactions from ICI therapy is limited because these morphologic types of cutaneous adverse reactions are more frequently associated with small molecule inhibitors (nibs) rather than with monoclonal antibody blockade with ICIs.[14,55] Keratoacanthoma-like irAE from ICI therapy rarely occurs; thus, a crateriform atypical squamous lesion encountered in a patient receiving ICI therapy will be in the differential diagnosis.[56]

Melanocyte-specific adverse skin reactions from ICI therapy may clinically manifest as hyperpigmentation or hypopigmentation of the skin. A completely regressed melanocytic lesion with macrophages containing melanin pigment require exclusion of hemosiderin and minocycline pigment. Prussian blue and Fontana-Masson stain may be useful in this scenario. The differential diagnosis of a regressed melanocytic lesion in the setting of ICI therapy includes a regressed nevus and regressed melanoma.[57] Histomorphologic features of residual banal nevi and melanoma provide diagnostic clues; however, further ancillary immunohistochemical studies (eg, HMB45 and Mart-1/Ki-67) may be necessary for this distinction. A dense lymphocytic infiltrate may be present in regressed nevi from ICI therapy, and a regressed halo nevus not associated with ICI therapy may show similar histopathologic features. Vitiligo-like irAE may show an identical histomorphology to de novo vitiligo not associated with ICI therapy, and clinical information is necessary for further distinction.[23,42]

PROGNOSIS

In general, early clinical studies suggest that patients with unresectable melanoma that developed irAEs in any organ from ICI therapy were associated with better outcome than were patients who did not develop irAEs during therapy.[58]

Furthermore, patients who developed more than 2 irAEs in any organ showed better overall survival than did patients with fewer than 2 irAEs.[58] Melanoma patients who developed cutaneous irAEs of any type had significantly better progression-free survival than did patients who did not develop cutaneous irAE from therapy.[59] In a meta-analysis of 137 studies with 139 treatment arms, including 28 ICI-based studies, patients with metastatic melanoma who developed vitiligo-like features during ICI therapy had improved overall survival compared with patients who did not develop vitiligo-like features during therapy.[60]

Cutaneous irAEs reported in many clinical trials include pruritis, rash not otherwise specified (NOS), and dermatitis. An in-depth examination of the histopathologic features of cutaneous irAEs reveals a spectrum of skin toxicities, listed in Table 1. Because most rash NOS and dermatitis reported in clinical trials are likely DHR, lichenoid, or spongiotic irAEs, umbrella classification of these specific types of cutaneous irAE as rash or dermatitis supports published findings that cutaneous irAEs correlate with good patient outcome. Although these studies look promising in that the irAEs could be a predictive prognostic marker of antitumor response to ICI therapy, in our experience, not all types of cutaneous irAEs are associated with good outcome. A cohort of patients with melanoma treated at MD Anderson who developed BP-irAE tended to have worse OS ($P<.06$) than did patients with LD-irAE (data not shown). Despite limited sample size and preliminary findings, the immunopathogenesis and management of LD-irAE and BP-irAE elucidate these observations. LD-irAE is a T helper (Th) 1–driven immune response from ICI therapy, in contrast with BP-irAE, which shows a Th2 immune profile. Furthermore, LD-irAE is primarily managed clinically with topical steroids and continuation of ICI therapy; in contrast, BP-irAE often requires systemic steroids and withholding of ICI therapy. Thus, the immune-activating benefits of ICI therapy in patients with BP-irAE are suppressed by systemic steroids and/or removed from cessation of ICI therapy. Further studies on the specific types of cutaneous irAEs and patient outcomes in a larger cohort of patients with different cancer types are needed.

IMMUNOPATHOGENESIS OF CUTANEOUS IMMUNE-RELATED ADVERSE EVENTS

Our knowledge of the immunopathogenesis and immune mechanisms that drive cutaneous irAEs from ICI therapy is limited, largely because they have only recently been recognized. Some early studies investigating the immune mechanisms of LD, psoriasiform, and BP irAEs from ICI therapy are provided later.

In the skin, LD-irAE is a frequently biopsied histopathologic type of irAE. LD-irAE and benign lichenoid keratosis (BLK) or LP-like keratosis not associated ICI therapy show near-identical histopathologic features; however, these diseases are clinically distinct. LD-irAE presents as diffuse papules and plaques, whereas BLK is a solitary lesion on the skin. Gene expression profiling of LD-irAE from ICI therapy compared with that of BLK identified a unique set of differentially expressed messenger RNAs (mRNAs) despite nearly identical histopathologic features.[61,62] LD-irAE from ICI therapy showed 74 significantly upregulated mRNA gene transcripts, and 93 mRNA gene transcripts were significantly downregulated.[61,62] Upregulated mRNA gene transcripts included chemokines CXCL12 and CCL14, which involve monocyte recruitment and regulation to the skin.[63,64] CD14, which is a surface marker of monocytes and coreceptor for Toll-like receptors (TLRs), was also upregulated in LD-irAE compared with BLK. In vivo studies confirmed that LD-irAE showed increased numbers of $CD14^+$ and $CD16^+$ monocytes in the skin.[61,62] Furthermore, TLRs 2 and 4 were upregulated in LD-irAE compared with BLK.[61,62] Collectively, LD-irAE showed activation of the cutaneous innate immune response. The immunopathogenesis of LD-irAE may involve recruitment of $CD14^+$ $CD16^+$ monocytes to the skin, CD14/TLR signaling, and a unique cutaneous microbiome in susceptible patients that drive LD-irAE from ICI therapy.[62] Additional studies on innate immune response and the role of the cutaneous microbiome in cutaneous irAEs are needed to further elucidate immune mechanisms involved in LD-irAE.

PD-irAE is an infrequent but recognized adverse reaction from ICI therapy.[8] PD-irAE shows similar clinical and histopathologic overlap with de novo psoriasis vulgaris.[8] The IL-17 pathway is critical in the immunopathogenesis of psoriasis vulgaris, and biologics with IL-17 blockade is an effective mode of therapy.[65,66] The innate immune responses in Th1 and Th17 cells are important in the immunopathogenesis of psoriasis vulgaris. The Th2 immune response is important in atopic dermatitis; however, some forms of atopic dermatitis show clinical and immunologic overlap with psoriasis vulgaris.[67–69] Furthermore, some forms of atopic dermatitis may show more hyperkeratosis and acanthosis, with overlap of histopathologic features of psoriasis vulgaris.[69] PD-irAE shows clinical and histologic features of psoriasis vulgaris

in addition to some features of spongiosis and eosinophilic inflammation. The immune profile of PD-irAE seems to show a Th17 and Th2 pattern similar to that of some forms of atopic dermatitis.[46,69] In our experience, treatment with an IL-17A inhibitor (secukinumab) in a patient who developed PD-irAE from ICI therapy resulted in dramatic improvement of the patient's skin toxicity without compromising the antitumor benefits of ICI therapy.[46] However, there was also a report of tumor progression in a patient receiving ICI therapy with IL-17 inhibition.[69,70] Further studies of the immunopathogenesis of PD-irAE and the use of biologic therapy to manage cutaneous irAE are critically needed.

BP-irAE shows identical clinical, histologic, and immunologic features to de novo BP not associated with ICI therapy.[25] The immunopathogenesis of BP-irAE is currently being investigated. Our preliminary studies show that BP-irAE is a Th2-driven immune response with greater numbers of Gata-3^+ immune cells (data not shown) compared with LD-irAE, which shows a Th1 immune profile and increased numbers of T-Bet$^+$ cells.[62] Despite identical clinical, histopathologic, and immunologic features of BP-irAE and de novo BP, gene expression profiling of BP-irAE revealed 119 differentially expressed mRNA gene transcripts compared with de novo BP.[71] Thirty mRNA transcripts were upregulated and included CCL18 chemokine, C1R, C1S complement, and TLR4. Genes related to Th17 activation and IL-23 signaling pathways were not upregulated in BP-irAE compared with de novo BP.[71] In our experience, early studies indicate that patients with BP-irAE develop immune serology targeted primarily against the BP180 antigen (data not shown). These studies suggest that BP-irAE shows a unique gene expression profile and immune mechanism driving BP-irAE via mediators of a classic complement pathway.[71] BP-irAE and herpes gestationis may show similar immune mechanisms, and the role of major histocompatibility complex proteins of the human leukocyte antigen system may influence susceptible patients in developing BP-irAE; however, more studies are critically needed. As more knowledge of the immune mechanisms of cutaneous irAEs is gathered, a proposed classification of cutaneous reactions may involve a predominant immune profile that involves skin toxicity reactions.

SUMMARY

Cutaneous irAEs pose off-target challenges in patients treated with ICI therapy. The breadth and diversity of the morphologic types of cutaneous irAEs have ushered dermatologists and dermatopathologists into the era of oncodermatopathology. Morphologic classification of cutaneous irAEs may be grouped into 3 main categories and 5 subcategories of the inflammatory reactions. An additional proposed classification may involve the type of immune response present in the types of cutaneous irAEs.

Future studies will increase the knowledge of the immune mechanisms that drive cutaneous irAEs, expose critically needed efficacious therapy to combat cutaneous irAEs, and unveil underlying mechanisms of morphologically related dermatologic disorders not associated with ICI therapy.

CLINICS CARE POINTS

- LD-irAE is the most frequently biopsied cutaneous irAE

- BP-irAE is the most frequently encountered autoimmune bullous irAE from ICI therapy

- Granulomatous/sarcoid-like irAE may clinically and radiographically mimic disease recurrence or sarcoidosis

- Vitiligo-like irAE is associated with improved clinical outcome

- Connective tissue disease–like irAE may be exacerbated with ICI therapy in patients with preexisting connective tissue disorders (eg, dermatomyositis)

ACKNOWLEDGEMENT

NIH/NCI. Grant number P30CA016672. The Department of Pathology Junior Faculty Award. The University of Texas MD Anderson Cancer Center Institutional Research Grant.

DISCLOSURE

The authors have nothing to disclose.

REFERENCES

1. Sanmamed MF, Chen L. A Paradigm Shift in Cancer Immunotherapy: From Enhancement to Normalization. Cell 2018;175(2):313–26.
2. Hodi FS, O'Day SJ, McDermott DF, et al. Improved survival with ipilimumab in patients with metastatic melanoma. N Engl J Med 2010;363(8):711–23.
3. Robert C, Long GV, Brady B, et al. Nivolumab in previously untreated melanoma without BRAF mutation. N Engl J Med 2015;372(4):320–30.
4. McDermott DF, Drake CG, Sznol M, et al. Survival, durable response, and long-term safety in patients with previously treated advanced renal cell carcinoma receiving nivolumab. J Clin Oncol 2015; 33(18):2013–20.
5. Puzanov I, Diab A, Abdallah K, et al. Managing toxicities associated with immune checkpoint inhibitors: consensus recommendations from the Society for Immunotherapy of Cancer (SITC) Toxicity Management Working Group. J Immunother Cancer 2017;5(1):95.
6. Minkis K, Garden BC, Wu S, et al. The risk of rash associated with ipilimumab in patients with cancer: a systematic review of the literature and meta-analysis. J Am Acad Dermatol 2013;69(3):e121–8.
7. Michot JM, Bigenwald C, Champiat S, et al. Immune-related adverse events with immune checkpoint blockade: a comprehensive review. Eur J Cancer 2016;54:139–48.
8. Kaunitz GJ, Loss M, Rizvi H, et al. Cutaneous eruptions in patients receiving immune checkpoint blockade: clinicopathologic analysis of the nonlichenoid histologic pattern. Am J Surg Pathol 2017; 41(10):1381–9.
9. Ng CY, Chen CB, Wu MY, et al. Anticancer drugs induced severe adverse cutaneous drug reactions: an updated review on the risks associated with anticancer targeted therapy or immunotherapies. J Immunol Res 2018;2018:5376476.
10. Mochel MC, Ming ME, Imadojemu S, et al. Cutaneous autoimmune effects in the setting of therapeutic immune checkpoint inhibition for metastatic melanoma. J Cutan Pathol 2016;43(9):787–91.
11. Wang LL, Patel G, Chiesa-Fuxench ZC, et al. Timing of onset of adverse cutaneous reactions associated with programmed cell death protein 1 inhibitor therapy. JAMA Dermatol 2018;154(9):1057–61.
12. Weber JS, Kahler KC, Hauschild A. Management of immune-related adverse events and kinetics of response with ipilimumab. J Clin Oncol 2012; 30(21):2691–7.
13. Sznol M, Ferrucci PF, Hogg D, et al. Pooled analysis safety profile of nivolumab and ipilimumab combination therapy in patients with advanced melanoma. J Clin Oncol 2017;35(34):3815–22.
14. Curry JL, Chu EY, Tetzlaff MT. Cutaneous drug eruptions, supplement. In: Barnhill R, editor. Barnhill's dermatopathology. 4th edition. New York: McGraw-Hill Education; 2020. p. 1–12.
15. Sibaud V. Dermatologic Reactions to Immune Checkpoint Inhibitors : Skin Toxicities and Immunotherapy. Am J Clin Dermatol 2018;19(3):345–61.
16. Naidoo J, Page DB, Li BT, et al. Toxicities of the anti-PD-1 and anti-PD-L1 immune checkpoint antibodies. Ann Oncol 2015;26(12):2375–91.
17. Sibaud V, Meyer N, Lamant L, et al. Dermatologic complications of anti-PD-1/PD-L1 immune checkpoint antibodies. Curr Opin Oncol 2016;28(4):254–63.

18. Belum VR, Benhuri B, Postow MA, et al. Characterisation and management of dermatologic adverse events to agents targeting the PD-1 receptor. Eur J Cancer 2016;60:12–25.

19. Shao K, McGettigan S, Elenitsas R, et al. Lupus-like cutaneous reaction following pembrolizumab: An immune-related adverse event associated with anti-PD-1 therapy. J Cutan Pathol 2018;45(1):74–7.

20. Sheik Ali S, Goddard AL, Luke JJ, et al. Drug-associated dermatomyositis following ipilimumab therapy: a novel immune-mediated adverse event associated with cytotoxic T-lymphocyte antigen 4 blockade. JAMA Dermatol 2015;151(2):195–9.

21. Uemura M, Faisal F, Haymaker C, et al. A case report of Grover's disease from immunotherapy-a skin toxicity induced by inhibition of CTLA-4 but not PD-1. J Immunother Cancer 2016;4:55.

22. Hua C, Boussemart L, Mateus C, et al. Association of vitiligo with tumor response in patients with metastatic melanoma treated with pembrolizumab. JAMA Dermatol 2016;152(1):45–51.

23. Mauzo SH, Tetzlaff MT, Nelson K, et al. Regressed melanocytic nevi secondary to pembrolizumab therapy: an emerging melanocytic dermatologic effect from immune checkpoint antibody blockade. Int J Dermatol 2017;58(9):1045–52.

24. Tetzlaff MT, Nelson K, Diab A, et al. Granulomatous/sarcoid-like lesions associated with checkpoint inhibitors: a marker of therapy response in a subset of melanoma patients. J Immunother Cancer 2018;6(1):14.

25. Jour G, Glitza IC, Ellis RM, et al. Autoimmune dermatologic toxicities from immune checkpoint blockade with anti-PD-1 antibody therapy: a report on bullous skin eruptions. J Cutan Pathol 2016;43(8):688–96.

26. Kwon CW, Land AS, Smoller BR, et al. Bullous pemphigoid associated with nivolumab, a programmed cell death 1 protein inhibitor. J Eur Acad Dermatol Venereol 2017;31(8):e349–50.

27. Chen WS, Tetzlaff MT, Diwan H, et al. Suprabasal acantholytic dermatologic toxicities associated checkpoint inhibitor therapy: A spectrum of immune reactions from paraneoplastic pemphigus-like to Grover-like lesions. J Cutan Pathol 2018;45(10):764–73.

28. Bhargava P, Flynt L, Marcal L. Nivolumab-induced subcutaneous fat necrosis: another FDG-avid immune-related adverse event. Clin Nucl Med 2020;45(2):125–6.

29. Chen CB, Wu MY, Ng CY, et al. Severe cutaneous adverse reactions induced by targeted anticancer therapies and immunotherapies. Cancer Manag Res 2018;10:1259–73.

30. Robinson S, Saleh J, Curry J, et al. Pembrolizumab-induced stevens-johnson syndrome/toxic epidermal necrolysis in a patient with metastatic cervical squamous cell carcinoma: a case report. Am J Dermatopathol 2020;42(4):292–6.

31. Curry JL, Tetzlaff MT, Nagarajan P, et al. Diverse types of dermatologic toxicities from immune checkpoint blockade therapy. J Cutan Pathol 2017;44(2):158–76.

32. Tetzlaff MT, Nagarajan P, Chon S, et al. Lichenoid dermatologic toxicity from immune checkpoint blockade therapy: a detailed examination of the clinicopathologic features. Am J Dermatopathol 2017;39(2):121–9.

33. Siegel J, Totonchy M, Damsky W, et al. Bullous disorders associated with anti-PD-1 and anti-PD-L1 therapy: A retrospective analysis evaluating the clinical and histopathologic features, frequency, and impact on cancer therapy. J Am Acad Dermatol 2018;79(6):1081–8.

34. Tetzlaff MT, Jazaeri AA, Torres-Cabala CA, et al. Erythema nodosum-like panniculitis mimicking disease recurrence: A novel toxicity from immune checkpoint blockade therapy-Report of 2 patients. J Cutan Pathol 2017;44(12):1080–6.

35. Rofe O, Bar-Sela G, Keidar Z, et al. Severe bullous pemphigoid associated with pembrolizumab therapy for metastatic melanoma with complete regression. Clin Exp Dermatol 2017;42(3):309–12.

36. Pintova S, Sidhu H, Friedlander PA, et al. Sweet's syndrome in a patient with metastatic melanoma after ipilimumab therapy. Melanoma Res 2013;23(6):498–501.

37. Naidoo J, Schindler K, Querfeld C, et al. Autoimmune bullous skin disorders with immune checkpoint inhibitors targeting PD-1 and PD-L1. Cancer Immunol Res 2016;4(5):383–9.

38. Boland P, Heath J, Sandigursky S. Immune checkpoint inhibitors and vasculitis. Curr Opin Rheumatol 2020;32(1):53–6.

39. Ravi V, Maloney NJ, Worswick S. Neutrophilic dermatoses as adverse effects of checkpoint inhibitors: A review. Dermatol Ther 2019;32(5):e13074.

40. Jonna S, Neiders M, Lakshmanan S, et al. Linear IgA disease of the gingiva following nivolumab therapy. J Immunother 2019;42(9):345–7.

41. Matsubara T, Uchi H, Haratake N, et al. Acute generalized exanthematous pustulosis caused by the combination of pembrolizumab plus chemotherapy in a patient with squamous-cell carcinoma. Clin Lung Cancer 2020;21(2):e54–6.

42. Coleman E, Ko C, Dai F, et al. Inflammatory eruptions associated with immune checkpoint inhibitor therapy: A single-institution retrospective analysis with stratification of reactions by toxicity and implications for management. J Am Acad Dermatol 2019;80(4):990–7.

43. Marques-Piubelli M, Tetzlaff MT, Nagarajan P, et al. Hypertrophic lichenoid dermatitis immune-related adverse event during combined immune checkpoint and exportin inhibitor therapy: A diagnostic pitfall for

superficially invasive squamous cell carcinoma. J Cutan Pathol 2020;47(10):954–9.

44. Li AW, Ko CJ, Leventhal JS. Generalized lichen nitidus-like eruption in the setting of mogamulizumab and tremelimumab. Eur J Dermatol 2017; 27(3):325–6.

45. Tetzlaff MT, Tang S, Duke T, et al. Lichenoid dermatitis from immune checkpoint inhibitor therapy: An immune-related adverse event with mycosis-fungoides-like morphologic and molecular features. J Cutan Pathol 2019;46(11):872–7.

46. Johnson D, Patel AB, Uemura MI, et al. IL17A blockade successfully treated psoriasiform dermatologic toxicity from immunotherapy. Cancer Immunol Res 2019;7(6):860–5.

47. Carlos G, Anforth R, Chou S, et al. A case of bullous pemphigoid in a patient with metastatic melanoma treated with pembrolizumab. Melanoma Res 2015; 25(3):265–8.

48. Morris LM, Lewis HA, Cornelius LA, et al. Neutrophil-predominant bullous pemphigoid induced by checkpoint inhibitors: a case series. J Cutan Pathol 2020;47(8):742–6.

49. Anhalt GJ. Paraneoplastic pemphigus. J Investig Dermatol Symp Proc 2004;9(1):29–33.

50. Richter MD, Crowson C, Kottschade LA, et al. Rheumatic syndromes associated with immune checkpoint inhibitors: a single-center cohort of sixty-one patients. Arthritis Rheumatol 2019;71(3):468–75.

51. Tomelleri A, Campochiaro C, De Luca G, et al. Anti-PD1 therapy-associated cutaneous leucocytoclastic vasculitis: A case series. Eur J Intern Med 2018;57: e11–2.

52. Curry JL, Tetzlaff MT, Nicholson K, et al. Histological features associated with vemurafenib-induced skin toxicities: examination of 141 cutaneous lesions biopsied during therapy. Am J Dermatopathol 2014; 36(7):557–61.

53. Antonov NK, Nair KG, Halasz CL. Transient eruptive keratoacanthomas associated with nivolumab. JAAD Case Rep 2019;5(4):342–5.

54. Ortega Sanchez G, Stenner F, Dirnhofer S, et al. Toxicity associated with PD-1 blockade after allogeneic haematopoietic cell transplantation. Swiss Med Wkly 2019;149:w20150.

55. Lacouture ME, Duvic M, Hauschild A, et al. Analysis of dermatologic events in vemurafenib-treated patients with melanoma. Oncologist 2013;18(3):314–22.

56. Bednarek R, Marks K, Lin G. Eruptive keratoacanthomas secondary to nivolumab immunotherapy. Int J Dermatol 2018;57(3):e28–9.

57. Staser K, Chen D, Solus J, et al. Extensive tumoral melanosis associated with ipilimumab-treated melanoma. Br J Dermatol 2016;175(2):391–3.

58. Freeman-Keller M, Kim Y, Cronin H, et al. Nivolumab in resected and unresectable metastatic melanoma:

characteristics of immune-related adverse events and association with outcomes. Clin Cancer Res 2016;22(4):886–94.

59. Sanlorenzo M, Vujic I, Daud A, et al. Pembrolizumab cutaneous adverse events and their association with disease progression. JAMA Dermatol 2015;151(11): 1206–12.

60. Teulings HE, Limpens J, Jansen SN, et al. Vitiligo-like depigmentation in patients with stage III-IV melanoma receiving immunotherapy and its association with survival: a systematic review and meta-analysis. J Clin Oncol 2015;33(7):773–81.

61. Curry JL, Tetzlaff MT, Reuben A, et al. Gene expression profiling of dermatologic toxicities from immune checkpoint therapy. J Immnotherapy Cancer 2017;5:523.

62. Curry JL, Reuben A, Szczepaniak-Sloane R, et al. Gene expression profiling of lichenoid dermatitis immune-related adverse event from immune checkpoint inhibitors reveals increased CD14(+) and CD16(+) monocytes driving an innate immune response. J Cutan Pathol 2019;46(9): 627–36.

63. Benarafa C, Wolf M. CXCL14: the Swiss army knife chemokine. Oncotarget 2015;6(33):34065–6.

64. Sanchez-Martin L, Estecha A, Samaniego R, et al. The chemokine CXCL12 regulates monocyte-macrophage differentiation and RUNX3 expression. Blood 2011;117(1):88–97.

65. Nickoloff BJ. Cracking the cytokine code in psoriasis. Nat Med 2007;13(3):242–4.

66. Blauvelt A, Reich K, Tsai TF, et al. Secukinumab is superior to ustekinumab in clearing skin of subjects with moderate-to-severe plaque psoriasis up to 1 year: Results from the CLEAR study. J Am Acad Dermatol 2017;76(1):60–69 e69.

67. Miossec P, Korn T, Kuchroo VK. Interleukin-17 and type 17 helper T cells. N Engl J Med 2009;361(9): 888–98.

68. Curry JL, Qin JZ, Bonish B, et al. Innate immune-related receptors in normal and psoriatic skin. Arch Pathol Lab Med 2003;127(2):178–86.

69. Guttman-Yassky E, Krueger JG. Atopic dermatitis and psoriasis: two different immune diseases or one spectrum? Curr Opin Immunol 2017;48:68–73.

70. Esfahani K, Miller WH Jr. Reversal of autoimmune toxicity and loss of tumor response by interleukin-17 blockade. N Engl J Med 2017; 376(20):1989–91.

71. Marques-Piubelli ML, Tetzlaff MT, Mudaliar K, et al. Differentially Expressed Genes in Bullous Pemphigoid Immune-related Adverse Event (BP-irAE) from Immune Checkpoint Inhibitor Therapy: Implications in the Immunopathogenic Mechanisms Driving BP-irAE Compared to de novo BP Control. Mod Pathol 2020;33:602–71.

Mucosal Melanomas of the Anogenital Tract

Clinical and Pathologic Predictors of Patient Survival

Priyadharsini Nagarajan, MD, PhD

KEYWORDS

• Anogenital • Melanoma • Anorectal • Vulvar • Pathology • Primary tumor • Staging

Key points

- Anogenital melanomas are rare and aggressive malignancies with high mortality rates; among anogenital melanomas, anorectal and vulvar melanomas are the most frequent types.

- In view of multifocal nature and advanced stage at diagnosis, these melanomas may require extensive surgical resections for control of primary tumor with potential for severe loss of function and morbidity.

- Because of the rarity of these tumors, site-specific staging systems do not exist for primary anogenital melanomas, and they are traditionally staged using criteria derived for primary cutaneous melanoma, based principally on tumor thickness and ulceration.

- However, compared with primary cutaneous melanomas, anogenital melanomas tend to be more frequently ulcerated, likely as a result of advanced stage at diagnosis and also because of external trauma related to normal physiologic functions, suggesting that ulceration may not be a robust histopathological indicator to predict outcome.

- Therefore, derivation of anatomic site-specific staging systems is critical for prognostication of patients with anorectal and vulvar melanomas.

ABSTRACT

Primary anogenital mucosal melanomas (AGMs) are rare aggressive malignancies that are typically diagnosed at an advanced stage. Ulceration is a common feature in AGMs and may not correlate with outcome. Therefore, staging of AGMs similar to primary cutaneous melanomas, based on tumor thickness and ulceration, may not robustly predict outcome. Derivation of site-specific staging systems is essential for prognostication and optimal management of these patients. To this end, recent retrospective studies have revealed tumor thickness (TT) and mitotic rate (MR) as features of most prognostic significance as follows: in anorectal (TT only) and vulvar (TT and MR) melanomas.

OVERVIEW

Primary mucosal melanomas (MMs) are primary melanomas arising from the mucosal epithelia lining the aerodigestive and anogenital tracts. They are extremely rare and comprise only 1.3% to 4% of all melanomas.[1–3] Although MMs and primary cutaneous melanomas (CMs) arise from malignant transformation of melanocytes, they are inherently different from each other in several aspects. Although CM is one of the most common

Pathology, The University of Texas MD Anderson Cancer Center, 1515 Holcombe Boulevard, B3-4621, Unit 85, Houston, TX 77030, USA
E-mail address: pnagarajan@mdanderson.org

Surgical Pathology 14 (2021) 225–235
https://doi.org/10.1016/j.path.2021.01.003
1875-9181/21/© 2021 Elsevier Inc. All rights reserved.

malignancies with an estimated incidence of 96,480 in 2019 (57,200 in men and 39,260 in women), non-cutaneous melanomas (including uveal melanoma and MM) accounted for only 7870 cases.[4] CM is most common among non-Hispanic whites.[5] Although the absolute number of MMs is highest among whites,[1] the relative proportion of MM in non-white populations is higher when compared with CM.[1,6] CM is more common among men (male-to-female ratio- 1.4:1), whereas there is a female predominance in MM (male-to-female ratio- 1:1.8), primarily because of vulvo-vaginal melanomas.[5,7,8] Although ultraviolet light exposure is the predominant cause of CM, the risk factors for the development of MM have not yet been elucidated.

Primary melanomas of the sinonasal tract are the most common type, accounting for approximately 55% of all MMs and are staged according the eighth edition American Joint Committee on Cancer (AJCC) staging system based on level of invasion and organs involved by the tumor.[9,10] In contrast, a specific staging system does not exist for anogenital melanomas (AGMs), of which anorectal and vulvo-vaginal melanomas are the most frequent types.[2] This article will focus on the prognostic value of clinical and histopathologic features of the primary tumor in pathologic staging of anorectal melanomas (ARMs) and vulvar melanomas (VMs).

ARM is the most common type of AGM, accounting for 0.4% to 1.6% of all melanomas, with an age-adjusted annual incidence of 0.343 cases per 1 million population in the United States.[11] There is a predominance in women (0.407 cases per 1 million population) compared with men (0.259 cases per 1 million population), with a male-to-female ratio of 1:1.56 to 1.7.[11,12] The mean age at presentation is 68.5 years (range: 26–89 years).[11,12] VM accounts for 1% to 7% of all melanomas, 4% to 10% of all gynecologic and approximately 5.3% of all vulvar malignancies in women.[13,14] The incidence is 1.08 to 1.36 cases per 1 million women per year in the United States.[14,15] It is most common among elderly and postmenopausal white women (mean: 61.6 years); however, the age at diagnosis ranges from 10 to 86 years.[14]

GROSS FEATURES

Similar to CM, AGMs present typically as irregular lesions with circumscribed or ill-defined borders and variable pigmentation.[6] Rarely, they may arise as a recent change or a new nodule in pre-existing melanosis or pigmented lesion. Nodular mass and unilateral vulvar lesion are common presenting features of ARM and VM, respectively. However, they are frequently multifocal in nature,[16] and may be amelanotic in many cases.[7] The most common presenting symptoms in patients with ARM are bleeding, mass or lesion (frequently mistaken to be hemorrhoids), pain/discomfort, change in bowel habits including diarrhea, abdominal fullness and ulcer. Lesion, bleeding, pruritus, pain/discomfort, irritation/discharge, foul odor, dyspareunia, and ulcer are frequent in VM.[12,17] Rarely, primary AGM can be completely asymptomatic and incidentally noticed during physical examination or may present as metastatic disease and detected in the course of evaluation for a primary site of origin. Bilateral vulvar involvement and midline tumors (clitoris or fourchette involvement) are often associated with a poor outcome.[17]

In contrast to sinonasal melanomas that are almost exclusively mucosal in origin, some AGMs of anorectal, vulvar, or penile origin may arise from mucosal, cutaneous (eg, anal verge, labia majora, penile shaft, and outer surface of foreskin) epithelia or from mucocutaneous transition zones. However, because of the delay in diagnosis, most of these tumors are large and multifocal at presentation, often spanning expansive areas, including cutaneous and mucosal surfaces, rendering accurate designation of epithelium of origin difficult to determine by clinical and histologic evaluation. Therefore, collaboration between the endoscopists, clinicians, and pathologists is essential to determine the anatomic site accurately, particularly in ARM, where the surgical, anatomic, and histologic extents of anal canal are distinct from each other.[18]

MICROSCOPIC FEATURES

Similar to CM, melanomas of all histologic patterns of growth including superficial spreading, nodular, and unclassified types can occur at mucosal sites. However, the most frequent histologic growth pattern is that of acral lentiginous or mucosal type,[12,17] in which the in situ component is composed of contiguous proliferation of single and nested atypical melanocytes along the basal layer of squamous, junctional, and columnar epithelia with frequent widespread extension far beyond the invasive component and/or grossly visible lesion. Ulceration is a common feature in AGM compared with CM, and up to 50% of VMs and 88% of ARMs are ulcerated,[12,17] which may be secondary to the advanced stage of melanoma at diagnosis and/or related to physiologic function-related external trauma.

DIFFERENTIAL DIAGNOSIS

Because of its rarity and innocuous and highly variable nature, AGM is often a diagnosis of exclusion in most patients. Several diseases can be pigmented or darker compared with the surrounding skin or mucosa and mimic MM: reactive conditions (eg, purpura, postinflammatory pigmentary alteration, and melanosis); infectious diseases (eg, tinea corporis); benign and malignant neoplastic conditions (eg, melanocytic-nevi: banal as well as other rare types and atypical genital nevi [AGN]; keratinocytic-lichen simplex chronicus, lichen sclerosis with pigment incontinence or hemorrhage, acanthosis nigricans, seborrheic keratosis, condyloma, mucosal melanotic macule or lentigo, basal cell carcinoma, squamous cell carcinoma in situ or high-grade intraepithelial lesion and paget disease; vascular-hemorrhoids, angiokeratoma, hemangioma; fibrohistiocytic-dermatofibroma) conditions.[19]

Occasionally, some of these entities may coexist with MM, incidentally or in close association. In fact, MM may be associated with pre-existing nevi, the frequency of which ranges from approximately 1.25% in ARM[12] to approximately 8% among VM, a feature correlating with improved overall survival (OS) among VM patients.[17]

Of these, distinction of melanoma from melanocytic nevi, which constitute approximately 2% of vulvar pigmented lesions,[20] in particular AGN,[21] can be challenging, especially on small biopsies. AGN can appear alarming with variable pigmentation clinically and with a confluence of melanocytic nests histologically. However, the small size (<1 cm), circumscription, symmetry, minimal single cell/lentiginous and pagetoid proliferation, low mitotic activity, and maturation of dermal component favor AGN, compared with MM, which is characterized by larger size (>1 cm), lack of circumscription or symmetry, lentiginous and pagetoid distribution of melanocytes, frequent ulceration, increased mitotic activity and lack of maturation of dermal component.[21] Moreover, *BRAF* V600E mutations are common among AGN,[22] while they are relatively rare among MM, the molecular alterations of which are *Richard A. Scolyer and colleagues article, "Mucosal Melanoma Molecular"*, in this issue.

DIAGNOSIS

Histopathologic evaluation is the gold standard for diagnosing MM. Therefore, biopsy should be considered in any mucocutaneous lesion that lacks a clear traumatic or reactive etiology, especially if it persists after conservative therapy. In most cases, evaluation of hematoxylin and eosin stained sections is sufficient for diagnosis of melanoma. Presence of a radial growth phase (ie, involvement of overlying epithelia by melanoma extending beyond the invasive or submucosal component and/or presence of lesional cells with more than 1 morphology) favors a primary tumor. However, metastatic melanoma should be excluded by comprehensive review of the patient's prior history and imaging studies. Excisional biopsies of smaller lesions and incisional biopsy of the thickest portions of larger lesions would be ideal. In the absence of obvious thick areas, multifocal sampling of large lesions to include periphery and center of the lesion (scouting biopsies) may become necessary for diagnosis and to assess the extent of tumor. Endoscopic evaluations and whole-body imaging including computed tomography (CT), positron emission tomography (PET), ultrasound, and MRI scans should be included in the initial work up to determine the local extent of disease and multifocality, as well as to identify metastatic disease, as up to 35% of MMs can present with metastatic disease compared with only 9% of CMs.[6,7]

ANCILLARY STUDIES, DIAGNOSTIC: IMMUNOHISTOCHEMISTRY

Histopathologic diagnosis is typically straightforward in most cases. However, it can become challenging because of small biopsy size, lack of cytoplasmic pigmentation, poor differentiation, and limited amount of evaluable tissue because of necrosis and/or cautery artifact. In these scenarios, judicial application of a panel of immunohistochemical studies including conventional melanocytic (HMB45, MART1/MelanA, S100, MITF), keratinocytic (keratin cocktail, p63) and vascular (ERG) markers may aid in defining the cell lineage.[23] In some occasions, the tumor cells can be poorly differentiated leading to loss of expression melanocytic markers mentioned previously, likely because of advanced stage at diagnosis.[24] This phenomenon may be seen in AGM and may be associated with aberrant expression of keratin, particularly keratin 18,[25] and in such cases, SOX10 might be the most sensitive immunohistochemical marker of melanocytic differentiation.

Although the expression patterns, diagnostic utility, and prognostic significance of *P*referentially expressed antigen in *m*elanoma (PRAME) has been evaluated to a greater extent in CM Cecilia Lezcano and colleagues' article, "PRAME Immunohistochemistry as an Ancillary Test for the Assessment of Melanocytic Lesions," in this issue,[26] little is known about its importance in MM. A recent study evaluating 29 MMs revealed that most MMs (83. 3%) showed immunohistochemical expression of PRAME in at least 55% of the tumor cells.[27] PRAME expression was higher among tumors with epithelioid cells and correlated with decreased OS.[27]

PROGNOSIS

MMs are typically associated with higher morbidity, often related to larger size and/or multifocal involvement of primary tumors, requiring extensive surgical procedures. Moreover, there is sometimes involvement of critical anatomic structures such as sphincters by melanoma, and the tumors may not be completely resectable without comprising the quality of life; thus, requiring local radiation therapy resulting in associated adverse effects.[28,29] In spite of local control of primary disease, MMs are typically associated with a worse prognosis when compared to CM,[6,7] with a 5-year survival of 27.6% and 76.3%, respectively, in MM and CM.[30] This poor prognosis is correlated with a propensity for developing metastasis among MM patients. In fact, up to 35% of all MM patients present with metastatic disease at the time of initial diagnosis, which correlates with poor outcome.[6,7] However, because of the rarity of MM, many of the studies frequently evaluate the various subtypes of MM together,[30–32] which precludes determination of unique characteristics of MM specific to a particular anatomic site and identification of type-specific clinical and pathologic prognostic features.

In retrospective studies of the Surveillance, Epidemiology, and End Results Program (SEER) database and smaller cohorts, several factors correlate with disease-specific survival (DSS), OS, and other measures of outcome by univariate analysis[13]: Increasing age[33–36] Ethnicity Central,[37,38] multifocal[38] or bilateral[17] vulvar involvement Clinical stage as defined by Ballantyne al (disease localized to the primary anatomic site vs regional metastasis vs distant metastasis),[33,39,40] seventh and eighth edition AJCC stage[13,41] Extent of regional metastases.[34,35,38,42–44]

Among histopathologic features of the primary tumor, ulceration,[17,33,36,42,45,46] mitotic rate,[17,33,47] and increasing tumor thickness,[17,34–36,41–51] lack of regression,[17] satellitosis,[17] lymphovascular invasion,[17,37,38,47] perineural invasion,[17,50] and positive margin status[46] have been shown to significantly correlate with DSS, OS and other measures of outcome by UV analysis. However, only clinical stage,[36] tumor thickness,[17,36] and mitotic rate[17] emerged as the most frequent prognostic features associating independently with outcome.

Similarly, a SEER database study of 640 cases of ARM has revealed that advanced clinical stage, rectal location of primary tumor, and lack of surgical intervention are associated with decreased OS by UV analysis.[11] However, only the presence of distant metastasis was an independent predictor

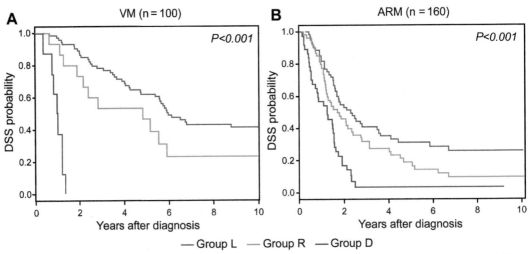

Fig. 1. Kaplan-Meier plots of disease-specific survival of (A) vulvar (VM, n = 100) and (B) anorectal (ARM, n = 160), according to the Ballantyne clinical staging system reflecting the extent of involvement by melanoma as follows: group L: localized disease, group R: regional metastases, and group D: distant metastases. (Adapted from Nagarajan P, Piao J, Ning J, et al. Prognostic model for patient survival in primary anorectal mucosal melanoma: stage at presentation determines relevance of histopathologic features. Modern pathology: an official journal of the United States and Canadian Academy of Pathology, Inc. 2020;33(3):496-513.)

Table 1
Univariate analysis of disease-specific survival of largest single institution cohorts of vulvar and anorectal melanoma according to Ballantyne stage at presentation (group L: localized disease, group R: regional metastasis, group D: distant metastasis)

Ballantyne Stage	Vulvar Melanoma			Anorectal Melanoma		
	n	HR (95% Confidence Interval (CI)	P-Value	n	HR (95% CI)	P-Value
All	100	-	<.001	160	-	<.001
Group L	76 (76%)	Reference	-	67 (42%)	Reference	-
Group R	16 (16%)	1.73 (0.89,3.35)	.104	55 (34%)	1.39 (0.91,2.11)	.124
Group D	8 (8%)	33.62 (11.37,99.38)	<.001	38 (24%)	3.45 (2.14,5.56)	<.001

of OS by multivariate analysis.[11] Studies evaluating smaller cohorts including one with the largest single institution cohort of ARM have revealed age,[52] clinical stage at presentation,[12] regional metastasis,[29,52] multifocality of primary tumor,[53] tumor size,[52,54] increasing tumor thickness,[12,29,31,52,53,55,56] level of colonic wall invasion,[52] histologic type,[12] lack of regression,[12] satellitosis,[12] presence of invasive melanoma at surgical margins,[12] and lymphovascular[12,52] and perineural[12,52] invasion to correlate with outcome. However, increasing age,[52] distant metastatic disease at presentation,[12] increasing thickness of primary tumor,[12,53] deeper invasion of colonic wall,[52] lack of regression,[12] and lymphovascular invasion[12] correlated independently and more frequently with DSS after multivariate analysis.

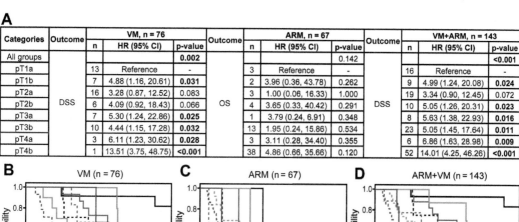

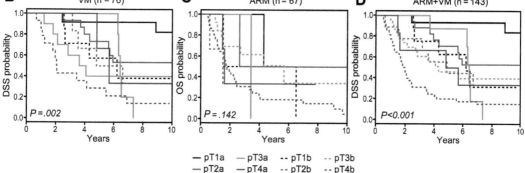

— pT1a — pT3a ·· pT1b -- pT3b
— pT2a — pT4a ·· pT2b -- pT4b

Fig. 2. Risk stratification of patients presenting with only localized disease at diagnosis according to the AJCC eighth edition cutaneous melanoma T-categories (pT1a: tumor thickness [TT] <0.8 mm, no ulceration; pT1b: TT <0.8 mm with ulceration and TT 0.8 to 1.0 mm irrespective of ulceration; pT2a: TT 1.1 to 2.0 mm, no ulceration; pT2b: TT 1.1 to 2.0 mm, with ulceration; pT3a: TT 2.1 to 4.0 mm, no ulceration; pT3b: TT 2.1 to 4.0 mm, with ulceration; pT4a: TT >4.0 mm, no ulceration; pT4b: TT >4.0 mm, with ulceration]. (*A*) Univariate analyses and (*B–D*) Kaplan Meier plots of (*B*) vulvar [VM, n = 76, DSS], (*C*) ARM (n = 67, OS), and (*D*) combined cohort of VM and ARM [n = 143, DSS]. (*Adapted from* Nagarajan P, Piao J, Ning J, et al. Prognostic model for patient survival in primary anorectal mucosal melanoma: stage at presentation determines relevance of histopathologic features. Modern Pathology: an official journal of the United States and Canadian Academy of Pathology, Inc. 2020;33(3):496-513.)

Table 2
Grouping of vulvar melanoma and anorectal melanoma patients presenting with only localized disease at diagnosis using the various T-categories and modifications of the American Joint Commission on Cancer eighth edition cutaneous melanoma and tumor thickness-mitotic rate staging systems and results of univariate analysis of overall survival and disease-specific survival

Categories	VM, n = 76				ARM, n = 67				VM + ARM, n = 143			
	Outcome	n	HR (95% CI)	P-Value	Outcome	n	HR (95% CI)	P-Value	Outcome	n	HR (95% CI)	P-Value
8th Edition AJCC Cutaneous Melanoma Stage												
I	DSS	36	Reference	-	DSS	8	Reference	-	DSS	44	Reference	-
II		40	2.58 (4.41,4.71)	.001		59	3.37 (0.81,13.97)	.095		99	3.06 (1.81,5.16)	<.001
Eighth Edition AJCC Cutaneous Melanoma T-category												
All groups	OS			.002	DSS			.142	DSS			<.001
pT1a		13	Reference	-		3	Reference	-		16	Reference	-
pT1b		7	4.88 (1.16,20.61)	.031		2	3.96 (0.36,43.78)	.262		9	4.99 (1.24,20.08)	.024
pT2a		16	3.28 (0.87,12.52)	.083		3	1.00 (0.06,16.33)	1.000		19	3.34 (0.90,12.45)	.072
pT2b		6	4.09 (0.92,18.43)	.066		4	3.65 (0.33,40.42)	.291		10	5.05 (1.26,20.31)	.023
pT3a		7	5.30 (1.24,22.86)	.025		1	3.79 (0.24,6.91)	.348		8	5.63 (1.38,22.93)	.016
pT3b		10	4.44 (1.15,17.28)	.032		13	1.95 (0.24,15.86)	.534		23	5.05 (1.45,17.64)	.011
pT4a		3	6.11 (1.23,30.62)	.028		3	3.11 (0.28,34.40)	.355		6	6.86 (1.63,28.98)	.009
pT4b		1	13.51 (3.75,48.75)	<.001		38	4.86 (0.66,35.66)	.120		52	14.01 (4.25,46.26)	<.001
Modified Tumor Thickness												
All groups	DSS			<.0001	DSS			.032	DSS			<.001
Thin		20	Reference	-		5	Reference	-		25	Reference	-
Intermediate		39	2.01 (0.90,4.50)	.089		21	2.36 (0.30,18.31)	.412		60	2.09 (1.00,4.38)	.050
Thick		17	5.41 (2.27,12.89)	.0001		41	4.98 (0.67,36.69)	.116		58	5.73 (2.74,11.94)	<.001
Tumor Thickness-Mitotic Rate												
pT1	OS	27	Reference	-	DSS	5	Reference	-	DSS	32	Reference	-
pT2		46	3.89 (1.92,7.88)	<.001		62	3.33 (0.80,13.80)	.097		108	4.64 (2.38,9.05)	<.001
N/A		3	-	-			-	-		3	-	-

STAGING

In contrast to head and neck MM, specific staging systems do not exist for AGM, with the exception of VM, for which the AJCC recommends use of the eighth edition CM staging system.[57] Although the AJCC eighth edition CM system may predict outcome for VM of cutaneous origin (lateral surfaces of labia majora), it is unclear if this system would also accurately prognosticate the VMs that originate from mucosal surfaces and/or mucocutaneous transitional epithelia. Given this lack of clarity, AGMs are traditionally staged using the Ballantyne clinical staging system[40] and/or the AJCC eighth edition CM staging system.[57]

CLINICAL STAGE PREDICTS OUTCOME IN VULVAR AND ANORECTAL MELANOMAS

Studies using the SEER database have revealed regional and distant metastasis in 24.9% and 6.7% in VM patients, respectively, at the time of diagnosis.[13] Moreover, higher burden of regional metastatic disease correlated with decreased DSS.[13] Similarly, evaluation of large single-institution cohorts of VM[17] revealed 24% of patients presenting with metastatic disease at diagnosis, of whom 16% had regional and 8% had distant metastasis (Nagarajan et al., 2020, **Fig. 1A**, **Table 1**). On the other hand, a greater proportion of ARM patients,

up to 52.2% to 59.6%%, present with metastatic disease at diagnosis, with almost equal distribution between those with regional (25.8% to 28.5%) and distant (26.4% to 31.2%) metastasis.[11,58] Evaluation of 160 ARM patients from a single institution revealed predominance of regional metastasis (34%) when compared with distant metastasis (24%) at presentation (adapted from Nagarajan and colleagues,[12] **Fig. 1B**, see **Table 1**). Presence of distant metastasis at the time of diagnosis correlated with worse DSS in both VM and ARM patients.[11–13,17,39]

RISK STRATIFICATION OF VULVAR AND ANORECTAL MELANOMA PRESENTING WITH LOCALIZED DISEASE AT DIAGNOSIS

Advanced clinical stage (ie, the presence of regional and/or distant metastatic disease) has been demonstrated to be the most robust predictor of outcome in VM and ARM. Conversely, the prognosis of VM and ARM patients that present with only localized disease is likely to be predicted by histopathologic parameters of the primary tumor. Prior studies have shown that tumor thickness, ulceration, and mitotic rate are most frequently and consistently associated with survival. Adapting from their previously published studies,[12] the author and colleagues re-evaluated the performance of various T-category systems

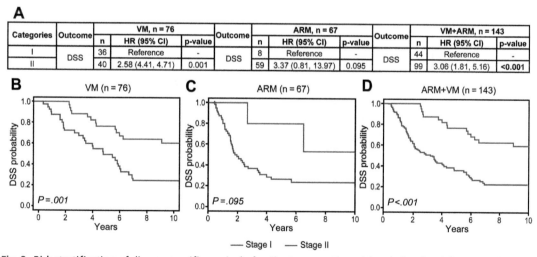

Categories	Outcome	VM, n = 76			Outcome	ARM, n = 67			Outcome	VM+ARM, n = 143		
		n	HR (95% CI)	p-value		n	HR (95% CI)	p-value		n	HR (95% CI)	p-value
I	DSS	36	Reference	-	DSS	8	Reference	-	DSS	44	Reference	-
II		40	2.58 (4.41, 4.71)	0.001		59	3.37 (0.81, 13.97)	0.095		99	3.06 (1.81, 5.16)	<0.001

Fig. 3. Risk stratification of disease-specific survival of patients presenting with only localized disease at diagnosis according to the AJCC eighth edition cutaneous melanoma stage (stage I: AJCC eighth cutaneous melanoma T-category T1a to T2a; stage II: T2b to T4b). (*A*) Univariate analyses and (*B–D*) Kaplan-Meier plots of (*B*) vulvar (VM, n = 76), (*C*) anorectal (ARM, n = 67) and (*D*) combined cohort of VM and ARM (n = 143). (*Adapted from* Nagarajan P, Piao J, Ning J, et al. Prognostic model for patient survival in primary anorectal mucosal melanoma: stage at presentation determines relevance of histopathologic features. Modern Pathology: an official journal of the United States and Canadian Academy of Pathology, Inc. 2020;33(3):496-513.)

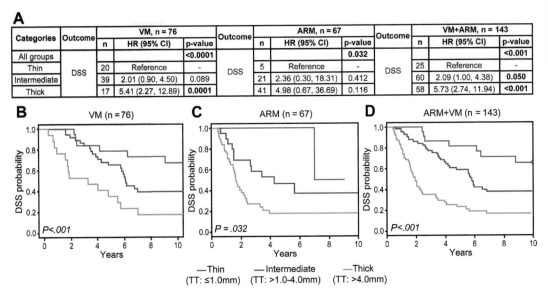

Fig. 4. Risk stratification of disease-specific survival of patients presenting with only localized disease at diagnosis according to the modified tumor thickness system (thin: TT ≤1.0 mm; intermediate: TT >1.0 to 4.0 mm; thick: TT >4.0 mm). (*A*) Univariate analyses and (*B–D*) Kaplan-Meier plots of (*B*) vulvar (VM, n = 76), (*C*) anorectal (ARM, n = 67), and (*D*) combined cohort of VM and ARM (n = 143). (*Adapted from* Nagarajan P, Piao J, Ning J, et al. Prognostic model for patient survival in primary anorectal mucosal melanoma: stage at presentation determines relevance of histopathologic features. Modern Pathology: an official journal of the United States and Canadian Academy of Pathology, Inc. 2020;33(3):496-513.)

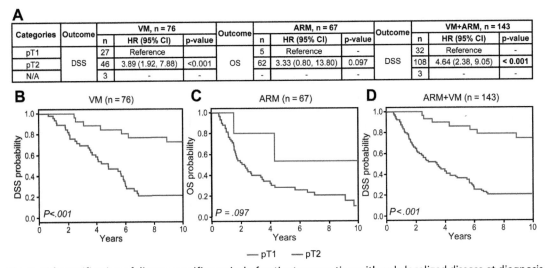

Fig. 5. Risk stratification of disease-specific survival of patients presenting with only localized disease at diagnosis according to the tumor thickness-mitotic rate system (pT1: TT ≤2.0 mm and mitotic rate <2/mm²; pT2: TT >2.0 mm and mitotic rate ≥2/mm²). (*A*) Univariate analyses and (*B–D*) Kaplan-Meier plots of (*B*) vulvar (VM, n = 76), (*C*) anorectal (ARM, n = 67), and (*D*) combined cohort of VM and ARM (n = 143). (*Adapted from* Nagarajan P, Piao J, Ning J, et al. Prognostic model for patient survival in primary anorectal mucosal melanoma: stage at presentation determines relevance of histopathologic features. Modern Pathology: an official journal of the United States and Canadian Academy of Pathology, Inc. 2020;33(3):496-513.)

that utilize tumor thickness, ulceration, and mitotic rate in risk stratifying localized VM and ARM.

Grouping of localized VM, ARM, and the combined VM + ARM cohort using the AJCC eighth edition CM system T-category system achieved statistically significant prediction of DSS for VM and the combined cohort (**Fig. 2, Table 2**, Nagarajan et al., 2020).[12,17] However, stratification of ARM could be achieved only for OS, due to too few events in some of the groups and was not statistically significant. However, although higher T-category (≥pT2b) correlated with decreased DSS (see **Fig. 2**A), there was considerable overlap of the Kaplan-Meier survival curves (**Fig. 2**B–D). Grouping of patients according to the AJCC 8th edition CM stage system delineated two groups of VM and combined cohort patients with statistically significant DSS probabilities (**Fig. 3, Table 2**, Nagarajan et al., 2020),[12,17] but did not achieve statistical significance in ARM. Grouping of patients using a modified tumor thickness system, revealed 3 well-delineated categories of VM, ARM and combined cohort patients of distinct DSS, particularly among patients with thick melanoma (**Fig. 4, Table 2**, Nagarajan et al., 2020).[12,17] In view increased frequency of ulceration and the consistent association of mitotic rate with outcome among AGM, we had proposed a T-categorization system using tumor thickness and mitotic rate for risk stratification of VM.[17] Application of this system significantly differentiated 2 groups of VM and combined cohort patients, but not among ARM patients with localized disease (**Fig. 5, Table 2**, Nagarajan et al., 2020).[12,17]

Performance of these T-categorization systems reveals that tumor thickness remains the most prognostically significant feature of primary tumor in AGM, particularly among ARM, whereas mitotic rate is also important in VM.[13,17] Although these T-categorization systems need to be validated using larger cohorts, they may reveal subgroups of VM and ARM patients presenting with localized disease who may benefit from increased surveillance and/or earlier adjuvant therapies.

SUMMARY

ARM and VM are the most common types of AGM, frequently affecting the elderly white population. Poor prognosis of AGM is related to advanced stage, including presence of metastatic disease at time of diagnosis. Clinical stage is the most significant feature predicting survival, whereas tumor thickness is the most robust primary tumor feature predicting survival among patients presenting with localized disease.

CLINICS CARE POINTS

- Anogenital mucosal melanomas can present innocuously mimicking several reactive and benign conditions.

- Close follow-up and prompt biopsy of persistent lesions may aid in early diagnosis of anogenital mucosal melanomas.

- Clinical stage at presentation is the most significant factor predicting outcome in AGM.

- Tumor thickness of the primary tumor followed by mitotic rate can aid in predicting survival among patients presenting with localized disease.

ACKNOWLEDGMENTS

The author thanks Jin Piao, PhD, and Jing Ning, PhD, for their exceptional assistance in statistical analysis and Kim Anh-Vu, BS, for her excellent assistance in preparing the figures. This publication is based on research supported by the Melanoma Research Alliance to PN (# 570806).

DISCLOSURE

The authors have nothing to disclose.

REFERENCES

1. Chang AE, Karnell LH, Menck HR. The National Cancer Data Base report on cutaneous and noncutaneous melanoma: a summary of 84,836 cases from the past decade. The American College of Surgeons Commission on Cancer and the American Cancer Society. Cancer 1998;83(8):1664–78.

2. McLaughlin CC, Wu XC, Jemal A, et al. Incidence of noncutaneous melanomas in the U.S. Cancer 2005; 103(5):1000–7.

3. Tacastacas JD, Bray J, Cohen YK, et al. Update on primary mucosal melanoma. J Am Acad Dermatol 2014;71(2):366–75.

4. Cancer Facts & Figures 2019. In: Atlanta: American Cancer Society.

5. Siegel RL, Miller DR, Jemal A. Cancer Statistics, 2019. CA Cancer J Clin 2019;69:7–34.

6. Ballester Sanchez R, de Unamuno Bustos B, Navarro Mira M, et al. Mucosal melanoma: an update. Actas Dermosifiliogr 2015;106(2):96–103.

7. Carvajal RD, Spencer SA, Lydiatt W. Mucosal melanoma: a clinically and biologically unique disease entity. J Natl Compr Canc Netw 2012;10(3):345–56.

8. Cancer facts & figures 2019. Atlanta (GA): American Cancer Society; 2019.

9. Williams MD, Franchi A, Helliwell T, et al. Data set for the reporting of mucosal melanomas of the head and neck: explanations and recommendations of the guidelines from the international collaboration on cancer reporting. Arch Pathol Lab Med 2019; 143(5):603–9.

10. Lydiatt WM, Brandwein-Gensler M, Kraus DH, et al. Mucosal melanoma of the head and neck. In: Amin MB, Gershenwald JE, Scolyer R, et al, editors. AJCC cancer staging manual. 8th edition. Switzerland: Springer Nature; 2017. p. 163–9.

11. Chen H, Cai Y, Liu Y, et al. Incidence, Surgical Treatment, and Prognosis of Anorectal Melanoma From 1973 to 2011: A Population-Based SEER Analysis. Medicine (Baltimore) 2016;95(7):1–8.

12. Nagarajan P, Piao J, Ning J, et al. Prognostic model for patient survival in primary anorectal mucosal melanoma: stage at presentation determines relevance of histopathologic features. Mod Pathol 2020;33(3):496–513.

13. Wohlmuth C, Wohlmuth-Wieser I, May T, et al. Malignant melanoma of the vulva and vagina: a US population-based study of 1863 patients. Am J Clin Dermatol 2020;21(2):285–95.

14. Boer FL, Ten Eikelder MLG, Kapiteijn EH, et al. Vulvar malignant melanoma: pathogenesis, clinical behaviour and management: review of the literature. Cancer Treat Rev 2019;73:91–103.

15. Weinstock MA. Malignant melanoma of the vulva and vagina in the United States: patterns of incidence and population-based estimates of survival. Am J Obstet Gynecol 1994;171(5):1225–30.

16. Lotem M, Anteby S, Peretz T, et al. Mucosal melanoma of the female genital tract is a multifocal disorder. Gynecol Oncol 2003;88(1):45–50.

17. Nagarajan P, Curry JL, Ning J, et al. Tumor thickness and mitotic rate robustly predict melanoma-specific survival in patients with primary vulvar melanoma: a retrospective review of 100 cases. Clin Cancer Res 2017;23(8):2093–104.

18. Shia J. An update on tumors of the anal canal. Arch Pathol Lab Med 2010;134(11):1601–11.

19. Heller DS. Benign tumors and tumor-like lesions of the vulva. Clin Obstet Gynecol 2015;58(3):526–35.

20. Rock B. Pigmented lesions of the vulva. Dermatol Clin 1992;10(2):361–70.

21. Ahn CS, Guerra A, Sangueza OP. Melanocytic nevi of special sites. Am J Dermatopathol 2016;38(12): 867–81.

22. Yelamos O, Merkel EA, Sholl LM, et al. Nonoverlapping clinical and mutational patterns in melanomas from the female genital tract and atypical genital nevi. J Invest Dermatol 2016;136(9): 1858–65.

23. Nagarajan P, Tetzlaff MT, Curry JL, et al. Use of new techniques in addition to IHC applied to the diagnosis of melanocytic lesions, with emphasis on CGH, FISH, and Mass Spectrometry. Actas Dermosifiliogr 2017;108(1):17–30.

24. Chang O, Argenyi Z. Loss of conventional melanocytic markers in malignant melanoma and lymph node metastasis; an uncommon but dangerous pitfall. Am J Dermatopathol 2017;39(10):760–3.

25. Chen N, Gong J, Chen X, et al. Cytokeratin expression in malignant melanoma: potential application of in-situ hybridization analysis of mRNA. Melanoma Res 2009;19(2):87–93.

26. Lezcano C, Jungbluth AA, Nehal KS, et al. PRAME expression in melanocytic tumors. Am J Surg Pathol 2018;42(11):1456–65.

27. Toyama A, Siegel L, Nelson AC, et al. Analyses of molecular and histopathologic features and expression of PRAME by immunohistochemistry in mucosal melanomas. Mod Pathol 2019;32(12):1727–33.

28. Ballo MT, Gershenwald JE, Zagars GK, et al. Sphincter-sparing local excision and adjuvant radiation for anal-rectal melanoma. J Clin Oncol 2002; 20(23):4555–8.

29. Kelly P, Zagars GK, Cormier JN, et al. Sphincter-sparing local excision and hypofractionated radiation therapy for anorectal melanoma: a 20-year experience. Cancer 2011;117(20):4747–55.

30. Altieri L, Eguchi M, Peng DH, et al. Predictors of mucosal melanoma survival in a population-based setting. J Am Acad Dermatol 2019;81(1):136–42.e2.

31. Heppt MV, Roesch A, Weide B, et al. Prognostic factors and treatment outcomes in 444 patients with mucosal melanoma. Eur J Cancer 2017;81:36–44.

32. Shi K, Zhu X, Liu Z, et al. Clinical characteristics of malignant melanoma in central China and predictors of metastasis. Oncol Lett 2020;19(2):1452–64.

33. Bradgate MG, Rollason TP, McConkey CC, et al. Malignant melanoma of the vulva: a clinicopathological study of 50 women. Br J Obstet Gynaecol 1990; 97(2):124–33.

34. Trimble EL, Lewis JL Jr, Williams LL, et al. Management of vulvar melanoma. Gynecol Oncol 1992;45(3):254–8.

35. Raber G, Mempel V, Jackisch C, et al. Malignant melanoma of the vulva. Report of 89 patients. Cancer 1996;78(11):2353–8.

36. Ragnarsson-Olding BK, Nilsson BR, Kanter-Lewensohn LR, et al. Malignant melanoma of the vulva in a nationwide, 25-year study of 219 Swedish females: predictors of survival. Cancer 1999;86(7):1285–93.

37. Phillips GL, Bundy BN, Okagaki T, et al. Malignant melanoma of the vulva treated by radical hemivulvectomy. A prospective study of the Gynecologic Oncology Group. Cancer 1994;73(10):2626–32.

38. Scheistroen M, Trope C, Koern J, et al. Malignant melanoma of the vulva. Evaluation of prognostic factors with emphasis on DNA ploidy in 75 patients. Cancer 1995;75(1):72–80.

39. Sanchez A, Rodriguez D, Allard CB, et al. Primary genitourinary melanoma: Epidemiology and

disease-specific survival in a large population-based cohort. Urol Oncol 2016;34(4):166.e7-14.

40. Ballantyne AJ. Malignant melanoma of the skin of the head and neck. An analysis of 405 cases. Am J Surg 1970;120(4):425–31.

41. Verschraegen CF, Benjapibal M, Supakarapongkul W, et al. Vulvar melanoma at the M. D. Anderson Cancer Center: 25 years later. Int J Gynecol Cancer 2001; 11(5):359–64.

42. Tasseron EW, van der Esch EP, Hart AA, et al. A clinicopathological study of 30 melanomas of the vulva. Gynecol Oncol 1992;46(2):170–5.

43. Raspagliesi F, Ditto A, Paladini D, et al. Prognostic indicators in melanoma of the vulva. Ann Surg Oncol 2000;7(10):738–42.

44. Tcheung WJ, Selim MA, Herndon JE 2nd, et al. Clinico-pathologic study of 85 cases of melanoma of the female genitalia. J Am Acad Dermatol 2012;67(4):598–605.

45. DeMatos P, Tyler D, Seigler HF. Mucosal melanoma of the female genitalia: a clinicopathologic study of forty-three cases at Duke University Medical Center. Surgery 1998;124(1):38–48.

46. Seifried S, Haydu LE, Quinn MJ, et al. Melanoma of the vulva and vagina: principles of staging and their relevance to management based on a clinicopatho-logic analysis of 85 cases. Ann Surg Oncol 2015; 22(6):1959–66.

47. Heinzelmann-Schwarz VA, Nixdorf S, Valadan M, et al. A clinicopathological review of 33 patients with vulvar melanoma identifies c-KIT as a prognostic marker. Int J Mol Med 2014;33(4):784–94.

48. Podratz KC, Gaffey TA, Symmonds RE, et al. Melanoma of the vulva: an update. Gynecol Oncol 1983;16(2):153–68.

49. Moxley KM, Fader AN, Rose PG, et al. Malignant melanoma of the vulva: an extension of cutaneous melanoma? Gynecol Oncol 2011;122(3):612–7.

50. Dias-Santagata D, Selim MA, Su Y, et al. KIT mutations and CD117 overexpression are markers of better progression-free survival in vulvar melanomas. Br J Dermatol 2017;177(5):1376–84.

51. Udager AM, Frisch NK, Hong LJ, et al. Gynecologic melanomas: a clinicopathologic and molecular analysis. Gynecol Oncol 2017;147(2):351–7.

52. Ren M, Lu Y, Lv J, et al. Prognostic factors in primary anorectal melanoma: a clinicopathologic study of 60 cases in China. Hum Pathol 2018;79:77–85.

53. Che X, Zhao DB, Wu YK, et al. Anorectal malignant melanomas: retrospective experience with surgical management. World J Gastroenterol 2011;17(4): 534–9.

54. Wang M, Zhang Z, Zhu J, et al. Tumour diameter is a predictor of mesorectal and mesenteric lymph node metastases in anorectal melanoma. Colorectal Dis 2013;15(9):1086–92.

55. Weyandt GH, Eggert AO, Houf M, et al. Anorectal melanoma: surgical management guidelines according to tumour thickness. Br J Cancer 2003;89(11):2019–22.

56. Wanebo HJ, Woodruff JM, Farr GH, et al. Anorectal melanoma. Cancer 1981;47(7):1891–900.

57. Gershenwald JE, Scolyer RA, Hess KR, et al. Melanoma staging: evidence-based changes in the American Joint Committee on Cancer eighth edition cancer staging manual. CA Cancer J Clin 2017;67(6):472–92.

58. Callahan A, Anderson WF, Patel S, et al. Epidemiology of anorectal melanoma in the United States: 1992 to 2011. Dermatol Surg 2016; 42(1):94–9.

Connective Tissue Diseases in the Skin
Emerging Concepts and Updates on Molecular and Immune Drivers of Disease

Carole Bitar, MD, May P. Chan, MD*

KEYWORDS

- Autoantibodies • Autoimmune • Lupus erythematosus • Dermatomyositis
- Mixed connective tissue disease • Plasmacytoid dendritic cells • Scleroderma • Systemic sclerosis

Key points

- Many autoimmune diseases demonstrate cutaneous manifestations that may be difficult to classify and that require careful correlation of clinical, histopathologic, and serologic findings for accurate diagnosis.

- Major advances have been made over the past decade in understanding the molecular and immune drivers of cutaneous lupus erythematosus, dermatomyositis, scleroderma/systemic sclerosis, and mixed connective tissue disease.

- Understanding the molecular and immunologic pathways involved in connective tissue diseases could lead to the development of new diagnostic tools and identification of potential therapeutic targets.

ABSTRACT

Cutaneous manifestations are common across the spectrum of autoimmune diseases. Connective tissue diseases manifesting in the skin are often difficult to classify and require integration of clinical, histopathologic, and serologic findings. This review focuses on the current understanding of the molecular and immune drivers involved in the pathogenesis of cutaneous lupus erythematosus, dermatomyositis, scleroderma/systemic sclerosis, and mixed connective tissue disease. Recent research advances have led to the emergence of new ancillary tools and useful diagnostic clues of which dermatopathologists should be aware to improve diagnostic accuracy for these diseases.

OVERVIEW

Connective tissue diseases (CTDs) are a heterogeneous group of autoimmune diseases that may be localized or systemic. The pathogenesis of these diseases is complex and involves an interplay of genetic, environmental, and immunologic factors. Cutaneous manifestations of CTDs are common and often display overlapping clinical and histopathologic features. A combination of clinical, histopathologic, and serologic studies is therefore required for precise diagnosis. In this article, the authors review the clinicopathologic findings of 4 major CTDs involving the skin, highlighting recent discoveries related to their pathogenesis and new pathologic tools that may aid in their diagnosis.

Department of Pathology, University of Michigan, 2800 Plymouth Road, NCRC Building 35, Ann Arbor, MI 48109, USA
* Corresponding author.
E-mail address: mpchan@med.umich.edu

Surgical Pathology 14 (2021) 237–249
https://doi.org/10.1016/j.path.2021.03.003
1875-9181/21/

CUTANEOUS LUPUS ERYTHEMATOSUS

Cutaneous lupus erythematosus (LE) may occur in the setting of systemic lupus erythematosus (SLE) or may be limited to the skin. These cutaneous lesions are divided into 3 clinical subtypes: acute cutaneous LE, subacute cutaneous lupus erythematosus (SCLE), and chronic cutaneous LE.[1] Of these, chronic cutaneous LE is further subclassified into discoid LE (DLE), tumid LE, LE panniculitis, hypertrophic/verrucous LE, and chilblain LE.[1,2] In addition, patients with LE may present with nonspecific findings, such as alopecia, vasculitis, livedo reticularis, neutrophilic dermatosis, and bullous lesions.[1,2] Many of these subtypes demonstrate significant histopathologic overlap; accurate diagnosis relies on careful correlation with clinical findings and laboratory testing. A summary of the clinical, histopathologic, and serologic findings of different cutaneous LE subtypes is provided in **Table 1**.[2,3]

PATHOGENESIS

Although the pathogenesis of cutaneous LE is not fully understood, human and animal studies have led to significant advances in the past decade. Of the many pathways and molecules implicated, type I interferon is thought to play a central role. In cutaneous LE, UV irradiation causes apoptosis of keratinocytes, which triggers the release of various cytokines, including interferons, interleukins, and tumor necrosis factor-α.[4,5] Release of type I interferons and nuclear debris from the dead keratinocytes stimulates plasmacytoid dendritic cells (PDCs), which aggregate near the dermoepidermal junction and release additional type I interferons as well as chemokines that recruit cytotoxic T cells.[6] The latter causes further damage of the basal keratinocytes. Together, keratinocytes, PDCs, and interferons constitute the most critical inflammatory pathway in the pathogenesis of cutaneous LE.

Another important pathway occurs through the effect of autoantigens released from the degenerated DNA and RNA of dead keratinocytes.[4,7] These autoantigens are phagocytosed by antigen-presenting cells, which in turn activate T cells, which subsequently attack more keratinocytes harboring the same autoantigens. These autoantigens also trigger autoantibody production by B cells, including various antinuclear antibodies (ANAs), such as anti-dsDNA, anti-ssDNA, anti-rRNP, anti-Ro, anti-La, and anti-Sm.[7] Different autoantibodies are associated with specific subtypes of LE (see **Table 1**).[2,3] It is noteworthy that although ANAs are essentially always present in

SLE, only a subset of patients with skin-limited cutaneous LE is found to have elevated ANAs, likely reflective of the correlation between ANAs and disease severity. Autoantibodies against type VII collagen may also develop in SLE, leading to bullous LE in these patients.

It is now known that neutrophils also play an important role in cutaneous LE. Neutrophil extracellular trap (NET) has been recently linked to various autoimmune diseases, including LE.[8] Activated neutrophils form an extracellular weblike "trap" by releasing various neutrophilic contents, such as DNA, histones, myeloperoxidase, and elastase. Although NET constitutes a crucial antimicrobial mechanism,[9] the nuclear antigens present in this structure may also trigger autoimmunity via activation of PDCs, upregulation of type I interferons,[10] as well as activation and expansion of autoreactive B cells.[11] A recent study of cutaneous LE revealed varying degrees of "NETosis" in different LE subtypes.[12] Interestingly, the neutrophils in DLE and LE panniculitis produced the largest amount of NETs compared with SCLE and chilblain LE, suggesting an association between NETosis and scarring in cutaneous LE.

Recent gene expression studies have identified the vestigial-like family member 3 (VGLL3) as a transcription cofactor responsible for the sex bias in LE.[13,14] VGLL3 is enriched in female skin and is an important regulator of female-biased genes. Animal models revealed that overexpression of epidermal VGLL3 resulted in a severe LE-like rash and a proinflammatory expression profile similar to that seen in SLE, thus supporting its pathogenetic role in LE.

HISTOPATHOLOGY

In most cutaneous LE subtypes (acute cutaneous LE, SCLE, DLE, hypertrophic LE, chilblain LE), the histopathologic hallmark is that of a vacuolar to sometimes lichenoid interface dermatitis involving the epidermis and adnexal epithelia (**Fig. 1**A, B). The interface change is a result of the collective actions of cytotoxic T cells, PDCs, and related cytokines. CD123, an immunohistochemical marker for PDCs, is now commonly used to support a diagnosis of cutaneous LE when clusters of CD123+ PDCs are found in skin biopsies. Although different studies have adopted slightly different definitions for a "PDC cluster," most require aggregation of at least 10 PDCs.[15,16] PDCs are found in perivascular locations and along the dermoepidermal junction (**Fig. 1**C, D). Prior studies have compared CD123 staining in cutaneous LE with numerous other dermatitides. The presence of PDC clusters is particularly helpful in distinguishing the above

Table 1
Clinical, histopathologic, and serologic findings in cutaneous lupus erythematosus

Cutaneous LE Subtype	Clinical Features	Histopathologic Findings	Association with SLE	Autoantibodies
Acute cutaneous LE	Nonscarring malar rash; widespread symmetric eruption of pruritic macules and papules	Interface dermatitis with thickening of basement membrane	+++	ANA Anti-dsDNA (SLE-specific) Anti-Sm (SLE-specific) Anti-rRNP (SLE-specific)
Subacute cutaneous LE	Annular or arcuate erythematous plaques with a predilection for upper trunk and other sun-exposed areas	Interface dermatitis with hyperkeratosis and thickening of basement membrane	+	ANA Anti-Ro Anti-La
Discoid LE	Well-demarcated scaly erythematous papules or plaques with a predilection for head and neck; scarring alopecia	Interface dermatitis with follicular plugging, thickening of basement membrane, pigment incontinence, and perivascular and periadnexal lymphocytic infiltrate	++	Negative in most cases
Tumid LE	Erythematous urticarial-like plaques with smooth surfaces and a predilection for head and neck and upper trunk	Superficial and deep perivascular and periadnexal lymphocytic infiltrate with abundant mucin	+/−	Negative
LE panniculitis	Indurated erythematous plaque with a predilection for head and neck and proximal extremities	Lobular lymphocytic panniculitis with hyaline fat necrosis, paraseptal lymphoid nodules, ± epidermal and dermal changes of discoid LE	+	Negative
Neonatal LE	Annular erythematous plaques with a predilection for the face and periorbital areas	Interface dermatitis	+/−	ANA Anti-Ro Anti-La
Chilblain LE	Painful violaceous macules on digits	Superficial to deep perivascular and periadnexal lymphocytic infiltrate with interface dermatitis and papillary dermal edema	++	ANA Anticardiolipin Anti-beta2-glycoprotein-I Lupus anticoagulant Anti-Ro Anti-La
Bullous LE	Nonscarring vesiculobullous eruption with a predilection for upper trunk and head and neck	Subepidermal blister with neutrophils; linear immune deposits on direct immunofluorescence	+++	ANA SLE-specific autoantibodies Autoantibodies against type VII collagen

Abbreviations: −, no association; +, rare association; ++, mild to moderate association; +++, strong association; dsDNA, double-stranded DNA; rRNP, ribosomal ribonucleoprotein; ssDNA, single stranded DNA.

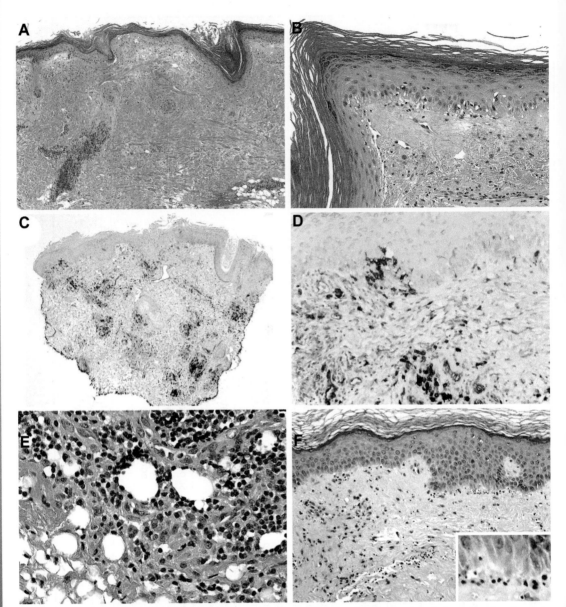

Fig. 1. Histopathologic features of cutaneous LE. (*A*) Follicular keratin plugging and periadnexal and perivascular lymphocytic inflammation in DLE. (*B*) Close examination reveals vacuolar interface change of the basal epidermis and follicular epithelium. A thickened basement membrane is also present. (*C*) CD123 shows many PDCs in the inflammatory infiltrate. (*D*) CD123+ PDCs aggregate at the dermoepidermal junction and in the dermis. (*E*) An example of LE panniculitis shows a lymphocytic lobular panniculitis with hyaline fat necrosis (*left lower corner*) and scattered plasma cells. (*F*) In nonbullous neutrophilic LE, a perivascular and interstitial neutrophilic infiltrate is present in the upper dermis. The neutrophils tend to tag the dermoepidermal junction, causing mild vacuolar change of the basal layer (*inset*). (hematoxylin-eosin [H&E], original magnifications: ×40 [*A*], ×200 [*B*], ×600 [*E*]; ×100 [*F*]; CD123, original magnifications: ×20 [*C*], ×400 [*D*].)

cutaneous LE subtypes from their histopathologic mimics, including but not limited to squamous neoplasms,[16,17] rosacea,[18] lichen planopilaris,[19,20] and mycosis fungoides.[21] However, CD123 did not seem to assist in the discrimination of chilblain LE and idiopathic perniosis.[22]

Increased numbers of PDCs are also found in cutaneous LE subtypes with little or no epidermal changes, rendering CD123 a useful tool in some notoriously difficult differential diagnoses. For example, the presence of CD123+ PDC clusters would support tumid LE over polymorphous light eruption,[23] and an increased percentage of CD123+ PDCs (≥20% of the total infiltrate) and the presence of CD123+ PDC clusters would favor LE panniculitis over subcutaneous panniculitis-like T-cell lymphoma (SPTCL).[21,24] In the latter differential diagnosis, the presence of readily identifiable plasma cells (**Fig. 1E**) together with changes typical of LE in the overlying dermis would also favor LE panniculitis over SPTCL, which typically lacks plasma cells and shows sharp restriction to the subcutis.[21] The presence of plasma cells in LE lesions underscores the important role of autoantibodies, which are secreted by plasma cells.

Despite the pathogenic role of NET in LE, neutrophils are usually inconspicuous in most cutaneous LE lesions, except in nonspecific lesions of SLE, such as nonbullous neutrophilic LE, bullous LE, leukocytoclastic vasculitis, and amicrobial pustulosis of the folds. In nonbullous neutrophilic LE, sometimes referred to as neutrophilic urticarial dermatosis associated with SLE, there is a predominance of neutrophils in the upper dermis, extending beyond the perivascular locations into the dermal interstitium. These neutrophils demonstrate leukocytoclasis and are frequently found near the dermoepidermal junction, causing mild vacuolation of the basilar keratinocytes (**Fig. 1F**).[25,26] In bullous LE, there is a subepidermal bulla with sparse neutrophils aggregating along the dermoepidermal junction. Autoantibodies responsible for this condition target type VII collagen, as evident by linear deposition of immunoglobulins, most commonly immunoglobulin G, along the basement membrane zone on direct immunofluorescence.[27]

DERMATOMYOSITIS

Dermatomyositis belongs to the spectrum of idiopathic inflammatory myopathies, which also encompasses polymyositis and inclusion body myositis. As its name implies, dermatomyositis primarily affects skin and muscles, although an amyopathic variant sparing the muscles exists.[28–30] Other organs, such as the lung, the heart, and the gastrointestinal system, may be infrequently involved. Cutaneous manifestations are diverse, with Gottron papules and heliotrope rash being the most characteristic and often the presenting signs of the disease.[28–30] In addition to timely treatment, which is crucial in preventing permanent tissue damage, accurate diagnosis of dermatomyositis also prompts appropriate clinical workup given its association with internal malignancy.[28–30]

PATHOGENESIS

The pathogenesis of dermatomyositis is complex and involves genetic, environmental, and immunologic factors. Polymorphisms of the HLA alleles in the major histocompatibility complex (MHC) are strongly associated with dermatomyositis.[31] MHC class I and II molecules are involved in antigen presentation and processing, and HLA polymorphism may confer a higher risk for autoimmune diseases by altering their ability to bind antigenic peptides.[32] Other potential risk factors include variants of non-HLA genes *GSDMB* and B lymphoid tyrosine kinase (*BLK*).[33]

Because T cells are stimulated by MHC class II molecules, a T-cell–driven mechanism is expected in dermatomyositis. As in LE, type I interferons produced by PDCs are upregulated in dermatomyositis and have been shown to correlate with disease activity.[34] Although type I interferon signaling was a common pathway shared by dermatomyositis and cutaneous LE, a recent study comparing the transcriptional profiles in both diseases found that interleukin-18 was distinctively upregulated in dermatomyositis, suggesting its role in the pathogenesis of this disease.[35] Also playing a role is the activation of complements, via either an antibody-dependent pathway or a classical complement cascade, which causes capillary destruction that results in tissue hypoperfusion and microinfarction in dermatomyositis.[29]

Another key mechanism is the production of autoantibodies by activated B cells. Although their pathogenic role is not fully elucidated, the identification of myositis-specific autoantibodies (MSAs) has contributed greatly to the understanding of the immunologic underpinnings of the different clinical phenotypes of dermatomyositis. Patients with *HLA-DRB1*03:02* and *HLA-DRB1*07:01* are predisposed to developing anti-Mi-2 antibodies, as these HLA molecules preferentially bind to the Mi-2 peptide,[36] a nuclear DNA helicase involved in transcription. Clinically, patients with anti-Mi-2 antibodies tend to have relatively mild disease with classic cutaneous findings and lower incidence of interstitial lung disease and malignancy.[37,38] In contrast, anti-TIF1-γ antibody is linked with cancer-associated dermatomyositis.[39] It is hypothesized that TIF1-γ mutation in some tumors may result in expression of tumor-specific antigens, which stimulate autoantibody production and consequent skin and muscle damage. Another important MSA is the anti-MDA-5 antibody. MDA-5 is an intracellular receptor for viral nucleic acids capable of triggering an innate antiviral response by promoting type I interferon production.[40,41] This antiviral function of MDA-5 lends support to the hypothesized causal relationship between viral infection and dermatomyositis, in that MDA-5 may be released from injured tissues following interaction with viral pathogens, resulting in formation of anti-MDA-5 autoantibodies. Patients harboring anti-MDA-5 antibodies are more likely to develop interstitial lung disease, mucocutaneous ulcers, amyopathic dermatomyositis, and inflammatory arthritis.[40,41] Clinical phenotypes associated with different MSAs are summarized in **Table 2**.[37]

HISTOPATHOLOGY

Histopathologic features vary depending on the types of cutaneous lesions biopsied. Heliotrope rash and erythematous macules and patches on the chest (V-neck sign), upper back (shawl sign), and lateral thigh (Holster sign) are characterized by epidermal atrophy, mild vacuolar interface dermatitis, sparse perivascular lymphocytic infiltrate, and increased interstitial dermal mucin (**Fig. 2**A, B). Mild hyperkeratosis is also common. The interface change may be subtle and focal, sometimes requiring multiple sections to identify. Overall, these changes are similar to but milder than those seen in cutaneous LE. As in LE, the interface change in dermatomyositis is mediated by cytotoxic T cells and PDCs. A prior study has shown preferential epidermal localization of CD123$^+$ PDCs in biopsies of dermatomyositis compared with LE.[42]

Gottron papules are hyperkeratotic papules located on the dorsal metacarpophalangeal and interphalangeal joints. These lesions typically show epidermal hyperplasia, hyperkeratosis, and vacuolar interface change. Although dermal mucin is an inconsistent finding, there is frequent lymphangiectasia, suggesting an element of localized lymphedema.[43] "Mechanic's hand" refers to hyperkeratotic plaques on the lateral aspects of the digits and hands. Histopathologically, these lesions resemble chronic eczematous dermatitis with acanthosis and hyperkeratosis; vacuolar interface dermatitis is variable. However, the presence of colloid bodies or dyskeratotic cells, typically located in the suprapapillary plates, would help exclude eczema.[44]

An uncommon variant is Wong-type dermatomyositis,[45] which is characterized by follicular and nonfollicular epidermal invaginations filled with keratin, clinically mimicking the follicular papules in pityriasis ruba pilaris. Histopathologically, these keratin plugs resemble cornoid lamellae seen in porokeratosis and are referred to as "columnar dyskeratosis" or "pseudocornoid lamellae" (**Fig. 2**C).[46]

Panniculitis is another rare cutaneous manifestation of dermatomyositis. A study of 18 cases of dermatomyositis panniculitis reported pathologic features identical to those of LE panniculitis, namely lymphocytic lobular panniculitis with lymphocyte "rimming" of adipocytes, clusters of CD123$^+$ PDCs, hyaline fat necrosis, mucin deposition, plasma cells, and calcification (**Fig. 2**D).[47] Correlation with history and other clinical stigmata of dermatomyositis is therefore key to the distinction of dermatomyositis panniculitis from LE panniculitis.

SCLERODERMA/SYSTEMIC SCLEROSIS

Scleroderma is a chronic fibrosing cutaneous disorder that may be localized and confined to the skin (morphea) or may be a manifestation of systemic sclerosis. The latter is further divided into (1) limited cutaneous systemic sclerosis (CREST syndrome) dominated by slowly progressive fibrosis of the skin, and (2) diffuse cutaneous systemic sclerosis characterized by rapidly progressive fibrosis of the skin, the lungs, and other internal organs.[48,49] Despite different clinical manifestations, all types of scleroderma demonstrate microvascular alteration and chronic inflammation in early stages, and sclerosis in late stages.[50]

PATHOGENESIS

The pathogenesis of scleroderma is a complex interplay of genetic, environmental, and immunologic factors as in other CTDs. Certain HLA haplotypes, such as *HLA-DRB1*11:04*, *HLA-DQB1*05:01*, and *HLA-DQB1*06:01*, are strongly linked to the disease.[51–53] Variants of non-HLA genes involved in cytokine signaling (*TNFAIP3*, *TNIP1*, *IRF5*, *STAT4*), T-cell activation (*CD247*), extracellular matrix deposition (*PPAR-gamma*), apoptosis (*DNASE1L3*), and autophagy (*ATG*) are additional risk factors for the disease.[54,55] In addition to genetic variants, a whole host of epigenetic mechanisms affecting genes involved in autoimmunity, T-cell function, TGF-β and Wnt pathways, and extracellular matrix also contribute to immune dysregulation, fibrosis, and abnormal angiogenesis in this disease.[54]

Genetically predisposed individuals require additional environmental triggers, such as exposure to silica, organic solvents, or certain viruses and drugs, to develop the disease.[54] Reactive oxygen species and reactive nitrogen species are thought to play a crucial role by inducing the production of proinflammatory and profibrotic cytokines, proliferation of fibroblasts, and oxidative damage of endothelial cells.[49,55] Recent studies have also highlighted the effects of "alarmins," a

Table 2
Association of myositis-specific autoantibodies with HLA haplotypes and clinical phenotypes of dermatomyositis

MSA	HLA Haplotype Associations	Clinical Phenotypes	Muscle Disease	Lung Disease	Malignancy Association
Anti-Mi-2	HLA-DRB1*03:02 HLA-DRB1*07:01	Classic DM (heliotrope rash, Gottron sign and papules, V-neck and shawl signs, cuticular overgrowth, punctate perionychium hemorrhage)	+++	+/–	+/–
Anti-MDA-5	HLA-DRB1*04:01 HLA-DRB1*12:02	Fever, alopecia, heliotrope rash, Gottron sign and papules, mechanic's hands, cutaneous ulcerations, painful palmar papules, calcinosis	+/–	+++ (ILD)	+/–
Anti-NXP2	–	Peripheral edema, calcinosis, intestinal vasculopathy, dysphagia	+++ (with distal muscle weakness)	+/–	+++
Anti-TIF-1γ	–	Classic DM, psoriasis-like lesions, red on white lesions, ovoid palatal patch	+	–	+++
Anti-SAE1/2	–	Classic DM, dysphagia, dark red/violaceous rash	+/–	+ (PAH)	+/–
Anti-synthetase	–	Fever, mechanic's hands, hiker's feet, arthritis	+++	+++ (ILD)	+/–

Abbreviations: DM, dermatomyositis; ILD, interstitial lung disease; MDA-5, melanoma differentiation-associated gene 5; NXP2, nuclear matrix protein 2; PAH, pulmonary arterial hypertension; SAE1/2, small ubiquitin-like modifier 1 activating enzyme; TIF-1γ, transcription intermediary factor 1γ.

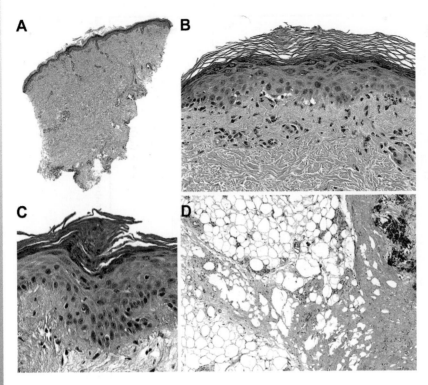

Fig. 2. Histopathologic features of dermatomyositis. (A) The histopathologic changes in dermatomyositis may be subtle, as seen in this biopsy from the lateral thigh (Holster sign), which shows minimal changes at scanning magnification. (B) High magnification reveals foci of vacuolar interface dermatitis with occasional cytoid bodies and superficial melanophages. (C) Pseudocornoid lamella is a feature of Wong-type dermatomyositis in which a focus of mild epidermal depression is associated with a small keratin plug. (D) Dermatomyositis panniculitis is histopathologically indistinguishable from LE panniculitis. A lobular lymphocytic panniculitis with hyalinized fat necrosis and dystrophic calcification is seen in this example. (H&E, original magnifications: ×20 [A], ×200 [B], ×400 [C], ×100 [D]).

heterogeneous group of cytokines functioning as endogenous danger signals. These alarmins have been found at elevated levels in lesional tissues of scleroderma.[49] Their activation leads to upregulation of fibrotic gene expression as well as proliferation and survival of fibroblasts and myofibroblasts as an attempt of tissue repair. These actions ultimately result in increased deposition of collagen and other extracellular matrix proteins in the skin and other vital organs.[49]

Although the role of ANAs in the pathogenesis of scleroderma remains unclear, up to 90% of these patients test positive for these antibodies. Similar to dermatomyositis, different scleroderma-related ANAs are associated with different clinical manifestations (Table 3).[56]

HISTOPATHOLOGY

The hallmark feature of scleroderma is thickening and hyalinization of dermal collagen bundles, often imparting a "square" appearance of the punch biopsy (Fig. 3A). Such hyalinization often begins in

the deep dermis and results in a sharply demarcated, straight horizontal dermosubcutaneous junction referred to as "line sign" (Fig. 3A, B).[57] Eccrine coils entrapped in the sclerotic dermis are notably devoid of perieccrine adipocytes (Fig. 3C). A perivascular and periadnexal lymphoplasmacytic infiltrate is usually present. Perineural inflammation has been described as a clue to subtle morphea.[58]

Corroborating the role of vascular damage in scleroderma, quantification of blood vessels revealed a lower density in the skin of systemic sclerosis patients compared with healthy subjects.[59] The number of dermal dendritic cells, as highlighted by factor XIIIa, is also decreased in systemic sclerosis.[59] That being said, although well-developed scleroderma is collagen rich and paucicellular, early scleroderma tends to show more subtle hyalinization with a normal or even slightly increased number of fibroblasts (see Fig. 3B). Dermal mucin is increased in all forms of scleroderma,[60] but tends to be more notable in early cases.

Table 3
Common scleroderma-related antinuclear autoantibodies and associated clinical phenotypes of systemic sclerosis

ANA	Cutaneous Involvement	Other Organ Involvement
Anti-Scl-70 (anti-topoisomerase I)	Diffuse	ILD, renal crisis
Anti-centromere	Limited	PAH
Anti-RNAP III	Diffuse	Renal crisis, gastric antral vascular ectasia
Anti-U3-RNP	Diffuse or limited	ILD, PAH, renal crisis, myocardial fibrosis, gastrointestinal involvement, myositis
Anti-U11/U12 RNP	Diffuse or limited	ILD, PAH

Abbreviations: ILD, interstitial lung disease; PAH, pulmonary arterial hypertension; RNAP, RNA polymerase; RNP, ribonucleoprotein.

Interestingly, a study has found that inflammation tended to be denser in morphea than in systemic sclerosis.[61] The same investigators also reported more diffuse thickening of collagen bundles with more frequent involvement of the papillary dermis in morphea compared with systemic sclerosis. In addition, morphea is more likely to involve the subcutis (morphea profunda). The latter is characterized by thickened and sclerotic pannicular septa (**Fig. 3**D, E), a feature that

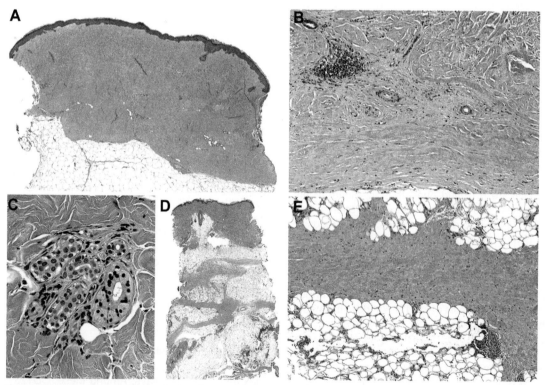

Fig. 3. Histopathologic features of scleroderma. (*A*) A "square" biopsy with extensive dermal sclerosis resulting in a sharp dermosubcutaneous interface referred to as a "line sign." (*B*) An example of early scleroderma in which hyalinized collagen bundles are limited to the deep dermis near the dermosubcutaneous junction (lower half of this field). There is also a mild increase in fibroblasts and a perivascular lymphocytic infiltrate. (*C*) An eccrine coil devoid of surrounding adipocytes is found in a sclerotic stroma. (*D*) An example of morphea profunda shows prominent thickening of the pannicular septa. (*E*) The thickened septa are composed of hyalinized collagen. A perivascular lymphocytic infiltrate is also present. (H&E, original magnifications: ×20 [*A*], ×100 [*B*], ×200 [*C*], ×10 [*D*], ×40 [*E*].)

overlaps with eosinophilic fasciitis. Distinction between morphea profunda and eosinophilic fasciitis is notoriously difficult and requires examination of the fascia, which is best sampled by incisional biopsy. The presence of eosinophils in the fascia would favor a diagnosis of eosinophilic fasciitis; however, up to 19% of cases may lack this feature.[62] Focal absence of fascial CD34 staining has been reported as a helpful feature in favoring eosinophilic fasciitis over morphea profunda.[62] Another immunohistochemical study reported a significantly higher CD4:CD8 ratio, a lower Th1:Th2 ratio, and lower percentage of Th17+ cells in morphea compared with eosinophilic fasciitis.[63] These results seem to argue against the hypothesis that eosinophilic fasciitis is a variant of morphea.

MIXED CONNECTIVE TISSUE DISEASE

Mixed connective tissue disease (MCTD) is now regarded as a unique entity that differs from other overlap syndromes and undifferentiated CTD.[64] It is defined by mixed clinical features of SLE, systemic sclerosis, polymyositis-dermatomyositis, and rheumatoid arthritis, as well as high titers of ANA and anti-U1-RNP autoantibodies.[65] Of note, MCTD is the first CTD for which a serologic test (anti-U1-RNP) constitutes one of the diagnostic criteria. The most common presentations of MCTD include polyarthritis, swelling of the hands, sclerodactyly, Raynaud phenomenon, esophageal dysmotility, and myositis.[64] It can progress to involve internal organs, such as the heart, the lung, the central nervous system, and, rarely, the kidneys.[64] The most common cutaneous manifestations are Raynaud phenomenon, digital ulcers, and nail fold capillary looping. Patients with MCTD may also develop rashes of cutaneous LE or dermatomyositis.[64]

PATHOGENESIS

Both genetic and immunologic factors contribute to the pathogenesis of MCTD. Various HLA haplotypes have been linked to this disease. For example, HLA-DRB1*15:01, HLA-DRB1*04, and HLA-DRB1*09:01 have been identified as risk alleles, whereas HLA-DRB1*07:01 has been found to be protective in a Polish population.[66]

Evidence suggested that impaired clearance of apoptotic cells and immune complexes play a role in the pathogenesis of MCTD. The U1 small nuclear ribonucleoprotein (U1-RNP) complex normally functions as part of the spliceosome.[65] U1-RNP consists of an RNA molecule and at least 10 RNA-binding proteins, including U1-70K.

During cell death, different components of this complex undergo apoptotic modifications, which alter the structure and antigenicity of the constituent proteins, allowing its RNA-binding domain and other epitopes to be recognized and targeted by autoreactive T cells, which in turn promote autoantibody production by B cells. U1-RNP also stimulates PDCs by binding to Toll-like receptors.[67] Subsequent type I interferon production likely leads to a cascade of inflammatory responses via the actions of proinflammatory cytokines.[65,68]

Another pathway for tissue injury in MCTD is via vascular damage. Anti-U1-RNP autoantibodies are known to activate endothelial cells, leading to intimal hyperplasia and obliterative vasculopathy. Vascular manifestations, such as vascular thrombosis, livedo reticularis, and pulmonary arterial hypertension, are particularly common in a subgroup of MCTD patients who also harbor antiphospholipid antibodies.[69] Other autoantibodies frequently identified in MCTD patients include anticyclic citrullinated peptides and rheumatoid factor.[70]

HISTOPATHOLOGY

The histopathologic features of the skin lesions of MCTD have not been well characterized. One study examined the cutaneous eruptions in 8 MCTD patients, including erythematous, annular, and/or papulosquamous lesions and an ill-defined, telangiectatic, scaly patch. All showed a vacuolar to lichenoid interface dermatitis reminiscent of SCLE.[71] However, unlike SCLE, there is also evidence of vasculopathy in the form of telangiectasia, hypovascularity, or thrombosis in the superficial vascular plexus. Granular vascular deposition of C5b-9 on direct immunofluorescence further serves as evidence of vascular damage.[71] In addition, sclerodermoid change was noted in 2 cases.[71] These histopathologic findings mirror the overlapping clinical features of LE, dermatomyositis, and scleroderma in MCTD.

SUMMARY

Research into the pathogenesis of CTDs has identified numerous immunologic mediators and complex molecular pathways. Among these, CD123+ PDCs, interferons, NETs, and "alarmins" are increasingly recognized as important drivers and potential therapeutic targets of these diseases. Major advances have also been made in understanding the actions of autoantibodies and their associations with specific clinical phenotypes. Recognition of the above will allow for better clinicopathologic correlation and improved understanding of the histopathologic changes in CTDs involving the skin, and development of new diagnostic tools for more precise classification of these diseases.

CLINICS CARE POINTS

- Vestigial-like family member 3 is enriched in female skin and contributes to the sex bias in connective tissue disease.

- Plasmacytoid dendritic cells and type I interferon play a central role in lupus erythematosus and dermatomyositis.

- NETosis occurs in cutaneous lupus erythematosus and is associated with scarring.

- Myositis-specific autoantibodies predict clinical phenotypes and prognosis of dermatomyositis.

- Oxidative stress and alarmins promote sclerosis in scleroderma.

- U1 small nuclear ribonucleoprotein is a key factor in the pathogenesis and diagnosis of mixed connective tissue disease.

DISCLOSURE

The authors have nothing to disclose.

REFERENCES

1. Walling HW, Sontheimer RD. Cutaneous lupus erythematosus: issues in diagnosis and treatment. Am J Clin Dermatol 2009;10:365–81.
2. Ribero S, Sciascia S, Borradori L, et al. The cutaneous spectrum of lupus erythematosus. Clin Rev Allergy Immunol 2017;53:291–305.
3. Didier K, Bolko L, Giusti D, et al. Autoantibodies associated with connective tissue diseases: what meaning for clinicians? Front Immunol 2018;9:541.
4. Li A, Wu H, Liao W, et al. A comprehensive review of immune-mediated dermatopathology in systemic lupus erythematosus. J Autoimmun 2018;93:1–15.
5. Little AJ, Matthew D, Vesely MD. Cutaneous lupus erythematosus: current and future pathogenesis-directed therapies. Yale J Biol Med 2020;93:81–95.
6. Yin Q, Xu X, Lin Y, et al. Ultraviolet B irradiation induces skin accumulation of plasmacytoid dendritic cells: a possible role for chemerin. Autoimmunity 2014;47:185–92.
7. Kim A, O'Brien J, Tseng LC, et al. Autoantibodies and disease activity in patients with discoid lupus erythematosus. JAMA Dermatol 2014;150:651–4.
8. Apel F, Zychlinsky A, Kenny EF. The role of neutrophil extracellular traps in rheumatic diseases. Nat Rev Rheumatol 2018;14:467–75.
9. Brinkmann V, Reichard U, Goosmann C, et al. Neutrophil extracellular traps kill bacteria. Science 2004;303:1532–5.
10. Lande R, Ganguly D, Facchinetti V, et al. Neutrophils activate plasmacytoid dendritic cells by releasing self-DNA-peptide complexes in systemic lupus erythematosus. Sci Transl Med 2011;3:73ra19.
11. Gestermann N, Domizio JD, Lande R, et al. Netting neutrophils activate autoreactive B cells in lupus. J Immunol 2018;200:3364–71.
12. Rafi R, Al-Hage J, Abbas O, et al. Investigating the presence of neutrophil extracellular traps in cutaneous lesions of different subtypes of lupus erythematosus. Exp Dermatol 2019;28:1348–52.
13. Liang Y, Tsoi LC, Xing X, et al. A gene network regulated by the transcription factor VGLL3 as a promoter of sex-biased autoimmune diseases. Nat Immunol 2017;18:152–60.
14. Billi AC, Gharaee-Kermani M, Fullmer J, et al. The female-biased factor VGLL3 drives cutaneous and systemic autoimmunity. JCI Insight 2019;4:e127291.
15. Tomasini D, Mentzel T, Hantschke M, et al. Plasmacytoid dendritic cells: an overview of their presence and distribution in different inflammatory skin diseases, with special emphasis on Jessner's lymphocytic infiltrate of the skin and cutaneous lupus erythematosus. J Cutan Pathol 2010;37:1132–9.
16. Walsh NM, Lai J, Hanly JG, et al. Plasmacytoid dendritic cells in hypertrophic discoid lupus erythematosus: an objective evaluation of their diagnostic value. J Cutan Pathol 2015;42:32–8.
17. Ko CJ, Srivastava B, Braverman I, et al. Hypertrophic lupus erythematosus: the diagnostic utility of CD123 staining. J Cutan Pathol 2011;38:889–92.
18. Brown TT, Choi EY, Thomas DG, et al. Comparative analysis of rosacea and cutaneous lupus erythematosus: histopathologic features, T-cell subsets, and plasmacytoid dendritic cells. J Am Acad Dermatol 2014;71:100–7.
19. Kolivras A, Thompson C. Clusters of CD123+ plasmacytoid dendritic cells help distinguish lupus alopecia from lichen planopilaris. J Am Acad Dermatol 2016;74:1267–9.
20. Rakhshan A, Toossi P, Amani M, et al. Different distribution patterns of plasmacytoid dendritic cells in discoid lupus erythematosus and lichen planopilaris demonstrated by CD123 immunostaining. An Bras Dermatol 2020;95:307–13.
21. Chen SJT, Tse JY, Harms PW, et al. Utility of CD123 immunohistochemistry in differentiating lupus

erythematosus from cutaneous T cell lymphoma. Histopathology 2019;74:908–16.

22. Wang ML, Chan MP. Comparative analysis of chilblain lupus erythematosus and idiopathic perniosis: histopathologic features and immunohistochemistry for CD123 and CD30. Am J Dermatopathol 2018; 40:265–71.

23. Wackernagel A, Massone C, Hoefler G, et al. Plasmacytoid dendritic cells are absent in skin lesions of polymorphic light eruption. Photodermatol Photoimmunol Photomed 2007;23:24–8.

24. Liau JY, Chuang SS, Chu CY, et al. The presence of clusters of plasmacytoid dendritic cells is a helpful feature for differentiating lupus panniculitis from subcutaneous panniculitis-like T cell lymphoma. Histopathology 2013;62:1057–66.

25. Gleason BC, Zembowicz A, Granter SR. Nonbullous neutrophilic dermatosis: an uncommon dermatologic manifestation in patients with lupus erythematosus. J Cutan Pathol 2006;33:721–5.

26. Brinster NK, Nunley J, Pariser R, et al. Nonbullous neutrophilic lupus erythematosus: a newly recognized variant of cutaneous lupus erythematosus. J Am Acad Dermatol 2012;66:92–7.

27. Contestable JJ, Edhegard KD, Meyerle JH. Bullous systemic lupus erythematosus: a review and update to diagnosis and treatment. Am J Clin Dermatol 2014;15:517–24.

28. Mainetti C, Beretta-Piccoli BT, Selmi C. Cutaneous manifestations of dermatomyositis: a comprehensive review. Clinic Rev Allerg Immunol 2017;53:337–56.

29. DeWane ME, Waldman R, Lu J. Dermatomyositis: clinical features and pathogenesis. J Am Acad Dermatol 2020;82:267–81.

30. Cobos GA, Femia A, Vleugels RA. Dermatomyositis: an update on diagnosis and treatment. Am J Clin Dermatol 2020;21:339–53.

31. Thompson C, Piguet V, Choy E. The pathogenesis of dermatomyositis. Br J Dermatol 2018;179:1256–62.

32. Raychaudhuri S, Sandor C, Stahl EA, et al. Five amino acids in three HLA proteins explain most of the association between MHC and seropositive rheumatoid arthritis. Nat Genet 2012;44:291–6.

33. Rothwell S, Lamb JA, Chinoy H. New developments in genetics of myositis. Curr Opin Rheumatol 2016; 28:651–6.

34. Crowson CS, Hein MS, Pendegraft RS, et al. Interferon chemokine score and other cytokine measures track with changes in disease activity in patients with juvenile and adult dermatomyositis. ACR Open Rheumatol 2019;1:83–9.

35. Tsoi L, Gharaee-Kermani M, Berthier CC, et al. IL-18-containing five-gene signature distinguishes histologically identical dermatomyositis and lupus erythematosus skin lesions. JCI Insight 2020;5:e139558.

36. O'Hanlon TP, Rider LG, Mamyrova G, et al. HLA polymorphisms in African Americans with idiopathic inflammatory myopathy: allelic profiles distinguish patients with different clinical phenotypes and myositis autoantibodies. Arthritis Rheum 2006;54: 3670–81.

37. Wolstencroft PW, Fiorentino DF. Dermatomyositis clinical and pathological phenotypes associated with myositis-specific autoantibodies. Curr Rheumatol Rep 2018;20:28.

38. Komura K, Fujimoto M, Matsushita T, et al. Prevalence and clinical characteristics of anti-Mi-2 antibodies in Japanese patients with dermatomyositis. J Dermatol Sci 2005;40:215–7.

39. De Vooght J, Vulsteke JB, De Haes P, et al. Anti-TIF1-γ autoantibodies: warning lights of a tumour autoantigen. Rheumatology (Oxford) 2020;59:469–77.

40. Fiorentino D, Chung L, Zwerner J, et al. The mucocutaneous and systemic phenotype of dermatomyositis patients with antibodies to MDA5 (CADM-140): a retrospective study. J Am Acad Dermatol 2011; 65:25–34.

41. Kurtzman DJB, Vleugels RA. Anti-melanoma differentiation-associated gene 5 (MDA5) dermatomyositis: a concise review with an emphasis on distinctive clinical features. J Am Acad Dermatol 2018;78:776–85.

42. McNiff JM, Kaplan DH. Plasmacytoid dendritic cells are present in cutaneous dermatomyositis lesions in a pattern distinct from lupus erythematosus. J Cutan Pathol 2008;35:452–6.

43. Fernandez-Flores A, Cassarino DS. Gottron papules show histopathologic features of localized lymphedema. Am J Dermatopathol 2017;39:518–23.

44. Concha JSS, Merola JF, Fiorentino D, et al. Re-examining mechanic's hands as a characteristic skin finding in dermatomyositis. J Am Acad Dermatol 2018;78:769–75.e2.

45. Mutasim DF, Egesi A, Spicknall KE. Wong-type dermatomyositis: a mimic of many dermatoses. J Cutan Pathol 2016;43:781–6.

46. Umanoff N, Fisher A, Carlson JA. Wong-type dermatomyositis showing porokeratosis-like changes (columnar dyskeratosis): a case report and review of the literature. Dermatopathology (Basel) 2015;2:1–8.

47. Santos-Briz A, Calle A, Linos K, et al. Dermatomyositis panniculitis: a clinicopathological and immunohistochemical study of 18 cases. J Eur Acad Dermatol Venereol 2018;32:1352–9.

48. Ferreli C, Gasparini G, Parodi A, et al. Cutaneous manifestations of scleroderma and scleroderma-like disorders: a comprehensive review. Clin Rev Allergy Immunol 2017;53:306–36.

49. Giovannetti A, Straface E, Rosato E, et al. Role of alarmins in the pathogenesis of systemic sclerosis. Int J Mol Sci 2020;21:E4985.

50. Rongioletti F, Ferreli C, Atzori L, et al. Scleroderma with an update about clinico-pathological correlation. G Ital Dermatol Venereol 2018;153:208–15.

51. Arnett FC, Gourh P, Shete S, et al. Major histocompatibility complex (MHC) class II alleles, haplotypes and epitopes which confer susceptibility or protection in systemic sclerosis: analyses in 1300 Caucasian, African-American and Hispanic cases and 1000 controls. Ann Rheum Dis 2010;69:822–7.

52. Furukawa H, Oka S, Kawasaki A, et al. Human leukocyte antigen and systemic sclerosis in Japanese: the sign of the four independent protective alleles, DRB1*13:02, DRB1*14:06, DQB1*03:01, and DPB1*02:01. PLoS One 2016;11:e0154255.

53. Rodriguez-Reyna TS, Mercado-Velazquez P, Yu N, et al. HLA class I and II blocks are associated to susceptibility, clinical subtypes and autoantibodies in Mexican systemic sclerosis (SSc) patients. PLoS One 2015;10:e0126727.

54. Tsou PS, Sawalha AH. Unfolding the pathogenesis of scleroderma through genomics and epigenomics. J Autoimmun 2017;83:73–94.

55. Sambo P, Baroni SS, Luchetti M, et al. Oxidative stress in scleroderma: maintenance of scleroderma fibroblast phenotype by the constitutive upregulation of reactive oxygen species generation through the NADPH oxidase complex pathway. Arthritis Rheum 2001;44:2653–64.

56. Stochmal A, Czuwara J, Trojanowska M, et al. Antinuclear antibodies in systemic sclerosis: an update. Clin Rev Allergy Immunol 2020;58:40–51.

57. Yang S, Draznin M, Fung MA. The "line sign" is a rapid and efficient diagnostic "test" for morphea: clinicopathological study of 73 cases. Am J Dermatopathol 2018;40:873–8.

58. Dhaliwal CA, MacKenzie AI, Biswas A. Perineural inflammation in morphea (localized scleroderma): systematic characterization of a poorly recognized but potentially useful histopathological feature. J Cutan Pathol 2014;41:28–35.

59. de-Sá-Earp AP, do Nascimento AP, Carneiro SC, et al. Dermal dendritic cell population and blood vessels are diminished in the skin of systemic sclerosis patients: relationship with fibrosis degree and disease duration. Am J Dermatopathol 2013;35:438–44.

60. Rongioletti F, Gambini C, Micalizzi C, et al. Mucin deposits in morphea and systemic scleroderma. Dermatology 1994;189:157–8.

61. Torres JE, Sánchez JL. Histopathologic differentiation between localized and systemic scleroderma. Am J Dermatopathol 1998;20:242–5.

62. Onajin O, Wieland CN, Peters MS, et al. Clinicopathologic and immunophenotypic features of eosinophilic fasciitis and morphea profunda: a comparative study of 27 cases. J Am Acad Dermatol 2018;78:121–8.

63. Moy AP, Maryamchik E, Nikolskaia OV, et al. Th1- and Th17-polarized immune infiltrates in eosinophilic fasciitis—a potential marker for histopathologic distinction from morphea. J Cutan Pathol 2017;44:548–52.

64. Pepmueller PH. Undifferentiated connective tissue disease, mixed connective tissue disease, and overlap syndromes in rheumatology. Mo Med 2016;113:136–40.

65. Paradowska-Gorycka A. U1-RNP and TLR receptors in the pathogenesis of mixed connective tissue disease. Part I. The U1-RNP complex and its biological significance in the pathogenesis of mixed connective tissue disease. Reumatologia 2015;53: 94–100.

66. Paradowska-Gorycka A, Stypinska B, Olesinska M, et al. Association of HLA-DRB1 alleles with susceptibility to mixed connective tissue disease in Polish patients. HLA 2016;87:13–8.

67. Paradowska-Gorycka A. U1-RNP and Toll-like receptors in the pathogenesis of mixed connective tissue disease. Part II. Endosomal TLRs and their biological significance in the pathogenesis of mixed connective tissue disease. Reumatologia 2015;53:143–51.

68. Hassan AB, Gunnarsson I, Karlsson G, et al. Longitudinal study of interleukin-10, tumor necrosis factor-α, anti-U1-snRNP antibody levels and disease activity in patients with mixed connective tissue disease. Scand J Rheumatol 2001;30:282–9.

69. Szodoray P, Hajas A, Kardos L, et al. Distinct phenotypes in mixed connective tissue disease: subgroups and survival. Lupus 2012;21:1412.

70. Tani C, Carli L, Vagnani S, et al. The diagnosis and classification of mixed connective tissue disease. J Autoimmun 2014;48-49:46–9.

71. Magro CM, Crowson AN, Regauer S. Mixed connective tissue disease: a clinical, histologic, and immunofluorescence study of eight cases. Am J Dermatopathol 1997;19:206–13.

Update on Molecular Genetic Alterations of Cutaneous Adnexal Neoplasms

Grace Hile, MD[a], Paul W. Harms, MD, PhD[a,b],*

KEYWORDS

• Cutaneous adnexal neoplasms • Genetics • Mutation • Sweat gland • Hair follicle • Oncogene
• Tumor suppressor

Key points

- Cutaneous adnexal tumors include benign tumors and aggressive carcinomas.
- Cutaneous adnexal tumors can be hallmarks of inherited tumor syndromes.
- Oncogenic drivers of adnexal neoplasms represent potential therapeutic targets.
- Molecular alterations can lead to expression of specific diagnostic markers.

ABSTRACT

Cutaneous adnexal tumors recapitulate follicular, sweat gland, and/or sebaceous epithelia, and range from benign tumors to aggressive carcinomas. Adnexal tumors can be hallmarks for inherited tumor syndromes. Oncogenic drivers of adnexal neoplasms modulate intracellular pathways including mitogen-activated protein kinase, phosphoinositide-3-kinase, Wnt/β-catenin, Hedgehog, nuclear factor κB, and Hippo intracellular signaling pathways, representing potential therapeutic targets. Malignant progression can be associated with tumor suppressor loss, especially *TP53*. Molecular alterations drive expression of specific diagnostic markers, such as CDX2 and LEF1 in pilomatricomas/pilomatrical carcinomas, and NUT in poromas/porocarcinomas. In these ways, improved understanding of molecular alterations promises to advance diagnostic, prognostic, and therapeutic possibilities for adnexal tumors.

OVERVIEW OF CUTANEOUS NEOPLASIA

Cutaneous adnexal neoplasms arise from, or recapitulate, hair follicle or gland-associated epithelial populations of the skin. These neoplasms arise sporadically or in the setting of inherited tumor syndromes. Evidence suggests that some forms of adnexal carcinoma can be among the most aggressive solid malignancies to arise in the skin. Although precise classification is critical for addressing these concerns, the diversity and rarity of adnexal tumors can raise diagnostic difficulties. In metastatic tumors of unknown primary, confirmation of cutaneous origin can be challenging. An improved understanding of the molecular features of adnexal tumors has the potential to improve the diagnosis, prognosis, and therapy for these tumors.[1–3]

Studies of squamous cell carcinoma (SCC) and basal cell carcinoma (BCC) indicate that

The authors have nothing to disclose.
a Department of Dermatology, University of Michigan, 1910 Taubman Center, 1500 East Medical Center Drive, Ann Arbor, MI 48109-5314, USA; b Department of Pathology, University of Michigan, 2800 Plymouth Road, Building 35, Ann Arbor, MI 48109 – 2800, USA
* Corresponding author.
E-mail address: paulharm@med.umich.edu

cutaneous carcinomas are characterized by the universal hallmarks of cancer: sustaining proliferative signaling, evading growth suppressors, resisting cell death, enabling replicative immortality, inducing angiogenesis, and activating invasion and metastasis.[4] Recent reports reveal

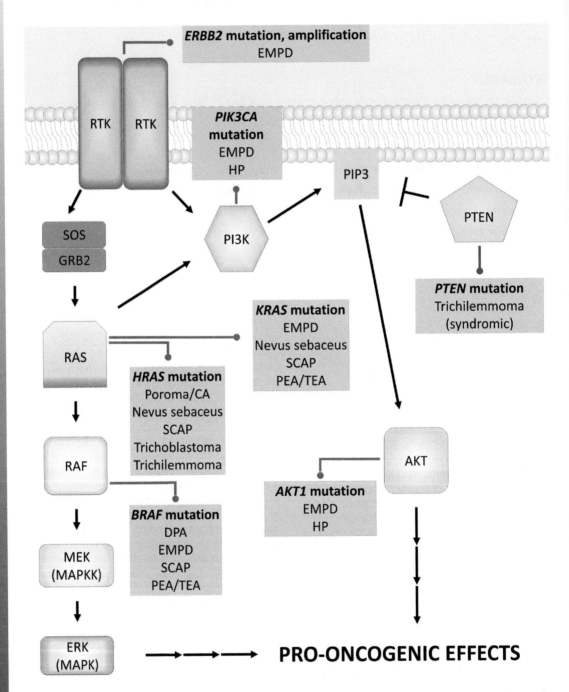

Fig. 1. Dysregulation of PI3K and mitogen-activated protein kinase (MAPK) pathways in adnexal neoplasms. Blue circle: activating event. Red circle: inactivating event. Gray box: genomic alteration (bold) and tumors in which that alteration has been reported for a subset of cases (may be a minority of cases). CA, carcinoma; DPA, digital papillary adenocarcinoma; EMPD, extramammary Paget disease; HP, hidradenoma papilliferum; PEA, papillary eccrine adenoma; RTK, receptor tyrosine kinase; SCAP, syringocystadenoma papilliferum; TAA, tubular apocrine adenoma.

Table 1
Molecular findings in cutaneous adnexal neoplasia

Differentiation	Diagnosis	Genetics (Sporadic)	Genetics (Syndromic)	References
Follicular, matrical	Pilomatricoma and pilomatrical carcinoma	Activating mutation: CTNNB1 (WNT/β-catenin signaling) Subclonal trisomy 18 (BCL2)	Numerous syndromes: for example, mismatch repair deficiency (somatic CTNNB1 accompany germline mismatch repair defects) Familial adenomatous polyposis (germline APC mutation)	9,12–14,16,17,87
Follicular, germinative	Trichoblastoma	Activating mutation: HRAS (minority)	ND	20
	Trichoepithelioma (trichoblastoma subtype)	Mutations: PTCH1, CTNNB1 (minority)	Brooke-Spiegler, Multiple familial trichoepitheliomas: CYLD Rombo: Unknown	16,26–29,54
Follicular, infundibulum/isthmus/outer root sheath	Basaloid follicular hamartoma	ND	Gorlin syndrome: PTCH1	3,88,89
	Fibrofolliculoma, trichodiscoma	ND	Birt-Hogg–Dube: FLCN (folliculin)	3
	Proliferating pilar tumor/Proliferating trichilemmal tumor	Malignant Aneuploidy		3,90
	Trichilemmoma Trichilemmal carcinoma	PIK3CA mutation Benign Mutation: HRAS Malignant Heterogeneous tumor suppressor mutations (especially TP53) and RTK/RAS activation	Cowden: PTEN	32–34

(continued on next page)

Table 1
(continued)

Differentiation	Diagnosis	Genetics (Sporadic)	Genetics (Syndromic)	References
Sweat gland	Adenoid cystic carcinoma	Fusion: *MYB-NFIB, MYBL1-NFIB*	ND	67,68
	Apocrine carcinoma	*ERBB2* (Her2/neu) amplification (single case) Most studies negative	ND	44
	Digital papillary adenocarcinoma	Mutation: *BRAF* V600E, *TP53* (minority of cases)	ND	44,45,70,71
	Endocrine mucin-producing sweat gland carcinoma	chr6 deletion (1 case)	ND	91
	Hidradenoma and hidradenocarcinoma	Benign and malignant *CRTC1-MAML2* and *CRTC3-MAML2* fusions (cAMP-CREB pathway) *EWSR1-POU5F1* fusion Malignant *TP53* mutation *ERBB2* (Her2/neu) amplification	ND	37–39,41–45
	Hidrocystoma	ND	Schopf-Schulz-Passarge: *WNT10 A*	92
	Mammary analog secretory carcinoma	Fusion: *ETV6-NTRK3* *NFIX-PKN1* (single case)	ND	93,94
	Microcystic adnexal carcinoma	Mutation: *TP53* Insertion: *JAK1* Deletion: *CDKN2A*, 6q	ND	5,43,73,74
	Poroma and porocarcinoma	Benign and malignant YAP/TAZ fusions (*YAP1-MAML2, YAP1-NUTM1, WWTR1-NUTM1*) *HRAS* activating mutation (minority) Malignant Tumor suppressor mutations: *CKDN2A, RB1, TP53, APC*	ND	7,42,43,45–47,49
	Primary cutaneous mucoepidermoid carcinoma	*CRTC1* rearrangement (cAMP/CREB pathway)	ND	95

Category	Tumor	Genetic alterations	Associated syndrome / notes	References
	lesions, and malignant counterparts	NF-κB pathway activation: *CYLD* inactivating mutations; *ALPK1* activating mutations; *MYB-NFIB* fusion (cylindroma); Other mutations: *AKT1, BCOR, DNMT3A*; Malignant *TP53* mutation	(may have superimposed somatic *DNMT3A, BCOR*)	
	Syringocystadenoma papilliferum and malignant counterpart	Benign: RAS/RAF activating mutations (*BRAF, HRAS, KRAS*); Malignant: Verrucous carcinoma in SCAP: *BRAF* mutation	Nevus sebaceus: *HRAS, PIK3CA*	20,62
	Syringoma	ND	Familial multiple syringomas: chr 16q22 (gene not identified)	96
	Syringofibroadenoma	ND	Nicolau–Balus syndrome (gene not identified); Schopf-Schulz-Passarge: *WNT10A*; Clouston: *GJB6* (Connexin 30)	3
	Tubular apocrine adenoma/papillary eccrine adenoma	RAS/RAF activating mutation (*BRAF, KRAS*)	ND	97
Mixed differentiation	Mixed tumor (chondroid syringoma) and malignant mixed tumor	Benign: *PLAG1* fusion; Malignant: *PLAG1* fusion; *PHF1-TFE3* fusion	ND	75,76
	Nevus sebaceus of Jadassohn	Postzygotic RAS mutations: *HRAS, KRAS*	Schimmelpenning (postzygotic *HRAS, KRAS* mutations)	77
Site-specific or unknown	Extramammary Paget's disease	Mutations activating RTK, MAPK, and PI3K signaling (*AKT1, BRAF* V600 E, *ERBB2, KRAS, NRAS, PIK3CA*); *FOXA1* promoter mutation, fusion; *TP53* mutation; Amplification: *ERBB2 (Her2/Neu)*	ND	79,80,82,84–86
	Hidradenoma papilliferum	PI3K activating mutation (*AKT1, PIK3CA, PIK3R1*)	ND	98,99

Abbreviations: cAMP, cyclic adenosine monophosphate; MAPK, mitogen-activated protein kinase; ND, no significant findings in literature; RTK, receptor tyrosine kinase.

mechanisms for these effects in cutaneous adnexal neoplasms. Often, activated oncogenes are downstream of receptor tyrosine kinases, activating the mitogen-activated protein kinase, and/or phosphoinositide-3-kinase (PI3K) pathways (**Fig. 1, Table 1**). Other dysregulated pathways include nuclear factor kappa-B (NF-κB), Hippo, cyclic adenosine monophosphate, and WNT/β-catenin pathways (see **Table 1**). Unlike BCC, the Hedgehog pathway is rarely altered genetically in cutaneous adnexal neoplasms. Progression of benign precursors to malignancy may be accompanied by inactivation of tumor suppressors, especially *TP53* (**Fig. 2**, see **Table 1**) Although UV-induced genomic damage plays a major role in SCC and BCC, the role for photodamage in cutaneous adnexal neoplasms is incompletely understood and likely varies by tumor type.[1–7]

Here, we review current knowledge regarding molecular pathogenesis of adnexal neoplasms within the hair follicle and sweat gland categories,

with implications for diagnosis and potential therapeutic targets. Sebaceous neoplasms are discussed in a companion article in this issue.[8]

LESIONS WITH PREDOMINANT FOLLICULAR DIFFERENTIATION

PILOMATRICOMA AND PILOMATRICAL CARCINOMA

Definition

Pilomatricoma (pilomatrixoma, calcifying epithelioma of Malherbe, benign calcifying epithelioma, trichomatricoma) is a common, benign adnexal neoplasm with differentiation toward the hair follicle matrix.[1–3]

Pilomatrical carcinoma (pilomatrix carcinoma, matrical carcinoma) is a rare neoplasm with less than 100 cases reported in the literature. Association with a precursor pilomatricoma is rare; the majority of cases arise de novo.[2]

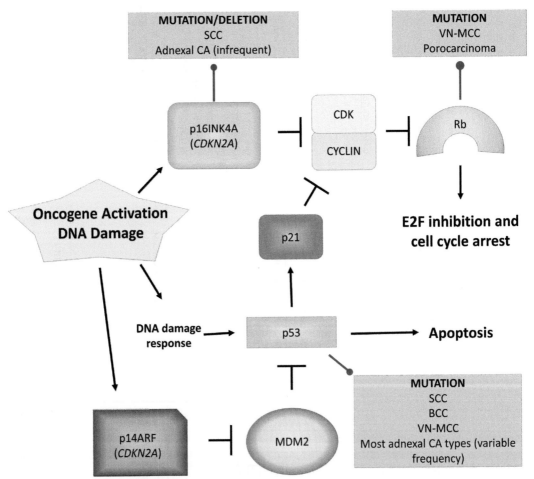

Fig. 2. Tumor suppressor inactivation in adnexal neoplasms. Red circle: inactivating event. CA, carcinoma; VN-MCC, virus-negative Merkel cell carcinoma.

Molecular Pathogenesis

Studies highlight a key role for Wnt/β-catenin signaling in the pathogenesis of pilomatricomas (see **Table 1**). Sporadic pilomatricomas are characteristically associated with activating mutations in the CTNNB1 gene.[9] The CTNNB1 gene encodes the protein β-catenin that is involved in intercellular adhesion, as well as in the Wnt signaling pathway that regulates cell proliferation, differentiation, and survival and is activated in normal hair follicle matrix cells to induce differentiation toward the hair shaft.[10] Transgenic mice expressing activated β-catenin develop skin tumors resembling pilomatricomas, supporting a functional role for activated β-catenin signaling in pilomatricoma formation.[11] Familial adenomatous polyposis (germline mutation of APC in the Wnt/β-catenin pathway) can demonstrate multiple pilomatricomas.[1] Multiple pilomatricomas also arise in association with inherited syndromes unrelated to the Wnt/β-catenin pathway, such as mismatch repair deficiency or myotonic dystrophy; in this context, pilomatricomas display somatic mutations of CTNNB1 similar to sporadic counterparts.[12,13]

An additional molecular aberration described in pilomatricomas is subclonal trisomy18, affecting the gene BCL2 involved in hair cycling.[14] Bone morphogenetic protein-2 is expressed in the shadow cells, and osteoblasts of ectopic bone within pilomatricomas, suggesting a role for this signaling factor in ectopic bone formation.[15]

In pilomatrical carcinoma, mutations in CTNNB1 also occur.[16,17] Thus far, the molecular basis of malignant progression from pilomatricoma has not been elucidated.[17] Pilomatrical carcinosarcoma displays shared chromosomal abnormalities between the carcinomatous and sarcomatous components.[18]

Clinical Features

Pilomatricoma classically presents as a slow-growing, asymptomatic, solitary, firm, 0.5 to 3.0-cm nodule. There is an increased frequency at younger ages and in females. Sites of predilection include the head and neck. Multiple pilomatricomas (5% of cases) can be familial, or associated with syndromes such as myotonic dystrophy, Gardner, and Sotos, among others. Recurrence after excision is rare for conventional pilomatricoma, but more frequent for the proliferating variant.[1–3]

Pilomatrical carcinoma typically presents as an asymptomatic solitary, large nodule on the face or scalp. There is increased frequency in middle-aged adults (5th decade) and men. Pilomatrical carcinomas have a risk of recurrence, regional metastasis, distant metastasis, and death from disease.[1,2]

Microscopic Features

Pilomatricomas are circumscribed tumors arranged as a single cystic nodule or multiple lobules. The tumor is centered in the deep dermis; extension to the subcutis may occur. The majority develop calcification or ossification. Two major cells types are found: basophilic cells and shadow (ghost) cells. Basophilic cells are small, monomorphous cells with darkly staining cytoplasm, indistinct cell borders, and a high nuclear:cytoplasmic ratio, positioned at the periphery of tumor lobules. Mitoses may be readily identifiable. Basophilic cells transition into large central aggregates of shadow cells: pale eosinophilic polygonal cells with well-defined borders and absence of nuclear staining. Variant forms include pigmented, anetodermic, bullous, proliferating, perforating, and superficial ("pilomatricomal horn").[1,2]

Pilomatricomal carcinomas are poorly circumscribed, asymmetric tumors in the dermis or subcutis. There is a predominance of atypical basophilic cells with pleomorphism, nucleoli, and frequent mitoses. Shadow cells are key to the diagnosis, but may be focal. Necrosis and ulceration may be present. Infiltrative growth can be accompanied by stromal desmoplasia.[1,2]

Immunohistochemistry

Nuclear and cytoplasmic β-catenin is present in basaloid cells of pilomatricomas (**Table 2**), with a loss of expression during maturation into shadow cells. The Wnt transcriptional targets CDX2 and LEF-1 are expressed in pilomatrical tumors.[9,19] Special AT-rich sequence-binding protein 2 (SATB2) is also expressed in a minority of pilomatrical carcinomas. BerEP4/EPCAM can assist with distinguishing pilomatrical carcinomas (negative) from BCC (positive).[2]

Differential Diagnosis

Shadow cells can rarely be seen in other cutaneous tumor types including BCC, panfolliculoma, trichoblastoma, and microcystic adnexal carcinoma (MAC). BCC with shadow cells may also harbor CTNNB1 mutation.[16] Matrical differentiation is seen in epithelial cysts associated with Gardner syndrome.[2] Although expression of CDX2 and SATB2 can also be seen in metastases of gastrointestinal origin, pilomatrical carcinomas lack glandular differentiation or CK20 expression, and express p63 and CK5/6.[18,19]

Table 2
Immunophenotypic findings in cutaneous adnexal neoplasia

Marker	Physiologic (Cutaneous Epithelial)	Tumor Expression (Cutaneous Epithelial)	Comments	Ref
Androgen receptor	Sebaceous, apocrine, eccrine (variable)	BCC (usually weak subset), sebaceous tumors, EMPD	Negative in trichoblastoma, trichoepithelioma	2,23
BCL-2	Some hair follicle populations	BCC (diffuse), pilomatricoma (basaloid), trichoblastoma/trichoepithelioma (peripheral)		2,23
Ber-EP4 (EpCAM)	Eccrine structures, telogen follicle	BCC, trichoblastoma/trichoepithelioma	Negative in pilomatricoma, poroma, MAC	2
β-Catenin (cytoplasmic, nuclear)	Hair matrix	Pilomatricoma and pilomatrical carcinoma	Membranous expression in most other epithelial tumors	2,9
BRAF(V600 E)	None	Digital papillary adenocarcinoma (minority), SCAP (subset), EMPD (minority), tubular apocrine adenoma/papillary eccrine adenoma (subset)		2,20,70,71,97
CD34	Outer root sheath	Trichilemmoma		2
CDX2	Unknown/none	Pilomatricoma and pilomatrical carcinoma		19
CEA	Eccrine duct, secretory	Ducts/glands of most sweat gland tumors	May be less sensitive than EMA	2
CK20	Merkel cells	EMPD (some cases), MCC, benign follicular tumors (colonizing Merkel cells)	BCC, MAC, other carcinomas lack colonizing Merkel cells	2,23,100
CK5/6	Epidermis, follicular epithelium (except matrix/IRS), glandular basal/myoepithelial	Diffuse in follicular tumors; basal or diffuse in sweat gland tumors	Negative in EMPD	2,100
CK7	Eccrine/apocrine/sebaceous secretory, myoepithelial; apocrine duct luminal	Hidradenoma (glands), spiradenoma, cylindroma, SCAP, ACC, mixed tumor, EMPD		2,100
c-Kit (CD117)	Eccrine/apocrine secretory (weak, subset)	ACC; variable expression in other sweat gland tumors		2,58

Marker	Cell type	Tumors	Notes	References
EMA	Eccrine duct/secretory, sebaceous	Ducts/glands of most sweat gland tumors		2
GATA3	Cutaneous epithelia except eccrine/apocrine	Most cutaneous epithelial tumors	May be less sensitive in eccrine/apocrine tumors	101
GCDFP-15	Apocrine	EMPD, apocrine tumors		2
Myb	Not defined	Spiradenoma, cylindroma, ACC; may be expressed in other sweat gland and follicular tumors	May be lost with malignant progression to spiradenocarcinoma	56,58,59,67,101
NUT	Absent	Poroma (24%), porocarcinoma (55%)		46
p63	Epidermis, follicular epithelium, glandular basal/myoepithelial	Diffuse in follicular tumors; basal or diffuse in sweat gland tumors	Negative in EMPD; may be less sensitive in apocrine	2,100,102
p75/NGFR	Outer root sheath; variable eccrine	Trichilemmoma		2
PHLDA1	Follicular stem cell	Trichoblastoma, trichoepithelioma, variable in MAC	Negative in BCC (exception may be micronodular BCC)	2
PLAG1	Not defined	Mixed tumor		75
S100	Eccrine secretory (weak, subset), myoepithelial	Spiradenoma, cylindroma, mixed tumor; myoepithelial layers		2
SOX10	Eccrine, myoepithelial	Hidradenoma (minority), spiradenoma, cylindroma; myoepithelial layers		58,103

Abbreviations: ACC, adenoid cystic carcinoma; CEA, carcinoembryonic antigen; CK, cytokeratin; EMA, epithelial membrane antigen; EMPD, extramammary Paget disease; MCC, Merkel cell carcinoma; NGFR, nerve growth factor receptor; SCAP, syringocystadenoma papilliferum.

TRICHOBLASTOMA

Definition

Trichoblastoma is a benign biphasic neoplasm with differentiation toward follicular germinative epithelium and follicular stroma. Trichoepitheliomas, considered a subtype of trichoblastoma, are discussed elsewhere in this article. Rarely, malignant transformation to trichoblastic carcinoma (non-BCC carcinoma arising in trichoblastoma) or trichoblastic carcinosarcoma has been described.[2]

Molecular Pathogenesis

The predominant driver for trichoblastoma remains unknown. A minority (11%) of sporadic trichoblastomas harbor activating mutations in HRAS (see Fig. 1, Table 1).[20] Trichoblastomas (with the exception of trichoepitheliomas) seem to lack PTCH1 mutations,[21] unlike BCC. Mutations in trichoblastic carcinoma remain unknown, although p53 overexpression has been reported.[22]

Clinical Features

Trichoblastoma presents as a solitary nodule, 0.5 to 3.0 cm in size. Tumors are generally asymptomatic, favor the head and neck, occur in the fifth or sixth decades of life, and have a female to male predominance of 2:1 to 5:1. Large nodular trichoblastoma is often associated with nevus sebaceus.[2,3] Trichoblastomas follow a benign course in the vast majority of cases. The clinical course of trichoblastic carcinoma and carcinosarcoma is not well-characterized.

Microscopic Features

Trichoblastomas are circumscribed deep dermal and subcutaneous tumors with varying proportions of follicular epithelial and stromal components. Classically, trichoblastomas consist of uniform basaloid cells with scant cytoplasm and peripheral palisading, arrayed in islands that interconnect in racemiform or retiform patterns. In some tumors, epithelial cells aggregate into large nodules. Abortive hair follicle structures may be present. The stroma recapitulates follicular mesenchyme, with abundant slender fibroblasts and delicate collagen fibers organized around epithelial islands. There is no significant tumor retraction, and cytologic atypia is absent.

Variant morphologies and unusual findings include adamantinoid/lymphadenoma (with central large cells displaying pale-staining cytoplasm and prominent nucleoli, and numerous interspersed lymphocytes), clear cell, rippled pattern, pigmented, focal sebaceous differentiation, and advanced follicular differentiation.[1,2]

Immunohistochemistry

Similar to other benign follicular tumors, trichoblastomas often display scattered small CK20+ cells, consistent with colonizing Merkel cells (see Table 2).[23]

Differential Diagnosis

The main differential diagnosis is BCC. Asymmetry, atypia, infiltrative growth, peripheral clefts around tumor nodules, and the presence of myxoid/inflammatory stroma are clues to the diagnosis of BCC. Unlike trichoblastoma, BCC express androgen receptor, Bcl-2 (diffuse), and CD10 (stromal).[23] PHLDA1 is expressed in most trichoblastomas and negative in BCC (with the possible exception of micronodular BCC).[2,24] CK20+ colonizing Merkel cells are absent in BCC, with the possible exception of infundibulocystic BCC.[23] BCC display frequent mutations of PTCH1 and/ or TP53. Of note, these mutations are absent in fibroepithelioma of Pinkus, raising the possibility that these tumors represent trichoblastomas or intermediate tumors rather than BCC.[25]

TRICHOEPITHELIOMA AND DESMOPLASTIC TRICHOEPITHELIOMA

Definition

Trichoepithelioma (cribriform trichoblastoma) and desmoplastic trichoepithelioma (columnar trichoblastoma) are uncommon benign neoplasms with differentiation toward follicular germinative epithelium and follicular stroma. There are 3 variants of trichoepithelioma: solitary, multiple, and desmoplastic.

Molecular Pathogenesis

The predominant driver in solitary and desmoplastic trichoepithelioma remains unknown. Inactivating PTCH1 mutations, similar to those in BCC, were reported in 2 of 21 trichoepitheliomas (see Table 1).[26] CTNNB1 mutation was found in 1 case of solitary trichoepithelioma.[16]

Multiple trichoepitheliomas occur in association with various syndromes including Brooke–Spiegler, multiple familial trichoepitheliomas, and Rombo. Of these, Brooke–Spiegler, and its phenotypic variant multiple familial trichoepitheliomas, are associated with germline loss-of-function mutations in the CYLD gene,[27–29] encoding a deubiquitinating enzyme that negatively regulates the NF-κB pathway.[30,31] Syndromic inactivating mutations of the CYLD gene correlate with upregulation of this pathway, resulting in proliferation, inhibition of apoptosis and tumorigenesis.[30]

Clinical Features

Solitary trichoepithelioma presents as a small papule or nodule on the face. Multiple trichoepitheliomas may coalesce into plaques. Syndromic lesions occur as bilateral, small, discrete, and/or confluent papules and nodules, preferentially involving the nasolabial folds.[1–3] Desmoplastic trichoepithelioma classically presents as a small solitary plaque with central dell on the face.[3]

Microscopic Features

Trichoepitheliomas are dermal tumors composed of follicular epithelial and stromal components. The epithelial component consists of small basaloid cells arranged in small nests and strands, classically in a cribriform pattern. Small horn cysts can be accompanied by foreign body giant cell reaction and calcification. Papillary–mesenchymal bodies (abortive attempts to form hair papillae) are characteristic. One-third of cases displays connection to the epidermis. There is no atypia. The stroma is fine and loose, similar to that of a trichoblastoma. Cleft retraction between tumor and stroma is absent.[1,2]

Desmoplastic trichoepithelioma displays strands and small nests of bland epithelial cells within a sclerotic stroma. Horn cysts, calcifications, and papillary mesenchymal bodies are diagnostic clues. Mitoses are rare to absent. Similar to conventional trichoepitheliomas, tumor clefting and atypia are absent.[1,2] Trichoadenoma may represent a variant of (desmoplastic) trichoepithelioma with a predominance of numerous large horn cysts.[3]

Immunohistochemistry

Immunohistochemical features resemble trichoblastoma (see **Table 2**).[23]

Differential Diagnosis

Desmoplastic trichoepithelioma raises a differential diagnosis of MAC, syringoma, and morpheaform BCC. The morphologic and immunophenotypic findings that distinguish BCC from trichoblastoma are also useful for trichoepithelioma (see **Table 2**).[2,23]

TRICHILEMMOMA

Definition

Trichilemmoma is a common benign lesion with differentiation toward the outer root sheath, with a component of infundibular/isthmic differentiation. The existence of the malignant counterpart, trichilemmal carcinoma, has been debated owing to substantial overlap with clear cell SCC.[2]

Molecular Pathogenesis

HRAS mutations are present in sporadic trichilemmomas (60%) and those associated with nevus sebaceous (92%) (see **Fig. 1**, **Table 1**).[32] Multiple trichilemmomas are a major diagnostic criterion for Cowden syndrome, part of the PTEN hamartoma tumor syndrome spectrum. By contrast, loss of PTEN expression is rare in sporadic tumors.[33] PTEN counteracts PI3-kinase by degrading its product phosphatidylinositol (3,4,5) trisphosphate (see **Fig. 1**).[4] Despite some morphologic overlap with viral verrucae, there is no definitive association of human papillomavirus with trichilemmoma.[2]

A sequencing study of 4 trichilemmal carcinomas described frequent TP53 mutations, with nonrecurrent alterations including mutations in NF1 and NRAS, PTEN deletion, TOP1 amplification, and fusions involving FGFR3 or ROS1.[34] Notably, many of these alterations (with the exception of TP53) are virtually absent in SCC.[35,36]

Clinical Features

Trichilemmoma presents as a small solitary papule on the head and neck, especially the central face. Multiple lesions are a cutaneous marker of Cowden syndrome. Trichilemmoma also is a common secondary neoplasm developing in nevus sebaceus.[2,3]

Microscopic Features

Trichilemmomas are lobular, dermal tumors with broad connection to the epidermis. The surface may display hypergranulosis and papillomatosis, similar to a verruca. The tumor consists of bland squamoid cells with variable glycogenation. In most cases, a subset of cells is optically clear with an eccentric nucleus, recapitulating the outer root sheath. Keratinization and squamous eddies may be present. At the periphery, small basaloid or columnar cells display subtle palisading. A thin cuticular basement membrane may be present. There is no atypia, nor is there clefting between the tumor and the stroma. Variant forms include desmoplastic trichilemmoma (with central desmoplastic changes) and trichilemmomal horn.[1,2]

Immunohistochemistry

Immunohistochemical features (see **Table 2**) include expression of CD34 and p75/NGFR, often in a peripheral/basal pattern corresponding to areas of most prominent outer root sheath differentiation.[2] Loss of PTEN expression is proposed to be a marker of Cowden syndrome.[3]

Differential Diagnosis

The differential diagnosis for trichilemmoma includes benign lesions (inverted follicular keratosis, viral verruca) and malignant (BCC, SCC, trichilemmal carcinoma). Inverted follicular keratosis lacks evidence of outer root sheath differentiation and has not been associated with Cowden syndrome. Circumscribed growth and absence of cytologic atypia distinguish trichilemmoma from carcinomas.[1,2]

NEOPLASMS WITH PREDOMINANT SWEAT GLAND DIFFERENTIATION

HIDRADENOMA AND HIDRADENOCARCINOMA

Definition

Hidradenoma (previously called eccrine acrospiroma or eccrine sweat gland adenoma) is a benign neoplasm corresponding to the secretory portion of sweat glands. Hidradenocarcinoma is the rare malignant counterpart of hidradenoma, in some cases arising within a precursor hidradenoma.[1,2]

Molecular Pathogenesis

Hidradenomas harbor a t(11;19) translocation in 50% of cases, resulting in fusion of CRTC1 (previously called MECT1) and MAML2, that drives transcriptional activation of cyclic adenosine monophosphate/CREB pathway targets (see Table 1).[37,38] CRTC3–MAML2 fusions are less common.[39] EWSR1-POU5F1 fusions have been described.[40]

Hidradenocarcinomas also harbor the CRTC1/MAML2 translocation, although at a lower frequency than the benign counterpart.[38] Mutations in TP53 occur (see Fig. 2).[41–45] Single cases of PIK3CA mutation, AKT1 mutation, and ERBB2 (Her2/neu) gene amplification have been described.[41,45]

Clinical Features

Hidradenomas typically present as large, solitary, asymptomatic nodules. Sites of predilection include the trunk, head, and neck, followed by extremities. Malignant progression is rare. Lymph node involvement without adverse outcome has been described in rare cases.[1,3] Hidradenocarcinoma typically present as a large solitary tumor occurring in the fifth to seventh decades. The overall rate of aggressive disease is unclear.[1,41]

Microscopic Features

Hidradenomas are dermal tumors with variable proportions of solid and cystic growth. Two cell morphologies predominate: polygonal eosinophilic cells and cells with clear or mucinous cytoplasm. Less common cell types include squamous, mucinous, goblet, signet ring, and oxyphilic. There is evidence of glandular differentiation, characterized by ducts and cysts with cuboidal lining. Tumor nodules are surrounded by prominent hyalinized basement membrane.[1,2] Clear cell hidradenoma is a major subtype of hidradenoma.

In poroid hidradenomas, small poroid cells predominate; these neoplasms likely represent a variant of eccrine poroma rather than hidradenoma.[39]

Hidradenocarcinomas are large, asymmetric tumors that display microscopic overlap with hidradenoma, accompanied by atypical features including infiltrative growth, stromal desmoplasia, deep extension, necrosis, perineural invasion, angiolymphatic invasion, pleomorphism, or frequent mitoses ($\geq$4/10 hpf). A precursor benign hidradenoma may be present. The risk of metastasis is independent of tumor grade.[2,41]

Immunohistochemistry

Immunophenotypic features are of eccrine and apocrine secretory epithelium (see Table 2).

Differential Diagnosis

Hidradenomas can be misinterpreted as mucoepidermoid carcinoma or SCC. The differential for clear cell hidradenomas may include sebaceous neoplasia, trichilemmoma (which lacks glands), and metastatic renal cell carcinoma (which expresses PAX8 and lacks glands).[1,2]

POROMA AND POROCARCINOMA

Definition and Molecular Pathogenesis

Poromas are benign neoplasms with differentiation toward the sweat gland duct. Porocarcinomas can develop de novo or evolve from a preexisting poroma.

Molecular Pathogenesis

Poromas are associated with dysregulation of the Hippo or RAS/mitogen-activated protein kinase pathways (see Fig. 1, Table 1). In most, Hippo pathway activity is dysregulated by fusion of YAP1 (YAP) to partners including MAML2 and NUTM1.[46] YAP is a transcriptional coactivator in the transcriptional enhanced associated domain family. The NUTM1 and MAML2 partners contribute to fusion protein activity via interaction with the transcriptional coactivators p300 and CBP. These fusions correlated with morphologic variants of poroma: *YAP1–MAML2* fusions predominated in hidroacanthoma simplex, whereas *YAP1–NUTM1* fusions were enriched in dermal duct tumor, poroid hidradenoma, and a subset of poromas.[46] Other studies found activating mutations in *HRAS* in a minority of tumors.[7,47] Rare drivers include the activating fusion of the YAP paralog TAZ (*WWTR1-NUTM1*), and activating *AKT1* mutation.[46] Although some reports found that tumor suppressors such as *TP53* are not altered in poromas, this point has been debated.[46–48]

Porocarcinomas display similar oncogenic drivers to poromas (*YAP-NUTM1* fusions in a majority, and *HRAS* mutations in a minority).[7,46,47] These are accompanied by inactivating mutation in tumor suppressor genes such as *TP53*, *CDKN2A*, and *RB1* (see **Fig. 2**, **Table 1**).[7,43,45–47,49] PI3K activating mutations (*PIK3CA*) have also been reported.[43–45] Single cases have demonstrated activating mutations of *ERBB2*, *KRAS*, *NRAS*, or *FGFR3*,[43,46] and *EWSR1* rearrangement.[50] UV mutations are present.[7]

Clinical Features

Poroma presents as a solitary, sessile nodule anywhere sweat glands are present, especially the palm and sole. Scalp lesions can arise in nevus sebaceus. Multiple lesions (eccrine poromatosis) rarely occur.[3]

Porocarcinoma presents as a plaque or nodule, often on the head and neck of elderly patients, in some cases within a preexisting poroma.[1,2] Porocarcinoma is associated with 17% to 22% local recurrence and regional metastatic rate, with distant metastasis and/or death in 11% to 12%.[51,52]

Microscopic Features

Poromas are lobular, circumscribed tumors with broad connection to the epidermis. Poroid cells are small and uniform, with round to oval nuclei, and amphophilic cytoplasm with variable amounts of glycogenation. Small lumina and variably sized cystic spaces are present. Variants include hidroacanthoma simplex (intraepidermal), dermal duct tumor (lacking connection to the epidermis), and poroid hidradenoma (overlapping with dermal duct tumor and hidradenoma). Syringoacanthoma may also be considered a poroma variant.

Porocarcinomas are malignant tumors with architectural and cytologic resemblance to poromas, accompanied by malignant features that can include cytologic atypia, infiltrative growth, and angiolymphatic invasion. Negative prognostic findings include high mitotic rate, lymphovascular invasion, and tumor depth of greater than 7 mm.[52]

Immunohistochemistry

There is immunophenotypic overlap with eccrine ductal epithelium (see **Table 2**). NUT expression (owing to *YAP–NUTM1* fusion) is present in a minority of poromas and approximately half of porocarcinomas.[46]

Differential Diagnosis

Porocarcinoma can be distinguished from poroma by atypia, infiltrative growth, necrosis, and altered expression of tumor suppressors (p53, Rb1, and p16).[48] Clear cell or squamoid areas can mimic SCC.[2] *NUTM1* fusions in poroma/porocarcinoma have a distinct partner from those in NUT carcinoma.[46]

SPIRADENOMA, CYLINDROMA, HYBRID LESIONS, AND MALIGNANT COUNTERPARTS

Definition

Spiradenoma, cylindroma, and spiradenocylindroma represent a continuum of sweat gland tumors. Malignant counterparts (also known as cylindroadenocarcinoma, malignant cylindroma, spiradenocarcinoma, malignant spiradenoma, or spiradenocylindrocarcinoma) are rare and arise in association with benign precursors.[1,2]

Molecular Pathogenesis

Genomic events predominantly involve activation of the NF-κB pathway, or the transcription factor Myb, which may act downstream of NF-κB (see **Table 1**). NF-κB is a critical component of the signaling cascade responsible for eccrine gland development during embryogenesis[53] and in cancer can promote tumorigenesis.[31] Inactivating mutations of the tumor suppressor *CYLD*, which represses NF-κB signaling, may be somatic or germline (Brooke–Spiegler syndrome).[54,55] A recent study revealed a recurrent hot spot mutation of the *ALPK1* gene in sporadic spiradenomas and spiradenocarcinomas, that activates the NF-κB pathway and is mutually exclusive from mutation of *CYLD*.[6] Sporadic cylindromas harbor *MYB–NFIB* fusions similar to ACC.[56] A subset of cylindromas have deleterious somatic mutations in the epigenetic modifier genes *DNMT3A* and *BCOR*, that coexist with somatic or germline *CYLD* mutations.[6,57] Cylindromas, but not spiradenomas or spiradenocarcinomas, display genomic UV damage.[6]

High-grade spiradenocarcinomas and cylindrocarcinomas carry loss-of-function *TP53* mutations not observed in matched precursors, implicating loss of this tumor suppressor in malignant progression (see **Fig. 2, Table 1**).[6,45]

Clinical Features

Cylindroma present as asymptomatic nodules in adults, with a predilection for head and neck, that may coalesce on the scalp ("turban tumor").[3]

Spiradenomas are typically painful dermal nodules with blue/gray coloration, with a predilection for head, neck, and upper trunk or upper extremities of young adults.[3]

Multiple tumors may be a manifestation of Brooke–Spiegler syndrome, together with other adnexal neoplasms such as trichoepithelioma.[2,3]

Malignant counterparts typically present as large solitary nodules on the head and neck of elderly adults. Malignant transformation occurs more frequently in the setting of multiple or syndromic lesions, and can manifest as new growth, ulceration, or bleeding in a preexisting lesion.[1,2] High-grade carcinomas are associated with aggressive disease, metastasis, and mortality. Low-grade and metaplastic carcinomas may recur locally but seem to lack metastatic potential.[1]

Microscopic Features

Spiradenomas and cylindromas exist on a morphologic spectrum. Classic spiradenomas are dermal or subcutaneous tumors, characterized by 1 or multiple round cellular nodules. Within tumor nodules, tumor cells form small interanastomosing cords. Two epithelial cell populations are noted: small cells with round nuclei and inconspicuous cytoplasm, and central cells with larger pale-staining nuclei. Infiltrating lymphocytes impart a distinctive "peppered" appearance. Small ductlike structures can often be identified. Hyaline droplets may be prominent. Variant forms and unusual findings include "giant vascular eccrine spiradenoma" (with prominent ectatic vessels), follicular differentiation, clear cell change, cystic change, adenomatous features, and sebaceous differentiation.[1,2]

Cylindromas are dermal tumors that display a "jigsaw puzzle'" configuration of interlocking epithelial islands rimmed by prominent hyaline basement membranes. There are 2 morphologic cell populations, similar to those described above for spiradenoma. Hyaline droplets and small ducts may be present. Tumor-infiltrating lymphocytes are not prominent. Spiradenocylindromas display hybrid features of cylindroma and spiradenoma.[1,2]

Malignant counterparts of spiradenomas and cylindromas arise in longstanding benign tumors and display features including infiltrative growth with desmoplasia, frequent mitoses, and cytologic atypia. Additional clues to malignant transformation include loss of the 2-cell population appearance, absence of lymphocytes (in a spiradenomatous tumor), and loss of hyaline sheath (in a cylindromatous tumor). Carcinoma subtypes are named after the analogous salivary gland tumors: basal cell adenocarcinoma-like pattern, low grade (mildly pleomorphic, small to medium-sized basaloid cells, in nodules and sheets); basal cell adenocarcinoma-like pattern, high grade (larger, more atypical basaloid cells with nucleoli and atypical mitoses); and invasive adenocarcinoma, not otherwise specified (large pleomorphic cells with abundant cytoplasm). Sarcomatoid (metaplastic) carcinomas display any of these 3 patterns, alongside a malignant spindled component.[1,2]

Differential Diagnosis

Trichilemmomas can have similar prominent basement membrane, but lack ducts and the jigsaw puzzle growth pattern. Malignant counterparts can be mistaken for cutaneous metastasis from visceral adenocarcinoma, or classified as adnexal carcinoma not otherwise specified; recognition of preexisting benign spiradenoma or cylindroma can be critical.

Immunohistochemistry

Immunohistochemical findings are similar to other sweat gland tumors (see **Table 2**) with expression of Myb in some cases.[56,58,59]

SYRINGOCYSTADENOMA PAPILLIFERUM AND MALIGNANT COUNTERPART

Definition

Syringocystadenoma papilliferum (SCAP) is a benign apocrine and squamous neoplasm that presents in isolation or as a secondary tumor in a nevus sebaceus. Malignant transformation in SCAP is extremely rare, and may involve the glandular component (syringocystadenocarcinoma papilliferum) or the squamous component (verrucous carcinoma).[1,2,60]

Molecular Pathogenesis

Activation of the RAS/RAF pathway is a consistent feature of SCAP (see **Fig. 1, Table 1**). *BRAF* V600E mutations are often present (52% in 1 study)[20] and are shared with contiguous verrucous proliferations, supporting a common clonal origin for the squamous and glandular components of SCAP.[61] Less frequent mutations include *HRAS* (26%)

and *KRAS* (rare).[20] SCAP arising in nevus sebaceus display matching *HRAS* mutations; in 1 case, an additional *PIK3CA* mutation was acquired in the SCAP component that was absent from the background nevus sebaceus.[62] Mutations in syringocystadenocarcinoma papilliferum have not been described. Verrucous carcinomas share *BRAF* mutations with the precursor SCAP, and lack evidence of human papillomavirus.[60]

Clinical Features

SCAP typically presents as a solitary papule/nodule in a child or young adult with a granular, moist-appearing surface. Alopecia accompanies lesions on the scalp. SCAP has a predilection for the head and neck, less commonly on the trunk and extremities.[3]

Syringocystadenocarcinoma papilliferum presents as a 2- to 6-cm nodule, inflammatory plaque, or tumor. The potential for metastasis and fatal course has been debated.[1]

Microscopic Features

SCAP is a dermal tumor with focal connection to the epidermis. Ductlike structures extend as invaginations from the surface. Superficially, these ducts are lined by keratinocytes, that transition to a 2-layered glandular epithelium with outer cuboidal cells and luminal columnar cells. Papillomatous projections may project into irregular cystic spaces. Plasma cells are a characteristic finding in tumor stroma. Dilated tubular glands may be present at the base. The zone of connection to the epidermis displays variable epidermal hyperplasia and may exhibit verrucous change.[1,2]

Syringocystadenocarcinoma papilliferum displays malignant cytologic atypia, as well as mitotic activity, loss of polarity, solid areas, and cribriform patterning. There may be retained myoepithelial layer (carcinoma in situ) or loss of the myoepithelial layer and frank invasion. Intraepidermal or intrafollicular pagetoid spread can occur.[1,2]

Immunohistochemistry

There are immunophenotypic findings of eccrine and apocrine epithelia (see **Table 2**).[63–65] Plasma cells express IgA (with a lesser component of IgG+ cells).[66]

Differential Diagnosis

Although the morphologic findings of SCAP are distinctive, there can be areas of morphologic resemblance to other adnexal apocrine neoplasms, such as tubular apocrine adenoma. Superficial biopsies of the verrucous surface might be mistaken for a squamous lesion.

ADENOID CYSTIC CARCINOMA

Definition

Adenoid cystic carcinoma (ACC) is a rare malignant tumor in the skin that is histologically identical to analogous tumors in the salivary gland and other sites.

Molecular Pathogenesis

Similar to ACC at other sites, cutaneous ACC harbors the t(6;9) (q22;p23) rearrangement resulting in the *MYB–NFIB* fusion (see **Table 1**).[67] The *MYBL1–NFIB* fusion has also been described.[68] Activating *NOTCH1* mutations have been associated with aggressive ACCs at other anatomic sites, but thus far have not been described in cutaneous ACC.[69]

Clinical Features

ACC presents as a solitary nodule in middle-age to elderly adults, often present for several years before diagnosis. There is a slight female predominance. Sites of predilection include the scalp, followed by the trunk and abdomen. ACC is characterized by frequent local recurrence.

Microscopic Features

ACC demonstrates cribriform, solid, and/or tubular growth patterns. At greater magnification, tumors demonstrate a mixture of true lumina and small round pseudocystic spaces with prominent basophilic mucin. Tumor cells are predominantly small hyperchromatic basaloid cells with minimal cytoplasm, accompanied by a subtle myoepithelial population. Perineural invasion is a common finding.

Immunohistochemistry

Immunohistochemical features (see **Table 2**) include consistent expression of c-Kit and Myb expression in most.[56,58,67]

Differential Diagnosis

ACC can resemble adenoid BCC. The differential diagnosis can also include spiradenoma, cylindroma, and cribriform carcinoma.[2] Myb and Kit expression are not specific for ACC (see **Table 2**).[56,58]

DIGITAL PAPILLARY ADENOCARCINOMA

Definition

Digital papillary adenocarcinoma is a very rare aggressive sweat gland malignancy.

Molecular Pathogenesis

Many tumors lack detectable mutations on targeted cancer panels. However, *TP53* mutations have been reported,[44,45] and *BRAF* V600E mutations can occur in a minority (see **Figs. 1** and **2**).[70,71] Overexpression of the receptor tyrosine kinase *FGFR2* has been demonstrated.[72]

Clinical Features

Digital papillary adenocarcinoma presents as a slow-growing nodule with a marked predilection for the fingers (80%) and toes, especially around the nails. These tumors have a strong male preponderance, and age range is from 14 to 83 years. There is significant potential for local recurrence and metastasis, especially to lymph node and lung, as well as death from disease. An aggressive course has not been linked to specific microscopic features. The treatment of choice is wide local excision or (partial) amputation.[1]

Microscopic Features

The classic appearance is a dermal tumor with papillary invaginations into the cystic spaces, with circumscribed or infiltrative borders. Solid areas or cribriform patterning can also be seen. Cytologic atypia is often low grade, characterized by hyperchromasia and nuclear enlargement. There can be mitotic activity and necrosis. Areas of clear cell change and squamous differentiation may be present.

Immunohistochemistry

Immunohistochemical features are summarized in **Table 2**.

Differential Diagnosis

Lesions with bland cytology mimic benign adnexal tumors or cysts. The presence of a dual cell population is not useful for this distinction. Many tumors on the differential (hidrocystoma, apocrine cystadenoma, and papillary eccrine adenoma) are uncommon to rare on the distal extremities. The diagnosis of hidradenoma should be applied with extreme caution on digital sites. Tubular papillary adenoma lacks solid growth and crowded glands. Metastatic carcinoma might be in the differential diagnosis for high-grade tumors.[1,2]

MICROCYSTIC ADNEXAL CARCINOMA

Definition

MAC is a low-grade, locally invasive malignant sweat duct tumor that has both sweat duct and follicular differentiation.

Molecular Pathogenesis

A recent study found that most MACs had few mutations and lacked a UV signature, suggesting that MACs originate from a relatively sun-protected niche in the dermis. The most recurrent mutation was *TP53* inactivation (22% of tumors) (see **Fig. 2**, **Table 1**). Frame-preserving insertions affecting the kinase domain of JAK1 (17% of cases) were mutually exclusive with *TP53* mutations, and correlated with increased phospho-STAT3 expression.[5] Single case reports have described *TP53* mutation, *CDKN2A* deletion,[43,73] and deletion on chromosome 6q.[74]

Clinical Features

MAC classically presents as a slow-growing firm plaque on the central face in the fifth to sixth decades of life. There is no sex predilection. MAC is locally destructive. Metastasis is rare, but has been reported. Recurrence is common, possibly owing to perineural extension. Management is by excision.[1,2]

Microscopic Features

Scanning magnification reveals a sclerosing tumor originating in the dermis, often with extension into the subcutis and deeper tissue planes. A focal connection to the epidermis may be present. Follicular differentiation is observed in the superficial portion of the tumor, in the form of basaloid keratinocytes forming horn cysts. The eccrine component consists of deeply infiltrating small strands of cuboidal cells with 2 cell layers and occasional lumen formation. The tumor is invested in a sclerotic or desmoplastic stroma. Mitoses are rare to absent. Cytologic atypia is not prominent. Perineural invasion occurs frequently. Variant forms and unusual findings include clear cell change, solid growth pattern (solid epithelial aggregates), and focal sebaceous differentiation.[1,2]

Immunohistochemistry

The immunohistochemical profile resembles sweat duct epithelium (see **Table 2**).

Differential Diagnosis

Owing to bland cytology, MAC raises a differential diagnosis including morpheaform BCC, desmoplastic trichoepithelioma, syringoma, and, in some cases, trichoadenoma or SCC. Infiltrative growth distinguishes MAC from benign lesions. There is increased phospho-STAT3 and p53 expression in MACs, unlike syringomas.[5] Morpheaform BCC and SCC generally have more cytologic atypia. Ber-EP4 is expressed in BCC, and not MAC (see **Table 2**).[23] The presence of follicular differentiation and minimal atypia distinguishes MAC from other sclerosing sweat gland carcinomas, such as syringoid carcinoma and squamoid eccrine ductal carcinoma.

TUMORS WITH MIXED DIFFERENTIATION

MIXED TUMOR (CHONDROID SYRINGOMA) AND MALIGNANT MIXED TUMOR

Definition

Mixed tumor is a benign sweat gland neoplasm composed of epithelial, myoepithelial, and mesenchymal elements and is the cutaneous analogue of pleomorphic adenoma.

Molecular Pathogenesis

Rearrangement of the gene *pleomorphic adenoma gene 1* (*PLAG1*), encoding a zinc finger transcription factor, is present in the majority of mixed tumors, and is accompanied by immunohistochemical expression of Plag1 (see **Tables 1** and **2**).[75] One case of malignant mixed tumor with *PHF1–TFE3* fusion has been described.[76]

Clinical Features

Mixed tumor typically presents as a solitary, slow-growing papule/nodule on the head and neck. Metastatic progression is extremely rare.

Malignant mixed tumor arises in a precursor mixed tumor, presenting as a large solitary nodule that may show rapid growth. Malignant mixed tumors can recur and metastasize to local nodes and distant sites. The risk of an aggressive course is unknown.

Microscopic Features

Mixed tumors are circumscribed tumors composed of glandular, myoepithelial, and stromal components. The glandular component may display small tubules reminiscent of syringoma (eccrine variant), or long branching tubules with 2 cell layers and more prominent cell lining (apocrine variant). The stromal component is chondromyxoid to cartilaginous. Variant forms and unusual findings include extensive fatty metaplasia (lipomatous change) and follicular/sebaceous differentiation.

Malignant mixed tumors demonstrate variable patterns, including adenocarcinoma, myoepithelial carcinoma, carcinoma not otherwise specified, and sarcomatoid carcinoma. By strict diagnostic criteria, the presence of a precursor mixed tumor is required for diagnosis.[2]

Immunohistochemistry

There is variable expression of apocrine, eccrine, and myoepithelial markers (see **Table 2**). PLAG1 is a sensitive marker.[75]

Differential Diagnosis

Owing to prominent chondroid, osseous, or lipomatous stroma, mesenchymal neoplasms can be a diagnostic consideration. Ductal elements in eccrine mixed tumor can resemble syringoma.

NEVUS SEBACEUS OF JADASSOHN (ORGANOID NEVUS)

Definition

Nevus sebaceus (organoid nevus) is a congenital hamartoma involving the epidermis and adnexal structures.

Molecular Pathogenesis

Nevus sebaceus is due to postzygotic mutation in the RAS pathway, specifically activating mutations in *HRAS* or *KRAS* (see **Fig. 1, Table 1**).[77] Secondary tumors arising in nevus sebaceus acquire additional mutations.[62]

Clinical Features

Nevus sebaceus presents at birth as a solitary, smooth, waxy plaque with overlying alopecia. There is a predilection for the scalp, face, and neck, but other areas can be involved, including the genital skin. Around puberty, lesions become more raised, papillated, and often acquire a more yellow color owing to sebaceous gland hyperplasia. Neoplasms arising in nevus sebaceus develop in adults, usually 40 to 50 years of age.[2]

Syndromic associations include didymosis aplasticosebacea, phakomatosis pigmentokeratotica, Schimmelpenning–Feuerstein–Mims syndrome, and SCALP (sebaceous nevus, central nervous system malformations, aplasia cutis congenital, limbal dermoid, and pigmented nevus) syndrome.[1,2]

Microscopic Features

In childhood, nevus sebaceus displays incompletely differentiated hair follicles and small sebaceous glands. At puberty, sebaceous glands become prominent, and papillomatous hyperplasia of the overlying epidermis develops. Hair follicles display incomplete and altered differentiation, including basaloid buds and dilated infundibular structures. The associated lack of mature terminal hair follicles results in alopecia. Ectopic apocrine glands and altered eccrine glands may be present. Over time, secondary neoplasms develop, most frequently SCAP and trichoblastoma; less common tumors include hidradenoma, syringoma, sebaceoma, mixed tumor, trichilemmoma, trichoadenoma, and other adnexal tumors. Malignant tumors arise less frequently, including BCC, SCC, and sebaceous carcinoma.[1,2,78]

Immunohistochemistry

Expression patterns correspond to the type of hamartomatous epithelia or secondary neoplasm (see **Table 2**).

Differential Diagnosis

The differential diagnosis of nevus sebaceus depends on sampling and clinical context. Sebaceous hyperplasia may be a consideration. Secondary neoplasms may be confused with their primary counterparts.[1,2]

SITE-SPECIFIC NEOPLASMS

EXTRAMAMMARY PAGET'S DISEASE

Definition

Extramammary Paget's disease (EMPD) is a rare adenocarcinoma characterized by intraepithelial growth of neoplastic cells, either originating in the skin without coexisting internal malignancy (primary EMPD), or in the setting of a visceral carcinoma of the urothelium, anorectal, gynecologic organs or other sites (secondary EMPD).[1,2]

Molecular Pathogenesis

EMPD displays diverse oncogenic drivers that activate receptor tyrosine kinase, mitogen-activated protein kinase, and/or PI3K signaling pathways (see **Fig. 1**, **Table 1**). *Her2/Neu* (*ERBB2*) amplification and activating mutations occur in approximately 10% of EMPD,[79-81] representing a potential therapeutic target. Additional abnormalities include RAS/RAF activating mutations (*BRAF* V600E, *KRAS*, and *NRAS*), PI3K pathway mutations (*PIK3CA*, *AKT1*), *TP53* mutation, mutations in chromatin remodeling genes, gain of chromosome 7, and loss of chromosome X.[80,82-86] A recent study revealed recurrent genomic alterations (promoter mutations or gene fusion) involving the transcription factor *FOXA1* (forkhead box A1, hepatocyte nuclear factor 3α) in 23% of EMPD, with potential oncogenic roles similar to those described in breast carcinoma and prostate carcinoma.[80] Multifocal EMPD demonstrates clonal identity between sites of involvement, consistent with a single transformation event.[83]

It is currently unknown whether secondary EMPD shares molecular changes with the associated internal malignancy. Interestingly, mammary Paget's disease has been reported to display distinct drivers from the underlying breast carcinoma.[83]

Clinical Features

EMPD most commonly presents as well-demarcated erythematous plaque on the genital skin of postmenopausal women. The lesion is often accompanied by pruritus or burning. Rare forms include hyperpigmentation or hypopigmentation and multicentric lesions. The treatment of choice for EMPD is surgical excision. Achieving negative margins and controlling local recurrences can be challenging. The 5-year survival of EMPD is estimated to be 75% to 91%, with invasive disease or associated malignancy having a shorter survival.

Microscopic Features

EMPD is a diffuse intraepidermal proliferation of large cells with pale-staining cytoplasm and large pleomorphic nuclei and (in some cases) prominent nucleoli. Lesional cells are scattered throughout all levels of the epidermis, with a predilection toward the lower epidermis. Occasional clusters with lumen formation may be observed. Neoplastic cells extend down the hair follicle epithelium and eccrine structures. Invasion occurs in a minority of cases, with rare metastasis to regional lymph nodes.

Immunohistochemistry

EMPD displays immunophenotypic evidence of apocrine differentiation (see **Table 2**). Mucicarmine and Alcian blue highlight cytoplasmic mucin. CK20 expression can be observed, especially in secondary EMPD.

Differential Diagnosis

The differential diagnosis of EMPD includes Bowen's disease and melanoma in situ. Many adnexal carcinomas can also display pagetoid scatter. EMPD lacks expression of CK5/6 and p63 (unlike Bowen's disease) and melanocytic markers (unlike melanoma in situ).

OTHER TUMORS

Molecular features of additional follicular and sweat gland tumors are included in **Table 1**. Some tumor types (eg, mucinous carcinoma) are not included owing to predominantly negative or absent genomic data.

SUMMARY

In recent years, substantial progress has been made toward defining genomic alterations in adnexal neoplasms, with potential diagnostic, prognostic, and therapeutic significance. In addition, molecular changes in adnexal neoplasms have revealed immunohistochemical markers with diagnostic usefulness. However, our knowledge remains limited. Most studies have focused on panels of cancer-related genes; for many tumor types, large exome- or genome-wide investigations are needed to define mutational signatures and novel drivers. The mutational signatures in non-UV tumors are not well-understood. Further investigations are needed to define the diagnostic specificity and sensitivity of specific molecular alterations (or their associated immunohistochemical markers) for challenging skin tumors and metastases of unknown primary. These efforts must be accompanied by more exact descriptions of clinical outcomes and prognostic features for specific tumor types. Finally, the therapeutic utility of targeted therapies such as BRAF, MEK, and PI3K inhibitors for aggressive adnexal neoplasms requires clinical validation. These insights will improve diagnosis and management of cutaneous adnexal neoplasms, and advance our understanding of tumor biology in general.

CLINICS CARE POINTS

- Cutaneous adnexal neoplasms display diversity in morphology, clinical behavior, and genetic alterations.
- Correct diagnosis of cutaneous adnexal neoplasms is essential to identify tumors with an aggressive course, or those that might be associated with inherited tumor syndrome.
- The diversity and rarity of adnexal tumors can raise diagnostic difficulties.
- Genetic alterations may be reflected in expression changes detectable by diagnostic immunohistochemistry.

REFERENCES

1. Elder DE, Massi D, Scolyer RA, et al, editors. WHO classification of skin tumors. 4 edition. Lyon, France: International Agency for Research on Cancer; 2018.
2. Kazakov D, McKee P, Michal M, et al. Cutaneous adnexal tumors. Philadelphia, United States: Lippincott Williams and Wilkins; 2012.
3. Bolognia JL, Schaffer JV, Cerroni L, editors. Dermatology. China: Elsevier; 2018.
4. Hanahan D, Weinberg RA. Hallmarks of cancer: the next generation. Cell 2011;144(5):646–74.
5. Chan MP, Plouffe KR, Liu CJ, et al. Next-generation sequencing implicates oncogenic roles for p53 and JAK/STAT signaling in microcystic adnexal carcinomas. Mod Pathol 2020;33(6):1092–103.
6. Rashid M, van der Horst M, Mentzel T, et al. ALPK1 hotspot mutation as a driver of human spiradenoma and spiradenocarcinoma. Nat Commun 2019; 10(1):2213.
7. Harms PW, Hovelson DH, Cani AK, et al. Porocarcinomas harbor recurrent HRAS-activating mutations and tumor suppressor inactivating mutations. Hum Pathol 2016;51:25–31.
8. North JP. Molecular genetics of sebaceous neoplasia. Surg Pathol Clin 2021;14(2):273–84.
9. Chan EF, Gat U, McNiff JM, et al. A common human skin tumour is caused by activating mutations in beta-catenin. Nat Genet 1999;21(4):410–3.
10. Kraft S, Granter SR. Molecular pathology of skin neoplasms of the head and neck. Arch Pathol Lab Med 2014;138(6):759–87.
11. Gat U, DasGupta R, Degenstein L, et al. De Novo hair follicle morphogenesis and hair tumors in mice expressing a truncated beta-catenin in skin. Cell 1998;95(5):605–14.
12. Chmara M, Wernstedt A, Wasag B, et al. Multiple pilomatricomas with somatic CTNNB1 mutations in children with constitutive mismatch repair deficiency. Genes Chromosomes Cancer 2013;52(7):656–64.
13. Rubben A, Wahl RU, Eggermann T, et al. Mutation analysis of multiple pilomatricomas in a patient with myotonic dystrophy type 1 suggests a DM1-associated hypermutation phenotype. PLoS One 2020;15(3):e0230003.
14. Agoston AT, Liang C, Richkind KE, et al. Trisomy 18 is a consistent cytogenetic feature in pilomatricoma. Mod Pathol 2010;23(8):1147.
15. Kurokawa I, Kusumoto K, Bessho K, et al. Immunohistochemical expression of bone morphogenetic protein-2 in pilomatricoma. Br J Dermatol 2000;143(4):754–8.
16. Kazakov DV, Sima R, Vanecek T, et al. Mutations in exon 3 of the CTNNB1 gene (beta-catenin gene) in cutaneous adnexal tumors. Am J Dermatopathol 2009;31(3):248–55.
17. Lazar AJ, Calonje E, Grayson W, et al. Pilomatrix carcinomas contain mutations in CTNNB1, the gene encoding beta-catenin. J Cutan Pathol 2005;32(2):148–57.
18. Luong TMH, Akazawa Y, Mussazhanova Z, et al. Cutaneous pilomatrical carcinosarcoma: a case report with molecular analysis and literature review. Diagn Pathol 2020;15(1):7.
19. Tumminello K, Hosler GA. CDX2 and LEF-1 expression in pilomatrical tumors and their utility in the diagnosis of pilomatrical carcinoma. J Cutan Pathol 2018;45(5):318–24.
20. Shen AS, Peterhof E, Kind P, et al. Activating mutations in the RAS/mitogen-activated protein kinase signaling pathway in sporadic trichoblastoma and syringocystadenoma papilliferum. Hum Pathol 2015;46(2):272–6.
21. Hafner C, Schmiemann V, Ruetten A, et al. PTCH mutations are not mainly involved in the pathogenesis of sporadic trichoblastomas. Hum Pathol 2007; 38(10):1496–500.

22. Fusumae T, Tanese K, Takeuchi A, et al. High-grade trichoblastic carcinoma arising through malignant transformation of trichoblastoma: immunohistochemical analysis and the expression of p53 and phosphorylated AKT. J Dermatol 2019;46(1):57–60.

23. Stanoszek LM, Wang GY, Harms PW. Histologic mimics of basal cell carcinoma. Arch Pathol Lab Med 2017;141(11):1490–502.

24. Yeh I, McCalmont TH, LeBoit PE. Differential expression of PHLDA1 (TDAG51) in basal cell carcinoma and trichoepithelioma. Br J Dermatol 2012; 167(5):1106–10.

25. Russell-Goldman E, Lindeman NI, Laga AC, et al. Morphologic, immunohistochemical, and molecular distinction between fibroepithelioma of Pinkus and "Fenestrated" basal cell carcinoma. Am J Dermatopathol 2020;42(7):513–20.

26. Vorechovsky I, Unden AB, Sandstedt B, et al. Trichoepitheliomas contain somatic mutations in the overexpressed PTCH gene: support for a gatekeeper mechanism in skin tumorigenesis. Cancer Res 1997;57(21):4677–81.

27. Hu G, Onder M, Gill M, et al. A novel missense mutation in CYLD in a family with Brooke-Spiegler syndrome. J Invest Dermatol 2003;121(4):732–4.

28. Salhi A, Bornholdt D, Oeffner F, et al. Multiple familial trichoepithelioma caused by mutations in the cylindromatosis tumor suppressor gene. Cancer Res 2004;64(15):5113–7.

29. Zhang XJ, Liang YH, He PP, et al. Identification of the cylindromatosis tumor-suppressor gene responsible for multiple familial trichoepithelioma. J Invest Dermatol 2004;122(3):658–64.

30. Brummelkamp TR, Nijman SM, Dirac AM, et al. Loss of the cylindromatosis tumour suppressor inhibits apoptosis by activating NF-kappaB. Nature 2003;424(6950):797–801.

31. King KE, George AL, Sakakibara N, et al. Intersection of the p63 and NF-kappaB pathways in epithelial homeostasis and disease. Mol Carcinog 2019; 58(9):1571–80.

32. Tsai JH, Huang WC, Jhuang JY, et al. Frequent activating HRAS mutations in trichilemmoma. Br J Dermatol 2014;171(5):1073–7.

33. Al-Zaid T, Ditelberg JS, Prieto VG, et al. Trichilemmomas show loss of PTEN in Cowden syndrome but only rarely in sporadic tumors. J Cutan Pathol 2012;39(5):493–9.

34. Ha JH, Lee C, Lee KS, et al. The molecular pathogenesis of Trichilemmal carcinoma. BMC Cancer 2020;20(1):516.

35. Pickering CR, Zhou JH, Lee JJ, et al. Mutational landscape of aggressive cutaneous squamous cell carcinoma. Clin Cancer Res 2014;20(24): 6582–92.

36. Lazo de la Vega L, Bick N, Hu K, et al. Invasive squamous cell carcinomas and precursor lesions on UV-exposed epithelia demonstrate concordant genomic complexity in driver genes. Mod Pathol 2020;33(11):2280–94.

37. El-Naggar AK. Clear cell hidradenoma of the skin–a third tumor type with a t(11;19)-associated TORC1-MAML2 gene fusion: genes chromosomes cancer. 2005;43:202-205. Adv Anat Pathol 2006;13(2):80–2.

38. Winnes M, Molne L, Suurkula M, et al. Frequent fusion of the CRTC1 and MAML2 genes in clear cell variants of cutaneous hidradenomas. Genes Chromosomes Cancer 2007;46(6):559–63.

39. Kuma Y, Yamada Y, Yamamoto H, et al. A novel fusion gene CRTC3-MAML2 in hidradenoma: histopathological significance. Hum Pathol 2017;70: 55–61.

40. Moller E, Stenman G, Mandahl N, et al. POU5F1, encoding a key regulator of stem cell pluripotency, is fused to EWSR1 in hidradenoma of the skin and mucoepidermoid carcinoma of the salivary glands. J Pathol 2008;215(1):78–86.

41. Kazakov DV, Ivan D, Kutzner H, et al. Cutaneous hidradenocarcinoma: a clinicopathological, immunohistochemical, and molecular biologic study of 14 cases, including Her2/neu gene expression/amplification, TP53 gene mutation analysis, and t(11;19) translocation. Am J Dermatopathol 2009; 31(3):236–47.

42. Biernat W, Peraud A, Wozniak L, et al. p53 mutations in sweat gland carcinomas. Int J Cancer 1998;76(3):317–20.

43. Cavalieri S, Busico A, Capone I, et al. Identification of potentially druggable molecular alterations in skin adnexal malignancies. J Dermatol 2019; 46(6):507–14.

44. Dias-Santagata D, Lam Q, Bergethon K, et al. A potential role for targeted therapy in a subset of metastasizing adnexal carcinomas. Mod Pathol 2011;24(7):974–82.

45. Le LP, Dias-Santagata D, Pawlak AC, et al. Apocrine-eccrine carcinomas: molecular and immunohistochemical analyses. PLoS One 2012; 7(10):e47290.

46. Sekine S, Kiyono T, Ryo E, et al. Recurrent YAP1-MAML2 and YAP1-NUTM1 fusions in poroma and porocarcinoma. J Clin Invest 2019;129(9):3827–32.

47. Bosic M, Kirchner M, Brasanac D, et al. Targeted molecular profiling reveals genetic heterogeneity of poromas and porocarcinomas. Pathology 2018; 50(3):327–32.

48. Zahn J, Chan MP, Wang G, et al. Altered Rb, p16, and p53 expression is specific for porocarcinoma relative to poroma. J Cutan Pathol 2019;46(9): 659–64.

49. Thibodeau ML, Bonakdar M, Zhao E, et al. Whole genome and whole transcriptome genomic profiling of a metastatic eccrine porocarcinoma. NPJ Precis Oncol 2018;2(1):8.

50. Antonescu CR, Zhang L, Chang NE, et al. EWSR1-POU5F1 fusion in soft tissue myoepithelial tumors. A molecular analysis of sixty-six cases, including soft tissue, bone, and visceral lesions, showing common involvement of the EWSR1 gene. Genes Chromosomes Cancer 2010;49(12):1114–24.

51. Nazemi A, Higgins S, Swift R, et al. Eccrine Porocarcinoma: new insights and a systematic review of the literature. Dermatol Surg 2018;44(10):1247–61.

52. Robson A, Greene J, Ansari N, et al. Eccrine porocarcinoma (malignant eccrine poroma): a clinicopathologic study of 69 cases. Am J Surg Pathol 2001;25(6):710–20.

53. Cui CY, Schlessinger D. Eccrine sweat gland development and sweat secretion. Exp Dermatol 2015;24(9):644–50.

54. Verhoef S, Schrander-Stumpel CT, Vuzevski VD, et al. Familial cylindromatosis mimicking tuberous sclerosis complex and confirmation of the cylindromatosis locus, CYLD1, in a large family. J Med Genet 1998;35(10):841–5.

55. Bignell GR, Warren W, Seal S, et al. Identification of the familial cylindromatosis tumour-suppressor gene. Nat Genet 2000;25(2):160–5.

56. Fehr A, Kovacs A, Loning T, et al. The MYB-NFIB gene fusion-a novel genetic link between adenoid cystic carcinoma and dermal cylindroma. J Pathol 2011;224(3):322–7.

57. Davies HR, Hodgson K, Schwalbe E, et al. Epigenetic modifiers DNMT3A and BCOR are recurrently mutated in CYLD cutaneous syndrome. Nat Commun 2019;10(1):4717.

58. Evangelista MT, North JP. MYB, CD117 and SOX-10 expression in cutaneous adnexal tumors. J Cutan Pathol 2017;44(5):444–50.

59. van der Horst MP, Marusic Z, Hornick JL, et al. Morphologically low-grade spiradenocarcinoma: a clinicopathologic study of 19 cases with emphasis on outcome and MYB expression. Mod Pathol 2015;28(7):944–53.

60. Alegria-Landa V, Jo-Velasco M, Santonja C, et al. Syringocystadenoma papilliferum associated with verrucous carcinoma of the skin in the same lesion: report of four cases. J Cutan Pathol 2020;47(1):12–6.

61. Friedman BJ, Sahu J, Solomides CC, et al. Contiguous verrucous proliferations in syringocystadenoma papilliferum: a retrospective analysis with additional evaluation via mutation-specific BRAFV600E immunohistochemistry. J Cutan Pathol 2018;45(3):212–6.

62. Kim JT, Newsom KJ, Shon W. Detection of somatic mutations in secondary tumors associated with nevus sebaceus by targeted next generation sequencing. Comment on Kitamura et al. Int J Dermatol 2018;57(1):120–2.

63. Kazakov DV, Requena L, Kutzner H, et al. Morphologic diversity of syringocystadenocarcinoma papilliferum based on a clinicopathologic study of 6 cases and review of the literature. Am J Dermatopathol 2010;32(4):340–7.

64. Huerre M, Bonnet D, Mc Carthy SW, et al. [Carcinosarcoma arising in eccrine spiradenoma. A morphologic and immunohistochemical study]. Ann Pathol 1994;14(3):168–73.

65. Bondi R, Urso C. Syringocystadenocarcinoma papilliferum. Histopathology 1996;28(5):475–7.

66. McKee PH, Fletcher CD, Rasbridge SA. The enigmatic eccrine epithelioma (eccrine syringomatous carcinoma). Am J Dermatopathol 1990;12(6):552–61.

67. North JP, McCalmont TH, Fehr A, et al. Detection of MYB alterations and other immunohistochemical markers in primary cutaneous adenoid cystic carcinoma. Am J Surg Pathol 2015;39(10):1347–56.

68. Kyrpychova L, Vanecek T, Grossmann P, et al. Small subset of adenoid cystic carcinoma of the skin is associated with alterations of the MYBL1 gene similar to their extracutaneous counterparts. Am J Dermatopathol 2018;40(10):721–6.

69. Ferrarotto R, Mitani Y, Diao L, et al. Activating NOTCH1 mutations define a distinct subgroup of patients with adenoid cystic carcinoma who have poor prognosis, propensity to bone and liver metastasis, and potential responsiveness to notch1 inhibitors. J Clin Oncol 2017;35(3):352–60.

70. Bell D, Aung P, Prieto VG, et al. Next-generation sequencing reveals rare genomic alterations in aggressive digital papillary adenocarcinoma. Ann Diagn Pathol 2015;19(6):381–4.

71. Trager MH, Jurkiewicz M, Khan S, et al. A case report of papillary digital adenocarcinoma with BRAFV600E mutation and quantified mutational burden. Am J Dermatopathol 2020;43(1):57–9.

72. Surowy HM, Giesen AK, Otte J, et al. Gene expression profiling in aggressive digital papillary adenocarcinoma sheds light on the architecture of a rare sweat gland carcinoma. Br J Dermatol 2019;180(5):1150–60.

73. Chen MB, Laber DA. Metastatic microcystic adnexal carcinoma with DNA sequencing results and response to systemic antineoplastic chemotherapy. Anticancer Res 2017;37(9):5109–11.

74. Wohlfahrt C, Ternesten A, Sahlin P, et al. Cytogenetic and fluorescence in situ hybridization analyses of a microcystic adnexal carcinoma with del(6)(q23q25). Cancer Genet Cytogenet 1997;98(2):106–10.

75. Bahrami A, Dalton JD, Krane JF, et al. A subset of cutaneous and soft tissue mixed tumors are genetically linked to their salivary gland counterpart. Gene Chromosome Canc 2012;51(2):140–8.

76. Panagopoulos I, Gorunova L, Lund-Iversen M, et al. Fusion of the genes PHF1 and TFE3 in malignant chondroid syringoma. Cancer Genomics Proteomics 2019;16(5):345–51.

77. Groesser L, Herschberger E, Ruetten A, et al. Postzygotic HRAS and KRAS mutations cause nevus sebaceous and Schimmelpenning syndrome. Nat Genet 2012;44(7):783–7.

78. Idriss MH, Elston DM. Secondary neoplasms associated with nevus sebaceus of Jadassohn: a study of 707 cases. J Am Acad Dermatol 2014;70(2):332–7.

79. Tanaka R, Sasajima Y, Tsuda H, et al. Human epidermal growth factor receptor 2 protein overexpression and gene amplification in extramammary Paget disease. Br J Dermatol 2013;168(6): 1259–66.

80. Takeichi T, Okuno Y, Matsumoto T, et al. Frequent FOXA1-activating mutations in extramammary Paget's disease. Cancers (Basel) 2020;12(4):820.

81. Fukuda K, Funakoshi T. Metastatic extramammary Paget's disease: pathogenesis and novel therapeutic approach. Front Oncol 2018;8:38.

82. Micci F, Teixeira MR, Scheistroen M, et al. Cytogenetic characterization of tumors of the vulva and vagina. Genes Chromosomes Cancer 2003;38(2): 137–48.

83. Zhang G, Zhou S, Zhong W, et al. Whole-exome sequencing reveals frequent mutations in chromatin remodeling genes in mammary and extramammary Paget's diseases. J Invest Dermatol 2019;139(4):789–95.

84. Kang Z, Xu F, Zhang QA, et al. Correlation of DLC1 gene methylation with oncogenic PIK3CA mutations in extramammary Paget's disease. Mod Pathol 2012;25(8):1160–8.

85. Kang Z, Xu F, Zhang QA, et al. Oncogenic mutations in extramammary Paget's disease and their clinical relevance. Int J Cancer 2013;132(4): 824–31.

86. Kiniwa Y, Yasuda J, Saito S, et al. Identification of genetic alterations in extramammary Paget disease using whole exome analysis. J Dermatol Sci 2019; 94(1):229–35.

87. Stevenson P, Rodins K, Susman R. The association between multiple pilomatrixomas and APC gene mutations. Australas J Dermatol 2018;59(4):e273–4.

88. Hahn H, Wicking C, Zaphiropoulous PG, et al. Mutations of the human homolog of Drosophila patched in the nevoid basal cell carcinoma syndrome. Cell 1996;85(6):841–51.

89. Johnson RL, Rothman AL, Xie J, et al. Human homolog of patched, a candidate gene for the basal cell nevus syndrome. Science 1996;272(5268):1668–71.

90. Gallant JN, Sewell A, Almodovar K, et al. Genomic landscape of a metastatic malignant proliferating tricholemmal tumor and its response to PI3K inhibition. NPJ Precis Oncol 2019;3:5.

91. Qin H, Moore RF, Ho CY, et al. Endocrine mucin-producing sweat gland carcinoma: a study of 11 cases with molecular analysis. J Cutan Pathol 2018;45(9):681–7.

92. Bohring A, Stamm T, Spaich C, et al. WNT10A mutations are a frequent cause of a broad spectrum of ectodermal dysplasias with sex-biased manifestation pattern in heterozygotes. Am J Hum Genet 2009;85(1):97–105.

93. Bishop JA, Taube JM, Su A, et al. Secretory carcinoma of the skin harboring ETV6 gene fusions: a cutaneous analogue to secretory carcinomas of the breast and Salivary Glands. Am J Surg Pathol 2017;41(1):62–6.

94. Kastnerova L, Luzar B, Goto K, et al. Secretory carcinoma of the skin: report of 6 cases, including a case with a novel NFIX-PKN1 translocation. Am J Surg Pathol 2019;43(8):1092–8.

95. Lennerz JK, Perry A, Dehner LP, et al. CRTC1 rearrangements in the absence of t(11;19) in primary cutaneous mucoepidermoid carcinoma. Br J Dermatol 2009;161(4):925–9.

96. Wu WM, Lee YS. Autosomal dominant multiple syringomas linked to chromosome 16q22. Br J Dermatol 2010;162(5):1083–7.

97. Liau JY, Tsai JH, Huang WC, et al. BRAF and KRAS mutations in tubular apocrine adenoma and papillary eccrine adenoma of the skin. Hum Pathol 2018;73:59–65.

98. Pfarr N, Sinn HP, Klauschen F, et al. Mutations in genes encoding PI3K-AKT and MAPK signaling define anogenital papillary hidradenoma. Genes Chromosomes Cancer 2016;55(2):113–9.

99. Pfarr N, Allgauer M, Steiger K, et al. Several genotypes, one phenotype: PIK3CA/AKT1 mutation-negative hidradenoma papilliferum show genetic lesions in other components of the signalling network. Pathology 2019;51(4):362–8.

100. Qureshi HS, Ormsby AH, Lee MW, et al. The diagnostic utility of p63, CK5/6, CK 7, and CK 20 in distinguishing primary cutaneous adnexal neoplasms from metastatic carcinomas. J Cutan Pathol 2004; 31(2):145–52.

101. Pardal J, Sundram U, Selim MA, et al. GATA3 and MYB expression in cutaneous adnexal neoplasms. Am J Dermatopathol 2017;39(4):279–86.

102. Mahalingam M, Nguyen LP, Richards JE, et al. The diagnostic utility of immunohistochemistry in distinguishing primary skin adnexal carcinomas from metastatic adenocarcinoma to skin: an immunohistochemical reappraisal using cytokeratin 15, nestin, p63, D2-40, and calretinin. Mod Pathol 2010; 23(5):713–9.

103. Cassarino DS, Su A, Robbins BA, et al. SOX10 immunohistochemistry in sweat ductal/glandular neoplasms. J Cutan Pathol 2017;44(6):544–7.

Molecular Genetics of Sebaceous Neoplasia

Jeffrey P. North, MD[a,b],*

KEYWORDS

- Sebaceous adenoma • Sebaceoma • Sebaceous carcinoma • Muir-Torre syndrome
- Sebaceous hyperplasia

Key points

- Both benign and malignant sebaceous neoplasms harbor multiple mutations in oncogenes and tumor suppressor genes with overlapping genetic profiles.
- Diagnosis of sebaceous tumors relies primarily on histopathologic assessment.
- Sebaceous adenomas typically have defects in DNA mismatch repair (*MLH1*, *MSH2*, *MSH6* mutations), as well as *TP53* and *RAS* mutations.
- Cutaneous sebaceous carcinomas show 3 genetic signature patterns: ultraviolet signature, defective DNA mismatch repair, and paucimutational patterns.
- Ocular sebaceous carcinomas harbor frequent *ZNF750* mutations and are divided into carcinomas with *TP53* and *RB1* mutations and *TP53/RB1* wild-type tumors that are associated with human papilloma virus infection.

ABSTRACT

Sebaceous neoplasia primarily includes sebaceous adenoma, sebaceoma, and sebaceous carcinoma (SC). Sebaceous adenoma, sebaceoma, and a subset of cutaneous SC are frequently associated with defective DNA mismatch repair resulting from mutations in *MLH1*, *MSH2*, or *MSH6*. These tumors can be sporadic or associated with Muir-Torre syndrome. SCs without defective DNA mismatch repair have ultraviolet signature mutation or paucimutational patterns. Ocular SCs have low mutation burdens and frequent mutations in *ZNF750*. Some ocular sebaceous carcinomas have *TP53* and *RB1* mutations similar to cutaneous SC, whereas others lack such mutations and are associated with human papilloma virus infection.

OVERVIEW

Tumors of the sebaceous glands are generally categorized into 3 main types: sebaceous hyperplasia; sebaceous adenoma, including sebaceoma; and sebaceous carcinoma (SC). Sebaceous differentiation can also be seen in a variety of other adnexal neoplasms (eg, basal cell carcinoma with sebaceous differentiation, reticulated acanthoma with sebaceous differentiation), but such tumors are not primary sebaceous neoplasms.

Sebaceous hyperplasia represents nonneoplastic enlargement of sebaceous glands and is typically found in regions of skin with the highest density of sebaceous glands, such as the face and scalp. Clinically, sebaceous hyperplasia presents as 2-mm to 6-mm yellowish, umbilicated papules with a peripheral crown of telangiectatic vessels that can be visualized by dermoscopy. It occurs sporadically in approximately 1% of the

Conflicts of interest: UpToDate author, cutaneous adnexal tumors article.
[a] Dermatopathology, Department of Dermatology, University of California San Francisco, School of Medicine, 1701 Divisadero Street, Room 280, San Francisco, CA 94115, USA; [b] Department of Pathology, University of California San Francisco, School of Medicine, 1701 Divisadero Street, Room 280, San Francisco, CA 94115, USA
* Dermatopathology, Department of Dermatology, University of California San Francisco, School of Medicine, 1701 Divisadero Street, Room 280, San Francisco, CA 94115.
E-mail address: Jeffrey.north@ucsf.edu

Surgical Pathology 14 (2021) 273–284
https://doi.org/10.1016/j.path.2021.03.005

population and in up to 30% of transplant patients on immunosuppressive medicines, particularly those taking cyclosporine.[1,2]

Sebaceous adenomas are benign neoplasms of sebaceous glands that have some overlapping clinical and histopathologic features with sebaceous hyperplasia. Clinically, sebaceous adenomas tend to be larger (5–15 mm) and lack the peripheral crown pattern of blood vessels. They are typically solitary, whereas sebaceous hyperplasia often presents with multiple papules. Early onset and/or multiple sebaceous adenomas are associated with Muir-Torre syndrome, particularly when arising on the trunk or extremities.[3]

SC is divided into ocular and cutaneous/extraocular subtypes. Ocular SC encompasses tumors arising on the conjunctiva and eyelid skin. Clinically, SC presents with progressively enlarging, reddish yellow papules/nodules. Epidemiologic studies for SC show an incidence rate of 0.11 to 0.23 per 100,000 person-years with a median age of 73 years and 90% of cases occurring in white people.[4,5] Age of onset before 50 years and extraocular location are associated with increased risk for development of additional cancers of the colon, pancreas, uterus, and ovaries, reflecting their likely association of SC with Muir-Torre syndrome. Approximately 70% to 90% of SCs occur on the head and neck.[6] Incidence of ocular SC seems to have stabilized in recent years, whereas cutaneous SC continues to increase in incidence.[4] SC has a low tumor-specific mortality, with a 5-year relative survival of 93%.[5]

MICROSCOPIC FEATURES

SEBACEOUS HYPERPLASIA AND SEBACEOUS ADENOMA

Sebaceous hyperplasia is characterized by multiple large sebaceous glands in the superficial dermis with a single peripheral layer of basaloid germinative cells and abrupt transition to mature lipidized sebocytes. Holocrine secretion is evident, and the sebaceous glands connect to a central follicular infundibulum (**Fig. 1**). Sebaceous adenomas also feature large lobules of predominantly mature lipidized sebocytes in the upper dermis, but show more disorganized maturation from the peripheral germinative cells to the inner lipidized sebocytes, including increasing thickness of the peripheral germinative cell layer greater than 2 cells. Sebaceous lobules in sebaceous adenoma also frequently connect directly to the epidermis rather than the normal connection to follicular infundibula seen in sebaceous hyperplasia and normal sebaceous glands (**Fig. 2**).

SEBACEOMA

Sebaceoma is a variant of sebaceous adenoma in which more than 50% of the neoplastic cells have basaloid germinative morphology (**Fig. 3**). Sebaceomas are often located deeper in the reticular dermis, although epidermal connection may be present. Mature lipidized sebocytes are present in more haphazard fashion, with single cells and small clusters of them scattered in the tumor. In some sebaceomas, lipidized sebocytes are only focally apparent, making it difficult to identify sebaceous lineage of the neoplasm without careful scrutiny of the entire neoplasm. Sebaceous ductal differentiation with the characteristic eosinophilic cuticular lining is often visible and can be a clue to the diagnosis in cases with few mature sebocytes. Mitotic figures are common in both sebaceous adenoma and sebaceoma, but atypical mitoses and significant cytologic atypia are absent.

Sebaceous adenomas and sebaceomas have well-circumscribed tumor architecture. Some sebaceomas show a palisaded architecture (ripple pattern sebaceoma), carcinoid-like pattern, labyrinthine/sinusoidal pattern, or petaloid pattern (see **Fig. 3C, D**).[7] These organoid patterns seem to have a low association with Muir-Torre syndrome, whereas cystic change within sebaceous neoplasms is highly associated with Muir-Torre syndrome and abnormality in DNA mismatch repair (MMR).[8]

SEBACEOUS CARCINOMA

SCs show malignant histopathologic features, including large size, asymmetry, irregular circumscription, high mitotic activity, nuclear crowding, and pleomorphism (**Figs. 4–6**). SC may have an intraepidermal component showing clusters and single atypical cells with pale/clear cytoplasm in the epidermis with pagetoid appearance (see **Fig. 5**). The invasive component of SC can vary from circumscribed basaloid tumor aggregates with scattered lipidized sebocytes to infiltrative clusters of more squamotized epithelial cells with pale cytoplasm. Adipophilin staining is sometimes required to confirm sebocytic lineage (see **Figs. 5–6**).

MOLECULAR PATHOLOGY FEATURES

MUIR-TORRE SYNDROME

Muir-Torre syndrome is an autosomal dominant cancer syndrome characterized by multiple tumors of the gastrointestinal tract, urogenital tract, and skin, including sebaceous tumors and

Fig. 1. Sebaceous hyperplasia. Multiple large sebaceous glands connect to central dilated follicular infundibula (*A*). The sebaceous glands in sebaceous hyperplasia show normal organization with a thin rim of basaloid germinative cells and ordered cytoplasmic lipidization culminating in holocrine secretion into the sebaceous duct (*B*). ([*A*] hematoxylin-eosin [H&E], original magnification ×20; [*B*] H&E, original magnification ×200 [*B*]).

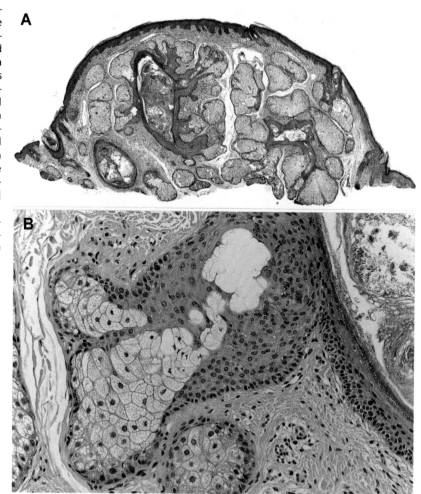

keratoacanthomas. It is a phenotypic variant of Lynch syndrome (hereditary nonpolyposis colon cancer syndrome). Early insights into the molecular features of sebaceous neoplasia came from the association of both benign and malignant sebaceous tumors with Muir-Torre syndrome.[9] Although mutations in 4 genes (*MLH1*, *MSH2*, *MSH6*, *PMS2*) encoding critical components for repair of DNA base pair mismatches cause Lynch syndrome, almost all patients with Muir-Torre syndrome harbor *MSH2* mutations (70%–90%), with *MLH1* mutation occurring in approximately 10% to 20%.[10–12] Mutations in *MSH6* also occur in a minority of patients with Muir-Torre, but study data range widely on the relative percentage.[13] An approximation of 10% seems reasonable.[14] In patients with germline mutations, tumors arise when the remaining wild-type allele of the affected MMR gene (*MLH1*, *MSH2*, *MSH6*) is lost through additional somatic mutation, loss of heterozygosity, or epigenetic silencing. Although *PMS2* mutations cause Lynch syndrome, they do not seem to be a significant cause of the Muir-Torre subtype that includes sebaceous tumors.

Muir-Torre Syndrome, Types 1 and 2

Approximately one-third of patients with Muir-Torre do not have detectable microsatellite instability (MSI), which has led to a proposed classification of 2 types of Muir-Torre syndrome.[15] Type 1 is the classic pattern with autosomal dominant inheritance and MSI. Patients with Muir-Torre type 2 lack MSI, show more variable genetic penetrance, and have later-onset tumors compared with patients with Muir-Torre type 1.

Mut Y Homolog–Associated Polyposis

Some patients showing a Muir-Torre phenotype lack mutations in the 4 MMR genes and do not

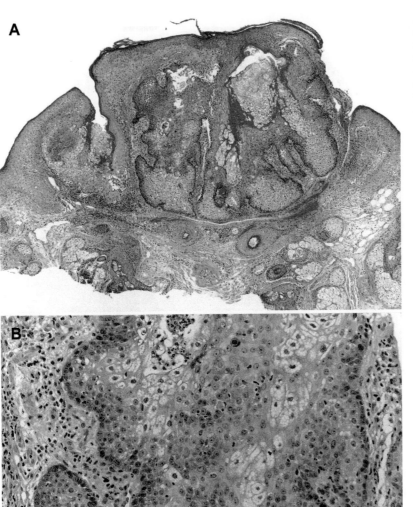

Fig. 2. Sebaceous adenoma. Sebaceous adenomas are well-circumscribed neoplasms in the upper dermis. Sebaceous adenomas frequently connect directly to the epidermis rather than to hair follicles (*A*). The peripheral rim of germinative cells is thicker (>2 cells) than in normal sebaceous glands (*B*). There is less orderly lipidization, but still greater than 50% of cells are mature lipidized sebocytes. ([*A*] H&E, original magnification ×20; [*B*] H&E, original magnification ×200).

show evidence of MSI. *MYH* mutations have been reported in such patients.[16] The diagnosis of Mut Y homolog (MYH)–associated polyposis has been used for these patients, but some investigators group these patients under the Muir-Torre type 2 category. *MYH* mutations should be screened for in patients with suspected Muir-Torre syndrome that have a negative work-up for *MLH1, MSH2,* and *MSH6* mutations, a lack of MSI, and an autosomal recessive familial inheritance pattern.

SEBACEOUS ADENOMA/SEBACEOMA

Besides the well-documented mutations in MMR genes *MSH2, MLH1,* and *MSH6,* limited study data are available for the molecular genetics of sebaceous adenomas. One study of whole-exome sequencing of sebaceous neoplasms included 4 sebaceous adenomas.[17] Three of the adenomas lacked mutations in MMR (MMR) genes, and 1 showed a *MSH2* mutation. The 3 non-MMR tumors had *HRAS* mutations and a mutation burden that was significantly lower than the *MSH2* mutant adenoma (1.2–2.7 vs 14.0 mutations/Mb). Mutations in epidermal growth factor receptor, *MET, RB1,* and *POLE* were detected in the non-MMR adenomas.

An additional study assessing sebaceous neoplasms with a targeted next-generation cancer

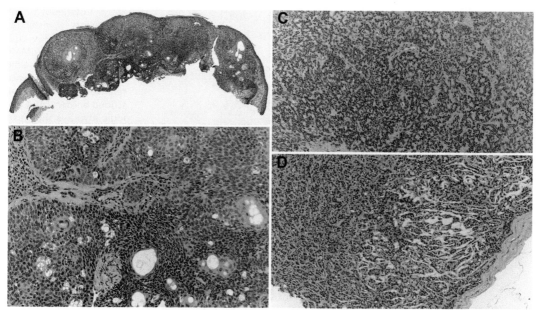

Fig. 3. Sebaceoma. Sebaceomas have well-circumscribed tumor aggregations in the reticular dermis that show a predominance of basaloid germinative cells (*A*). Mature lipidized sebocytes are scattered throughout the tumor with concurrent areas of sebaceous ductal differentiation (*B*). Lipidized sebocytes are inconspicuous in some cases (*C*). A palisaded or ripple pattern can be seen (*C*), as well as a labyrinthine/sinusoidal pattern (*D*) ([*A*] H&E, original magnification ×20; [*B*] H&E, original magnification ×200; [*C*, *D*] H&E, original magnification ×100).

sequencing panel assessed 9 sebaceous adenomas and 7 sebaceomas.[18] *RAS* mutations were also found in this investigation (*HRAS* and *KRAS* in 2 out of 9 sebaceous adenomas and sebaceomas each, and in 2 out of 7 and 3 out of 7 sebaceomas respectively). *TP53* mutations were the most common finding (7 out of 9 sebaceous adenomas, 4 out of 7 sebaceomas), followed by *CDKN2A* mutations. *EGFR* and *CTNNB1* mutations were identified in 5 out of 9 and 6 out of 9 sebaceous adenomas respectively, and in 2 out of 7 sebaceomas each. Two sebaceous adenomas without *CTNNB1* mutation had mutations in the *APC* gene, suggesting the Wnt signaling pathway is important in the development of sebaceous neoplasms.

CUTANEOUS/EXTRAOCULAR SEBACEOUS CARCINOMA

Similar to sebaceous adenomas/sebaceomas, *TP53* mutations occur commonly in all types of cutaneous SC.[18,19] *NOTCH1/2* and *FAT3* mutations are also frequent in cutaneous SCs.[19] These 3 genes encode important tumor suppressors and are mutated frequently in multiple cancer types, including squamous cell carcinoma.[20] Recent genomic profiling of SC with exome sequencing reveals that 3 distinct genetic patterns occur among SCs, including tumors with ultraviolet (UV)

signature mutation profiles, MSI/MMR profiles, and paucimutational profiles (**Table 1**).[19]

Sebaceous Carcinoma, Mismatch Repair, or Microsatellite Instability Pattern

MMR/MSI pattern SCs show high numbers of DNA insertion/deletion mutations (indels) that are characteristic of neoplasms with impaired DNA MMR. These SCs typically have mutations in MLH1, MSH2, or MSH6, and may be related to Muir-Torre syndrome or may be sporadic. The inability to repair DNA mismatches leads to replicative errors in areas of repetitive DNA sequences (MSI), which is characteristic of this SC type. *HRAS* and *KRAS* mutations are also common in MMR/MSI SCs, as are *RREB1* and *KMT2D* mutations.[19] These SCs are found more frequently on the trunk and proximal extremities than other SC types. Histopathologically they tend to be well or moderately differentiated and have circumscribed collections of tumor cells (see **Fig. 4**).

Sebaceous Carcinoma, Ultraviolet Signature Pattern

As expected, UV signature SCs are found in areas of chronic sun exposure such as the face and occur at a later age than the other types of SC (mean age, 83 years).[19] This group shows the greatest mutation burden of all SC types (15–586

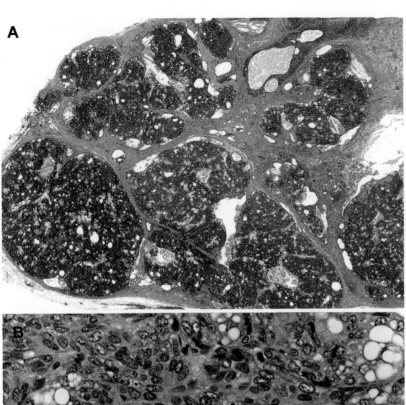

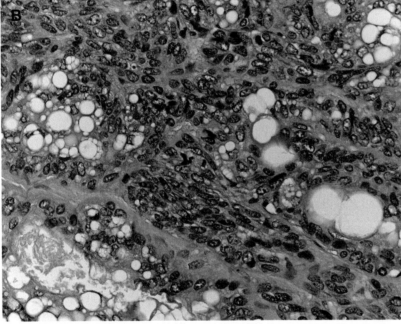

Fig. 4. Cutaneous SC, microsatellite instability (MSI) pattern. SCs with impaired DNA MMR (MSI type) show basaloid tumor aggregates with relatively smooth/circumscribed borders (*A*). Cytologic atypia is shown by increased nuclear size with pleomorphism, and scattered mitotic figures are present (*B*) ([*A*] H&E, original magnification ×20; [*B*] H&E, original magnification ×200).

mutations/Mb) with a predominance of somatic single nucleotide variant mutations and high levels of pyrimidine dimer-type mutations. In contrast with other cutaneous SC types, *RAS* mutations are uncommon in UV signature SCs. RNA sequencing shows transcriptome similarities between UV signature SCs and cutaneous squamous cell and basal cell carcinomas, whereas MMR/MSI SCs have distinct transcription profiles.[19] Histopathologically, UV signature SCs seem to be more poorly differentiated than other SC types and have more infiltrative tumor architecture (see **Fig. 5**). Squamous differentiation can be seen in UV signature SCs.

Sebaceous Carcinoma, Paucimutational Pattern

As opposed to UV and MSI SCs, which have high tumor mutation burdens, there is a group of SCs with low tumor mutation burden (1–5 mutations/Mb). This paucimutational SC group is found

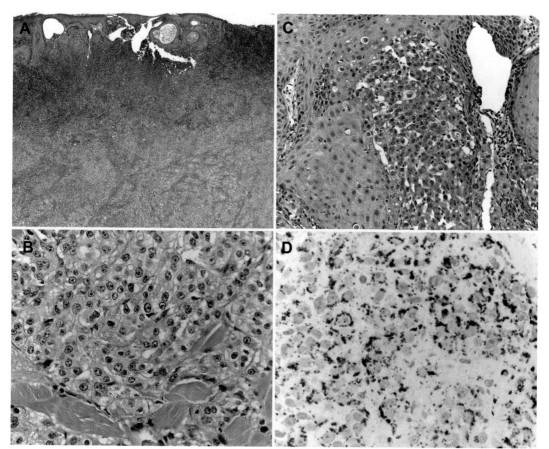

Fig. 5. Cutaneous SC, ultraviolet (UV) pattern. SCs with UV signature patterns tend to have more infiltrative (*A*) and poorly differentiated (*B*) histopathologic features. They may also show an intraepidermal component with pagetoid features (*C*). A vesicular pattern of adipophilin staining helps confirm sebocytic differentiation (*D*) ([*A*] H&E, original magnification ×20; [*B*, *C*] H&E, original magnification ×400; [*D*] adipophilin, original magnification ×400).

primarily on the face and includes both cutaneous and ocular SCs. The cutaneous paucimutational SCs lack distinct mutational profiles, whereas ocular SCs have frequent *ZNF750* and *TP53* mutations[19] and are discussed in greater detail below.

OCULAR SEBACEOUS CARCINOMA

As more molecular data has become available for SC, it is clear that cutaneous and ocular SCs are genetically distinct. Ocular SCs lack mutations in DNA MMR genes and MSI and are thus not associated with Muir-Torre syndrome. Histopathologically, ocular SC can show features of both MSI and UV pattern cutaneous SC with basaloid tumor aggregates and infiltrative architecture (see **Fig. 6**). An initial sequencing study of 27 SCs (23 ocular, 4 cutaneous) with a 409-gene panel found *TP53* and *RB1* mutations are common in ocular SC (66% and 48% of SCs respectively).[21] Mutations affecting the phosphatidylinositol-4,5-

bisphosphate 3-kinase (PI3K) signaling pathway (eg, *PIK3CA* and *PTEN* mutations) were also frequent. *HER2* gene amplifications have been reported in 2 studies of ocular SC, with 1 showing 7% of tumors with *HER2* amplification and the other with 57% showing *HER2* amplification.[22,23]

Further study of ocular SC with whole-exome analysis of 9 ocular and 23 cutaneous SCs found ZNF750 mutations to be the most common mutation in ocular SC (8 out of 9), whereas only 4 out of 23 cutaneous SCs had ZNF750 mutations.[19] A subsequent sequencing study of 53 ocular SCs from Chinese patients also found a high percentage of *ZNF750* mutations (73%), as well as frequent *TP53* (85%), and *RB1* (37%) mutations.[24] A study of ZNF750 immunohistochemical staining in benign and malignant sebaceous tumors found complete loss of ZNF750 expression in a subset of ocular SC (4 out of 11), but retained expression in all other sebaceous tumors.[25] Complete loss was

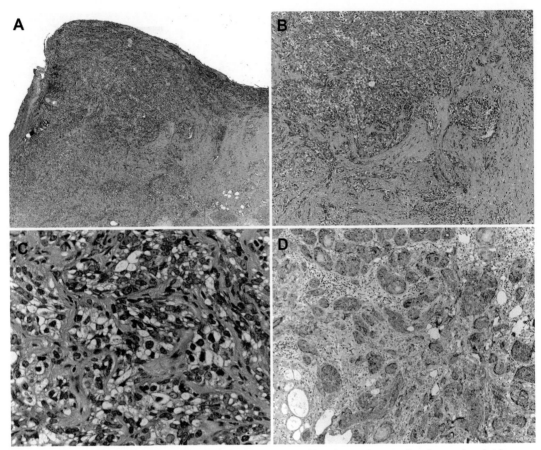

Fig. 6. Ocular SC. Ocular SCs tend to have low tumor mutational burden and most often have a basaloid appearance (*A*). They can have both rounded and infiltrative tumor aggregates (*B*). Basaloid germinative sebocytes mix haphazardly with lipidized sebocytes (*C*). Adipophilin staining highlights the sebocytic differentiation (*D*). ([*A*] H&E stain, original magnification ×20; [*B*] original magnification ×100; [*C*] 400; [*D*] adipophilin, original magnification ×100).

found in both ocular SCs with *ZNF750* mutations and in cases without them, indicating that ZNF750 may be lost through mutations or other mechanisms such as epigenetic silencing.

These mutations were further confirmed in an additional exome sequencing study of 31 ocular SCs with frequent *ZNF750* (42%), *TP53* (71%), and *RB1* (39%) mutations.[26] In addition, mutations in *NOTCH1* and *PCDH15* were detected in 26% and 16% respectively in this cohort. *PCDH15* mutations were highly associated with metastasis. Specifically, *PCDH15* mutations were found in 50% (4 out of 8) of metastatic SCs, whereas only 4% (1 out of 23) of SCs without evidence of metastasis had a *PCDH15* mutation.

Human Papilloma Virus and Ocular Sebaceous Carcinoma

Studies assessing involvement of human papilloma virus (HPV) in SC have yielded disparate

Table 1
Recurring mutations in cutaneous sebaceous carcinoma by mutation signature type

MMR Defective	UV Signature	Paucimutational
MSH2 (most), MLH1, MSH6	*TP53*	*HRAS*
HRAS, KRAS	RREB1	*NOTCH1*
TP53, RB1	*NOTCH1/2*	—
RREB1	*FAT3*	—
NOTCH1/2	KMT2D	—
FAT3	—	—
KMT2D	—	—

findings. Some have not found evidence of HPV infection,[22,27,28] whereas others report high percentages of detectable HPV infection by in situ hybridization in up to 62% of cases.[29] A high percentage of ocular SCs have *TP53* and/or *RB1* mutations, indicating the importance of these tumor suppressors in SC. To determine whether HPV infection may be responsible for inactivation of these tumor suppressor proteins in *TP53/RB1* wild-type SCs, Tetzlaff and colleagues[30] used a combination of whole-transcriptome sequencing and RNA in situ hybridization and found high-risk HPV infection in 44% (4 out of 9) of wild-type *TP53/RB1* cases. HPV infection was not found in any tumors with *TP53* and/or *RB1* mutations. They proposed 2 types of ocular SC based on *TP53/RB1* mutation and HPV status. Type 1 tumors have *TP53* and/or *RB1* mutations and occur in older patients. When mutations in both *RB1* and *TP53* were present, the SCs were more prone to aggressive behavior such as local recurrence. Type 2 patients are younger and lack *TP53* or *RB1* mutations, but have high-risk HPV infection in which viral E6 and E7 proteins disable p53 and Rb tumor suppressor functions. Similar results with HPV infection detected in only wild-type TP53/RB1 SCs were found in a later study by the same group.[26]

DIAGNOSIS

The diagnosis of sebaceous tumors relies predominantly on tumor characteristics visualized by routine hematoxylin-eosin (H&E)–stained sections (discussed earlier, and see **Figs. 1–6**). Immunostaining with adipophilin, epithelial membrane antigen, and factor13A can help confirm the sebocytic lineage of a tumor.

SEBACEOUS NEOPLASMS WITH AMBIGUOUS HISTOPATHOLOGY

Although many sebaceous adenomas and SCs have clearly benign or malignant histopathologic features, there is a subset of intermediate neoplasms in which there is marked interobserver variability in the diagnosis of sebaceous adenoma versus SC.[31] These neoplasms have circumscribed architecture but atypical cytologic features with nuclear crowding and pleomorphism, as well as brisk mitotic activity. Terminology such as SC in situ has been proposed for such tumors.[32] Because mutations in *TP53* and *CDKN2A* have been detected in both sebaceous adenomas and SCs, it is not surprising that immunostains for p53, p16, and bcl-2 have minimal benefit in this differential diagnosis.[18] Mitotic rate does show

some discriminatory power, but, given significant overlap between benign and malignant sebaceous neoplasms, mitotic rate is not completely reliable in such cases. Although there is high variability in the diagnosis of these tumors, available clinical follow-up data for such lesions in the skin suggest they are low-risk neoplasms.[18,33]

IMMUNOHISTOCHEMICAL STAINING FOR THE DIAGNOSIS OF MUIR-TORRE SYNDROME

Immunoperoxidase stains for MLH1, MSH2, MSH6, and PMS2 are widely available to assess for loss of MMR protein expression. There are numerous publications on the topic of use of immunostaining in sebaceous tumors to assist in the diagnosis of Muir-Torre syndrome, some of which report positive predictive values as high as 100%.[15] Such studies have led to widespread adoption of this technique. However, given the frequent loss of MMR proteins in spontaneous sebaceous tumors, immunostaining as a screening tool is prone to a high number of false-positive tests, up to 56% in 1 study with a specificity of only 48%.[14]

The appropriate use committee of the American Society of Dermatopathology indicated that immunostaining to screen for Muir-Torre syndrome is typically unnecessary in patients more than 60 years of age with a periocular SC or single sebaceous neoplasm on the head/neck region.[34] Patients with any of the following are more likely to associated with Muir-Torre syndrome, and immunostaining could be considered appropriate:

- Age less than 60 years with a sebaceous neoplasm
- Multiple sebaceous neoplasms and/or keratoacanthomas
- Cystic sebaceous neoplasm
- Sebaceous neoplasm on the trunk or extremities
- Sebaceous neoplasm in a patient with a history of another Muir-Torre–related malignancy

MMR proteins form dimers to perform their function in DNA repair. MSH2 dimerizes with and stabilizes MSH6. When MSH2 is lost, expression of both MSH2 and MSH6 is typically lost. Similarly, MLH1 dimerizes with PMS2. Given these dimer relationships, a 2-stain antibody screen for MSH2 and MLH1 is a more cost-effective tool than the 4-antibody panel approach. Given the low sensitivity and specificity of immunostaining for Muir-Torre syndrome, such testing should only serve as a diagnostic adjunct in the work-up of this disease. The use of risk-factor assessments such as the Mayo Muir-Torre syndrome risk score algorithm, which incorporates personal and family history of malignancy and sebaceous neoplasms, can better help estimate the likelihood of Muir-Torre syndrome.[14]

SUMMARY

The diagnosis of sebaceous tumors relies fundamentally on architectural and cytologic assessment with routine H&E and immunoperoxidase stains. A subset of well-circumscribed sebaceous neoplasms show overlapping features of sebaceous adenoma and SC and generate significant variability in their diagnoses. In the past 5 years, multiple studies have helped unravel the complexity of the genetic landscape of sebaceous neoplasia. However, given wide-ranging mutation burdens and overlapping mutational profiles in both benign and malignant sebaceous neoplasms, current genetic assessments cannot reliably distinguish between sebaceous adenomas and SCs. However, they do provide valuable insights into the pathology and potential treatments of these tumors. Genetically, sebaceous neoplasms are divided into 3 main groups:

- Sebaceous adenomas, including sebaceoma, and SCs with defects in DNA MMR
  - Mutations in *MLH1*, *MSH2*, or *MSH6* and potential Muir-Torre association
  - Frequent *HRAS*, *KRAS*, *TP53*, *RREB1*, and *KMT2D* mutations
  - *MYH* mutations in cases that lack MSI
  - Occur more frequently on the trunk/extremities than other SC types, particularly in patients with Muir-Torre
- SCs with UV signature mutation profiles
  - Older patients in areas of chronic sun exposure on head/neck
  - Highest mutational burden of all SCs with predominance of UV signature mutations
  - Histopathologically more likely to be poorly differentiated and infiltrative and can display squamous differentiation
  - Frequent *TP53*, *NOTCH1/2*, *FAT3*, *RREB1*, and *KMT2D* mutations
  - Expression profile resembling cutaneous squamous cell and basal cell carcinomas
- SCs with low mutation burden, including both cutaneous and ocular SCs
  - Cutaneous SC with low mutation rates occur on the head/neck and lack recurrent mutation profiles
  - Ocular SCs are within the low-mutation pattern, have frequent *ZNF750* mutations, and can be further subdivided into 2 types

- *TP53/RB1* wild-type tumors associated with HPV infection
- SCs with *TP53* and/or *RB1* mutations that are not associated with HPV infection
  - Older patients with higher likelihood of recurrence
- *PCDH15* mutations associated with metastasis

CLINICS CARE POINTS

- Sebaceous tumors with a predominance of germinative cells, such as sebaceoma, can mimic other basaloid adnexal neoplasms (eg, spiradenoma, basal cell carcinoma). Recognition of subtle solitary lipidized sebocytes and sebaceous ductal differentiation, as well as immunostaining with adipophilin facilitates correct diagnosis.

- Mitotic activity is common in benign sebaceous neoplasms. A diagnosis of SC requires cytologic atypia, infiltrative growth, and/or large tumor size.

- SC can be divided into cutaneous and ocular variants. Ocular SC is not associated with Muir-Torre syndrome.

- Molecular testing can characterize different pathways of sebaceous neoplasia (paucimutational, UV signature, and MMR defect types), but has limited ability to distinguish adenomas from carcinomas.

- HPV-associated ocular SCs lack *TP53* and *RB1* mutations and have lower likelihood for recurrence.

REFERENCES

1. de Berker DA, Taylor AE, Quinn AG, et al. Sebaceous hyperplasia in organ transplant recipients: shared aspects of hyperplastic and dysplastic processes? J Am Acad Dermatol 1996;35(5 Pt 1):696–9.
2. Salim A, Reece SM, Smith AG, et al. Sebaceous hyperplasia and skin cancer in patients undergoing renal transplant. J Am Acad Dermatol 2006;55(5):878–81.
3. Bhaijee F, Brown AS. Muir-Torre syndrome. Arch Pathol Lab Med 2014;138(12):1685–9.
4. Dores GM, Curtis RE, Toro JR, et al. Incidence of cutaneous sebaceous carcinoma and risk of associated neoplasms. Cancer 2008;113(12):3372–81.

5. Tripathi R, Chen Z, Li L, et al. Incidence and survival of sebaceous carcinoma in the United States. J Am Acad Dermatol 2016;75(6):1210–5.

6. Wu A, Rajak SN, Chiang C-J, et al. Epidemiology of cutaneous sebaceous carcinoma. Australas J Dermatol 2020. https://doi.org/10.1111/ajd.13387.

7. Wiedemeyer K, Kyrpychova L, Isikci ÖT, et al. Sebaceous neoplasms with rippled, Labyrinthine/Sinusoidal, petaloid, and carcinoid-like patterns: a study of 57 cases validating their occurrence as a morphological spectrum and showing no significant association with muir–torre syndrome or DNA mismatch repair protein deficiency. Am J Dermatopathol 2018;40(7):479–85.

8. Rütten A, Burgdorf W, Hügel H, et al. Cystic sebaceous tumors as marker lesions for the Muir-Torre syndrome: a histopathologic and molecular genetic study. Am J Dermatopathol 1999;21(5):405–13.

9. Lee BA, Yu L, Ma L, et al. Sebaceous neoplasms with mismatch repair protein expressions and the frequency of co-existing visceral tumors. J Am Acad Dermatol 2012;67(6):1228–34.

10. Kruse R, Rütten A, Lamberti C, et al. Muir-Torre phenotype has a frequency of DNA mismatch-repair-gene mutations similar to that in hereditary nonpolyposis colorectal cancer families defined by the Amsterdam criteria. Am J Hum Genet 1998; 63(1):63–70.

11. Mangold E, Pagenstecher C, Leister M, et al. A genotype-phenotype correlation in HNPCC: strong predominance of msh2 mutations in 41 patients with Muir-Torre syndrome. J Med Genet 2004;41(7):567–72.

12. Jessup CJ, Redston M, Tilton E, et al. Importance of universal mismatch repair protein immunohistochemistry in patients with sebaceous neoplasia as an initial screening tool for Muir-Torre syndrome. Hum Pathol 2016;49:1–9.

13. Mahalingam M. MSH6, past and present and Muir–Torre Syndrome—Connecting the Dots. Am J Dermatopathology 2017;39(4):239–49.

14. Roberts ME, Riegert-Johnson DL, Thomas BC, et al. A clinical scoring system to identify patients with sebaceous neoplasms at risk for the Muir–Torre variant of Lynch syndrome. Genet Med 2014;16(9): 711–6.

15. John AM, Schwartz RA. Muir-Torre syndrome (MTS): an update and approach to diagnosis and management. J Am Acad Dermatol 2016;74(3):558–66.

16. Ponti G, Leon MP de, Maffei S, et al. Attenuated familial adenomatous polyposis and Muir–Torre syndrome linked to compound biallelic constitutional MYH gene mutations. Clin Genet 2005;68(5):442–7.

17. Georgeson P, Walsh MD, Clendenning M, et al. Tumor mutational signatures in sebaceous skin lesions from individuals with Lynch syndrome. Mol Genet Genomic Med 2019;7(7):e00781.

18. Harvey NT, Tabone T, Erber W, et al. Circumscribed sebaceous neoplasms: a morphological, immunohistochemical and molecular analysis. Pathology 2016;48(5):454–62.

19. North JP, Golovato J, Vaske CJ, et al. Cell of origin and mutation pattern define three clinically distinct classes of sebaceous carcinoma. Nat Commun 2018;9(1):1894.

20. Sato K, Komune N, Hongo T, et al. Genetic landscape of external auditory canal squamous cell carcinoma. Cancer Sci 2020. https://doi.org/10.1111/cas.14515.

21. Tetzlaff MT, Singh RR, Seviour EG, et al. Next-generation sequencing identifies high frequency of mutations in potentially clinically actionable genes in sebaceous carcinoma. J Pathol 2016;240(1):84–95.

22. Kwon MJ, Shin HS, Nam ES, et al. Comparison of HER2 gene amplification and KRAS alteration in eyelid sebaceous carcinomas with that in other eyelid tumors. Pathol Res Pract 2015;211(5):349–55.

23. Na HY, Choe J-Y, Shin SA, et al. Proposal of a provisional classification of sebaceous carcinoma based on hormone receptor expression and HER2 Status. Am J Surg Pathol 2016;40(12):1622–30.

24. Bao Y, Selfridge JE, Wang J, et al. Mutations in TP53, ZNF750, and RB1 typify ocular sebaceous carcinoma. J Genet Genomics 2019;46(6):315–8.

25. North JP, Solomon DA, Golovato J, et al. Loss of ZNF750 in ocular and cutaneous sebaceous carcinoma. J Cutan Pathol 2019;46(10):736–41.

26. Xu S, Moss TJ, Laura Rubin M, et al. Whole-exome sequencing for ocular adnexal sebaceous carcinoma suggests PCDH15 as a novel mutation associated with metastasis. Mod Pathol 2020;33(7): 1256–63.

27. Gonzalez-Fernandez F, Kaltreider SA, Patnaik BD, et al. Sebaceous carcinoma. Tumor progression through mutational inactivation of p53. Ophthalmology 1998;105(3):497–506.

28. Stagner AM, Afrogheh AH, Jakobiec FA, et al. p16 expression is not a surrogate marker for high-risk human papillomavirus infection in periocular Sebaceous Carcinoma. Am J Ophthalmol 2016;170: 168–75.

29. Hayashi N, Furihata M, Ohtsuki Y, et al. Search for accumulation of p53 protein and detection of human papillomavirus genomes in sebaceous gland carcinoma of the eyelid. Virchows Arch 1994;424(5):503–9.

30. Tetzlaff MT, Curry JL, Ning J, et al. Distinct biological types of ocular adnexal sebaceous carcinoma: HPV-driven and virus-negative tumors arise through nonoverlapping molecular-genetic alterations. Clin Cancer Res 2019;25(4):1280–90.

31. Harvey NT, Budgeon CA, Leecy T, et al. Interobserver variability in the diagnosis of circumscribed sebaceous neoplasms of the skin. Pathology 2013;45(6):581–6.

32. Kramer JM, Chen S. Sebaceous carcinoma in situ. Am J Dermatopathol 2010;32(8):854–5.

33. Kazakov DV, Kutzner H, Spagnolo DV, et al. Discordant architectural and cytological features in cutaneous sebaceous neoplasms–a classification dilemma: report of 5 cases. Am J Dermatopathol 2009;31(1):31–6.

34. Task Force/Committee Members, Vidal CI, Sutton A, Armbrect EA, et al. Muir-Torre syndrome appropriate use criteria: effect of patient age on appropriate use scores. J Cutan Pathol 2019;46(7):484–9.

Pigmented Epithelioid Melanocytoma
Morphology and Molecular Drivers

Sarah Benton, BA[a], Jeffrey Zhao, BA[a],
Sepideh Asadbeigi, MD[a], Daniel Kim, BS[a], Bin Zhang, MS[a],
Pedram Gerami, MD[a,b,*]

KEYWORDS

- Pigmented epithelioid melanocytoma • PRKAR1A mutation • PRKCA fusion • Melanocytoma
- Molecular pathology • Epithelioid

Key points

- Advances in molecular diagnostics have allowed for more precise and consistent classification and subclassification of pigmented epithelioid melanocytoma (PEM).
- These tumors typically have a component of epithelioid melanocytes with vesicular nuclei, prominent nucleoli, and heavily pigmented cytoplasm.
- Specific morphologic subtypes of PEM have distinct characteristic molecular findings. Cases with a combined pattern of conventional nevi and larger pigmented epithelioid melanocytes typically have *BRAF* mutations accompanied by mutations in *PRKAR1*. This is the variant of PEM most often seen in patients with Carney complex.
- PEMs with monomorphic epithelioid melanocytes with sheetlike growth pattern frequently have *PRKCA* fusion.
- As with Spitz tumors, sentinel lymph node involvement from PEMs is common but distant metastasis or death of disease is extremely rare.

ABSTRACT

Pigmented epithelioid melanocytoma (PEM) was originally described based on keen morphologic analysis identifying a group of melanocytic tumors sharing heavily pigmented epithelioid melanocytes. It is defined as heavily pigmented epithelioid, spindled, and dendritic melanocytes with characteristic vesicular nuclei, prominent nucleoli, and melanophages. PEM often involves regional lymph nodes. Recent advances in molecular analysis have allowed for subclassification of PEM into more specific subsets of melanocytic tumors. The most common subsets include *PRKCA* fusions, which result in pure PEMs with sheets of monomorphic epithelioid melanocytes, and PEMs with combined pattern and mutations in both *PRKAR1A* and *BRAF*.

OVERVIEW

In 2004, Zembowicz and colleagues[1] described a new category of melanocytic neoplasm that they referred to as pigmented epithelioid melanocytoma (PEM). In their seminal paper, the

---

Authors S. Benton and J. Zhao contributed equally to this article.

[a] Department of Dermatology, Feinberg School of Medicine, Northwestern University, 676 North St Clair Street, Suite 1765, Chicago, IL 60611, USA; [b] Robert H. Lurie Cancer Center, Feinberg School of Medicine, Northwestern University, 676 North St Clair Street, Suite 1765, Chicago, IL 60611, USA
* Corresponding author. Department of Dermatology, Feinberg School of Medicine, Northwestern University, 676 North St Clair Street, Suite 1765, Chicago, IL 60611.
E-mail address: pedram.gerami@nm.org

Surgical Pathology 14 (2021) 285–292
https://doi.org/10.1016/j.path.2021.01.004
1875-9181/21/© 2021 Elsevier Inc. All rights reserved.

surgpath.theclinics.com

investigators describe recognizing this distinct subgroup of melanocytic tumors during the course of a study of borderline melanocytic tumors.[1] It was noted that the tumors had significant morphologic overlap with animal-type melanoma and the epithelioid blue nevus (EBN) of Carney complex (CC).[2–6] Characteristic clinical behavior included involvement of sentinel lymph nodes in 40% to 50% of cases with only rare reported cases resulting in distant metastasis. In the past 10 years, the capability for genomic analysis of melanocytic tumors has greatly expanded.[7–12] Genomic analysis now reveals that these tumors identified by keen morphologic analysis can be further subdivided into several distinct genomic subtypes.[7,13,14] In this review, we discuss recent revelations regarding the genomics of PEM and how the genomics delineates the specific morphologic patterns.

GROSS FEATURES

Early studies on PEM describe a tendency for younger populations with a median age of 20 to 27 years and some cases occurring in infants and children.[1,15] Lesions may occur in a wide body distribution, including the head and neck region and the trunk, but the extremities are most frequently involved.[15] Compared with melanoma, there is less frequent predilection for fair-skinned individuals with lesions occurring in all Fitzpatrick subtypes. Clinically, the lesions are blue to blue-black papules or nodules.[16] Ulceration is not uncommon, as it was described in 7 of 41 cases in the original study describing them.[1]

MICROSCOPIC FEATURES

There is a spectrum of possible morphologic features in PEM. Characteristic features include the presence of epithelioid or mixed epithelioid and spindle-shaped melanocytes with vesicular nuclei and heavily pigmented cytoplasm.[17] Typically, many accompanying melanophages are also seen. PEM can be a pure lesion (pure PEM) or associated with a more conventional nevus component (combined PEM).[18] Pure lesions most frequently are entirely confined to the dermis and have a sheetlike proliferation of monomorphic-appearing epithelioid melanocytes with vesicular nuclei and pigmented cytoplasm. In the periphery, there may be some spindle and dendritic melanocytes and many melanophages. Less frequently, a pure PEM may have mostly spindle cytology. These lesions are typically compound symmetric lesions having surmounting epidermal hyperplasia. Nests of monomorphic, heavily pigmented spindle-shaped melanocytes

can be seen in the epidermis and dermis with many associated melanophages. The nests can have some expansile features but typically lack the solid sheetlike appearance seen in the purer epithelioid cases.

In combined PEM, the lesion may be compound or dermal. If there is a junctional component, it usually consists of the more conventional nevus component. The dermal component may have a plexiform arrangement with distinct nests often consisting of intermixed aggregates of conventional nevus cells near aggregates of larger pigmented melanocytes which may vary from epithelioid to oval or spindle in shape. Melanophages are also frequently interspersed between and around nests. This subtype shares many common features with deep penetrating nevus such as combined pattern, plexiform arrangement of nests, and frequent aggregation of nests around the adnexa and neurovascular structures. Combined cases typically occur with conventional acquired nevi, but rare cases occurring as a combined lesion within congenital nevi have also been described.

Nuclear atypia can vary from mild to severe. In some cases, large epithelioid cells can be multinucleated and may appear similar to a Reed-Sternberg cell. Mitotic activity of up to 2/mm^2 is not uncommon.[1,19] Ulceration is not infrequent, and in the original study describing PEM was present in 7 of 41 cases.[1]

GENOMIC STUDIES

Advances in genomics have revealed that there are distinct genomic patterns correlating with the various morphologic patterns that have been observed. Two studies to date have assessed larger series of PEM cases with next generation sequencing (NGS) looking at both DNA and mRNA sequencing (**Table 1**). In these 2 series by Cohen and colleagues[20] and Isales and colleagues[19] consisting of 13 and 16 cases, respectively, the most common aberrations identified included mutations in *PRKAR1A* in association with mutations in *BRAF*, *PRKCA* fusions, *MAP2K1* in-frame deletions, and *GNAQ* mutations. The 2 overall most common aberrations involved either (1) a *PRKAR1A* mutation in association with a *BRAF* mutation or (2) a *PRKCA* fusion. Further, these studies suggest that these 2 most common aberrations correlate with specific morphologic subtypes. Specifically, *PRKCA* fusion PEMs tend to be pure PEMs with monomorphic-appearing sheetlike growth of epithelioid melanocytes in the dermis, as shown in **Fig. 1**. *PRKCA* is adjacent to *PRKAR1A* on the long arm of

Table 1
Summary of pigmented epithelioid melanocytoma (PEM) studies using next generation sequencing with DNA and RNA sequencing

Previous Studies with Both DNA and mRNA Sequencing on PEM Tumors	PRKCA Fusions	PRKAR1A Mutations	MAP2K1 In-Frame Deletions	GNAQ Mutations
Total (n = 30)	8	4	3	3
Isales (n = 16)[19]	5	1	1	1
Cohen (n = 13)[20]	2	3	2	2
Bahrami (n = 1)[43]	1			

chromosome 17.[21] *PRKCA* codes for protein kinase C alpha (PKCα), which is involved in activating tyrosinase in melanosomes to regulate the rate-limiting step in melanin synthesis.[22]

Conversely, PEMs with mutations in *PRKAR1A* and *BRAF* tend to be the combined pattern PEM. These may have nests of conventional nevus cells in the epidermis. The dermis may have both the conventional nevus cells with some larger heavily pigmented epithelioid to oval melanocytes with vesicular nuclei. This is the pattern of PEM that tends to occur in patients with CC, as shown in **Fig. 2** of a patient with suspected CC. A clinical photo of this patient's multiple blue nevi and

epithelioid blue nevi is shown in **Fig. 3**. Because the patients have a germline mutation in *PRKAR1A*, they are prone to developing this subset of combined melanocytic nevus.

Not surprisingly, those cases with *GNAQ* mutations have many common features with conventional blue nevi but with some of the cells having more epithelioid morphology. Too few cases of PEMs with *MAP2K1* in-frame deletion have been described to be able to characterize a specific morphology, but the cases reported thus far were pure PEMs without a conventional nevus component.[19,20] Last, we have observed a unique subtype of melanocytic neoplasm that

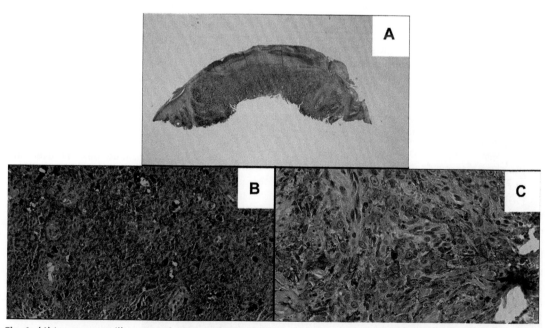

Fig. 1. (*A*) Low-power silhouette of a PRKCA fusion PEM shows a compound melanocytic proliferation with sheet-like growth of pigmented epithelioid melanocytes in a 12-year old child (hematoxylin-eosin [H&E], ×2). (*B*) At medium power, one can see the solid cellular growth of the PEMs with very little intervening stroma (H&E, ×20). (*C*) Higher magnification shows characteristic cytologic features of PEM with cells with large vesicular nuclei, prominent nucleoli, and heavily pigmented cytoplasm (H&E, ×40).

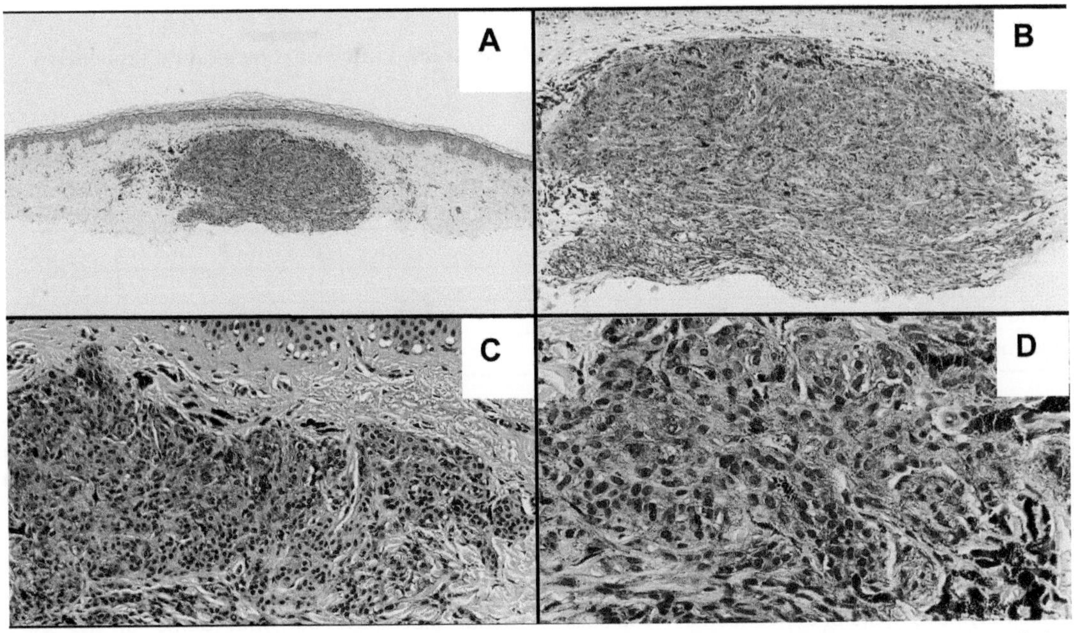

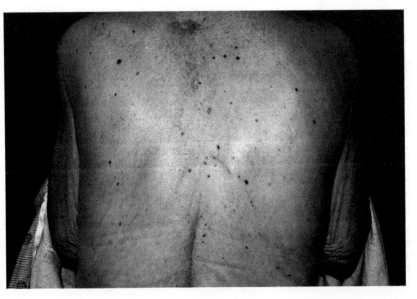

Fig. 2. (*A*) Low-power silhouette shown of a PEM/EBN in a patient with likely CC. This variant of PEM typically has a BRAF mutation followed by a PRKAR1A mutation. Low power shows a heavily pigmented dermal-based melanocytic neoplasm (H&E, ×4). (*B*) The epithelioid melanocytes have pigmented cytoplasm, and there are many surrounding melanophages (H&E, ×10). (*C*) PEMs are present with adjacent aggregates of more conventional nevomelanocytes (H&E, ×20). (*D*) The PEMs are seen in small aggregates separated by melanophages and thin bands of fibrous collagen. The cells lack high-grade nuclear atypia or significant mitotic activity (H&E, ×40).

can be classified as PEM, which has a combination of both genomic fusions characteristic of Spitz, such as *NTRK1* or *MAP3K8*, with a *PRKAR1A* mutation. The *NTRK1* fusion cases with *PRKAR1A* mutation PEMs observed are symmetric with epidermal hyperplasia with a compound proliferation of heavily pigmented spindle-shaped to oval-shaped melanocytes. **Fig. 4** shows a PEM characterized by *NTRK3* fusion and *PRKAR1a* mutation with a predominance of spindle cell morphology, a common finding in *NTRK3* fusions. Some cases from both genomic studies were unable to identify any specific genomic aberrations.

Fig. 3. The clinical image of a patient with suspected CC shows many blue nevi all over and multiple epithelioid blue nevi typical of CC.

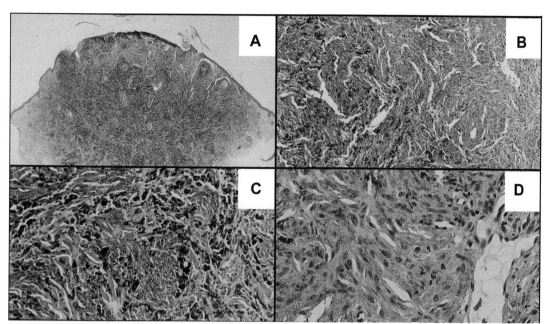

Fig. 4. (*A*) This variant of PEM was characterized by NTRK3 fusion and a PRKAR1A mutation. The section shows a compound, heavily pigmented melanocytic neoplasm with overlying epidermal hyperplasia (H&E, ×2x). (*B*) Unlike other variants of PEM, this lesion has a predominance of spindle cell morphology, a common finding in NTRK3 fusions (H&E, ×10). (*C*) The nests and fascicles of spindle cells are separated by thin fibrous bands of collagen and melanophages (H&E, ×20). (*D*) Higher power morphology shows that although the cells are predominantly spindle in shape, they also have vesicular nuclei, prominent nucleoli, and pigmented cytoplasm (H&E, 40x).

IMMUNOHISTOCHEMISTRY

Immunohistochemical studies may show loss of R1α expression in *PRKAR1A* mutated PEMs as well as some PEM cases with mutations other than *PRKAR1A* (i.e., *MAP2K1*) and cases without identified initiating genetic alteration.[20] Hence, in these latter cases, *PRKAR1A* may be inactivated by a different mechanism, for example, epigenetics or other. *PRKAR1A* encodes for protein kinase A regulatory subunit type 1alpha (R1α), which regulates intracellular cyclic AMP (cAMP) signaling pathways involved in melanocyte proliferation and melanin synthesis. Fusion PEM cases typically do not show loss of R1α expression.

DIFFERENTIAL DIAGNOSIS

The differential diagnosis may include several benign as well as malignant entities.[23–33] Other benign entities with overlapping morphology include conventional *GNAQ* mutation or *CYSLTR2* mutated blue nevi. However, these cases typically have a more prominent conventional dendritic to spindle-shaped blue nevus component with more limited epithelioid component. It is important not to confuse the many accompanying epithelioid-shaped melanophages with EBN cells. Bleaching a slide before immunohistochemistry (IHC) can help more definitively differentiate the melanophages from melanocytes. Deep penetrating nevi may have many overlapping architectural features with the combined pattern PEM because it is also a subset of combined nevus most frequently having a *BRAF* and a *CTNNB1* mutation. However, the larger epithelioid cells in these cases are less heavily melanized. Genetic analysis can easily allow for distinction among these entities.

The most important distinction is differentiating PEM from pigment synthesizing melanoma. Generally, pigment synthesizing melanomas occur in older patients, median age 38, compared with PEM.[34] There is also a greater predilection for sun-exposed sites. Subtle histologic clues might include background solar damage, the presence of an atypical lentiginous or pagetoid junctional component extending laterally in the epidermis far beyond the dermal component, prominent areas of melanocytes with high-grade nuclear atypia, expansile growth, and mitotic activity greater than 2/mm.[2]

Genomic studies have shown that pigment synthesizing melanomas similar to many combined pattern PEMs lack PRKAR1A expression. In a small series of 8 cases studied by NGS, all had genomic alterations in *PRKAR1A* and the 2 in which such mutations were not identified demonstrated loss of heterozygosity of the *PRKAR1A* locus. Four cases also had *hTERT* promoter mutations and *BRAF* mutations were also common. Hence these cases share many genomic features with the combined pattern of PEM, which also has *BRAF* and *PRKAR1A* mutations. Hence, the combined pattern of PEM can exist on a spectrum with pigment synthesizing melanoma. It may be the addition of the *hTERT* promoter mutation in some of these cases which transforms them to malignancy. However, significantly more cases and exploration into this is required for any definitive conclusions. Also importantly, *PRKCA* fusions are exceedingly rare in melanoma. This suggests that this variant of PEM is an extremely stable nevus with exceedingly low risk for malignant transformation.

PROGNOSIS

The original studies of PEM described the presence of involvement of sentinel lymph nodes in 40% to 50% of PEMs. A single case with distant metastatic disease was noted.[1] These cases likely consisted of a diverse genomic background including cases with *PRKAR1A* and *BRAF* mutations, *PRKCA* fusions, and some of the other genomic aberrations described in this article. The data show that similar to Spitz tumors, sentinel node involvement does not predict distant metastatic disease.[15,35–38] Most PEMs are stable melanocytic neoplasms with low risk for transformation, particularly pure PEMs with a *PRKCA* fusion. Combined PEMs with *BRAF* mutations in conjunction with *PRKAR1A* mutations may exist on a spectrum with pigment synthesizing melanomas. Hence in differentiating the combined pattern of PEM from pigment synthesizing melanoma, additional molecular tests, such as fluorescence in situ hybridization (FISH) or comparative genomic hybridization (CGH) to look for chromosomal copy number aberrations, or DNA to look for *hTERT* promoter mutations, may also be of utility. If pigment synthesizing melanoma is excluded, aggressive behavior is unlikely.

EPITHELIOID BLUE NEVUS OF CARNEY COMPLEX

In patients with the combined pattern of PEM, we recommend a thorough clinical history and physical examination to assess for other possible stigmata of CC. If other features are identified, then genetic assessment for a germline mutation in *PRKAR1A*

should be considered.[39] CC is an autosomal dominant syndrome involving multiple neoplasms including endocrine tumors, myxomas, psammomatous melanotic schwannomas, and PEMs/EBN.[40–42] Identification of 2 or more major criteria is an indication for additional one-time screening including possible thyroid ultrasound, testicular ultrasound for males, transabdominal ultrasound in females, and follow-up consultation with a clinical geneticist. Additional surveillance for sequelae including myxomas may be warranted for patients with PEM/EBN suspected to have CC.[41]

SUMMARY

Keen morphologic assessment allowed for the identification of a subset of heavily pigmented melanocytic tumors of atypical cytology with a limited number of distinct genetic aberrations. Genetic studies have shown that there are distinct subtypes of PEM with specific morphologic features. The combined pattern of PEM most commonly has mutations in *BRAF* and *PRKAR1A*. This is the pattern of PEM also referred to as epithelioid blue nevi and seen in patients with CC. For the most part, these are stable nevi. However, these lesions may have some overlapping features with pigment synthesizing melanomas. Many pigment synthesizing melanomas also have *TERT* promoter mutations. In diagnostically challenging cases, FISH or CGH to look for chromosomal copy number aberrations or sequencing to look for *TERT* promoter mutations can be of diagnostic utility. All of these cases may have loss of R1α expression by immunohistochemistry. Pure PEMs with a solid and cellular proliferation of monomorphic pigmented epithelioid cells commonly have a PRKCA fusion. PRKCA fusions are exceedingly rare in melanoma, and PEMs with this aberration are typically benign, stable nevi. This subtype of PEM does not show loss of R1α expression by IHC.

CLINICS CARE POINTS

- Morphologic molecular correlation can allow for subtyping of pigmented epithelioid melanocytomas (PEMs) into more specific subsets of melanocytic tumors.

- Combined PEMs are typically *PRKAR1A*-mutated PEMs and are the subtype of PEM seen in patients with Carney complex (CC). The identification of these lesions may be an indication for further assessment for the possibility of CC.

- *PRKAR1A* mutated PEMs may be part of a spectrum with pigment synthesizing melanomas and may have some shared molecular and morphologic features.

- *PRKCA* fusion PEMs are mostly stable nevi with low risk for malignant transformation and conservative re-excision is typically adequate treatment.

- Both subtypes of PEM may show involvement of sentinel lymph nodes, though as in Spitz tumors, this does not indicate a higher likelihood of distant metastasis.

ACKNOWLEDGEMENT

This study was supported by the IDP Foundation, Inc.

DISCLOSURE

Dr P. Gerami has served as a consultant for Myriad Genomics, DermTech Int., Merck, and Castle Biosciences, and has received honoraria for all. All other authors report no relevant conflicts of interest. This work is original and has not been previously published.

REFERENCES

1. Zembowicz A, Carney JA, Mihm MC. Pigmented epithelioid melanocytoma: a low-grade melanocytic tumor with metastatic potential indistinguishable from animal-type melanoma and epithelioid blue nevus. Am J Surg Pathol 2004;28(1):31–40.

2. Darier J. Le melanome malin mesenchymateux ou melano-sarcome. Bull Assoc Fr Cancer 1925;14: 221–49.

3. Brenn T. Pitfalls in the evaluation of melanocytic lesions. Histopathology 2012;60(5):690–705.

4. Crowson AN, Magro CM, Mihm MC Jr. Malignant melanoma with prominent pigment synthesis: "animal type" melanoma–a clinical and histological study of six cases with a consideration of other melanocytic neoplasms with prominent pigment synthesis. Hum Pathol 1999;30(5):543–50.

5. Howard B, Ragsdale B, Lundquist K. Pigmented epithelioid melanocytoma: two case reports. Dermatol Online J 2005;11(2):1.

6. Levene A. Disseminated dermal melanocytosis terminating in melanoma. A human condition resembling equine melanotic disease. Br J Dermatol 1979;101(2):197–205.

7. Scolyer AR, Thompson FJ, Warnke WK, et al. Pigmented epithelioid melanocytoma. Am J Surg Pathol 2004;28(8):1114–5.

8. Ito K, Mihm MC. Pigmented epithelioid melanocytoma: report of first Japanese cases previously diagnosed as cellular blue nevus. J Cutan Pathol 2009; 36(4):439–43.

9. Blebea C, Li D, Castelo-Soccio L, et al. Generalized congenital epithelioid blue nevi (pigmented epithelioid melanocytomas) in an infant: Report of case and review of the literature. J Cutan Pathol 2019; 46(12):954–9.

10. Wiesner T. Genomic rearrangements in unusual and atypical melanocytic neoplasms. JAMA Dermatol 2016;152(3):260–2.

11. Donati M, Kastnerova L, Cempirkova D, et al. Vulvar pigmented epithelioid melanocytoma with a novel HTT-PKN1 fusion: a case report. Am J Dermatopathol 2020;42(7):544–6.

12. Friedman BJ, Hernandez S, Fidai C, et al. A pediatric case of pigmented epithelioid melanocytoma with chromosomal copy number alterations in 15q and 17q and a novel NTRK3-SCAPER gene fusion. J Cutan Pathol 2020;47(1):70–5.

13. Zembowicz A, Knoepp SM, Bei T, et al. Loss of expression of protein kinase A regulatory subunit 1α in pigmented epithelioid melanocytoma but not in melanoma or other melanocytic lesions. Am J Surg Pathol 2007;31(11):1764–75.

14. Williams EA, Shah N, Danziger N, et al. Clinical, histopathologic, and molecular profiles of PRKAR1A-inactivated melanocytic neoplasms. J Am Acad Dermatol 2020. https://doi.org/10.1016/j.jaad.2020.07.050.

15. Mandal RV, Murali R, Lundquist KF, et al. Pigmented epithelioid melanocytoma: favorable outcome after 5-year follow-up. Am J Surg Pathol 2009;33(12): 1778–82.

16. Moscarella E, Ricci R, Argenziano G, et al. Pigmented epithelioid melanocytoma: clinical, dermoscopic and histopathological features. Br J Dermatol 2016;174(5):1115–7.

17. Zembowicz A, Cohen JN, LeBoit PE. Pigmented epithelioid melanocytoma. In: Busam KJ, Gerami P, Scolyer RA, editors. Pathology of melanocytic tumors. Philadelphia, PA: Elsevier; 2019. p. 124–9.

18. Jurakic Toncic R, Murat Susic S, Curkovic D, et al. Pigmented epithelioid melanocytoma in congenital nevus of medium size in children. Dermatol Pract Concept 2020;10(3):e2020067.

19. Isales MC, Mohan LS, Quan VL, et al. Distinct genomic patterns in pigmented epithelioid melanocytoma. Am J Surg Pathol 2019;43(4):480–8.

20. Cohen JN, Joseph NM, North JP, et al. Genomic analysis of pigmented epithelioid melanocytomas reveals recurrent alterations in PRKAR1A, and PRKCA Genes. Am J Surg Pathol 2017;41(10):1333–40.

21. Zembowicz A, Scolyer RA. Nevus/Melanocytoma/Melanoma: an emerging paradigm for classification of melanocytic neoplasms? Arch Pathol Lab Med 2011;135(3):300–6.

22. Quan VL, Panah E, Zhang B, et al. The role of gene fusions in melanocytic neoplasms. J Cutan Pathol 2019;46(11):878–87.

23. Lim C, Murali R, McCarthy SW, et al. Pigmented epithelioid melanocytoma: a recently described melanocytic tumour of low malignant potential. Pathology 2010;42(3):284–6.

24. Smith KJ, Barrett TL, Skelton HG 3rd, et al. Spindle cell and epithelioid cell nevi with atypia and metastasis (malignant Spitz nevus). Am J Surg Pathol 1989;13(11):931–9.

25. Carney JA, Gordon H, Carpenter PC, et al. The complex of myxomas, spotty pigmentation, and endocrine overactivity. Medicine (Baltimore) 1985;64(4):270–83.

26. Zembowicz A, Phadke PA. Blue nevi and variants: an update. Arch Pathol Lab Med 2011;135(3):327–36.

27. Requena L, de la Cruz A, Moreno C, et al. Animal type melanoma: a report of a case with balloon-cell change and sentinel lymph node metastasis. Am J Dermatopathol 2001;23(4):341–6.

28. Dick W. Melanosis in men and horses. Lancet 1832; 19(479):192.

29. Groben PA, Harvell JD, White WL. Epithelioid blue nevus: neoplasm Sui generis or variation on a theme? Am J Dermatopathol 2000;22(6):473–88.

30. Ferrara G, Zalaudek I, Savarese I, et al. Pediatric atypical spitzoid neoplasms: a review with emphasis on 'red' ('spitz') tumors and 'blue' ('blitz') tumors. Dermatology 2010;220(4):306–10.

31. Goto K, Pissaloux D, Paindavoine S, et al. CYSLTR2-mutant cutaneous melanocytic neoplasms frequently simulate "pigmented epithelioid melanocytoma," expanding the morphologic spectrum of blue tumors. Am J Surg Pathol 2019;43(10):1368–76.

32. Cohen JN, Spies JA, Ross F, et al. Heavily pigmented epithelioid melanoma with loss of protein kinase a regulatory subunit-α Expression. Am J Dermatopathol 2018;40(12):912–6.

33. Motaparthi K, George EV, Guo R. Distant metastasis due to heavily pigmented epithelioid melanoma with underlying BRAF V600E, NOTCH1, ERBB3, and PTEN mutations. J Cutan Pathol 2019;46(8):613–8.

34. Cohen NJ, Yeh WI, Mully ET, et al. Genomic and clinicopathologic characteristics of PRKAR1A-inactivated melanomas: toward genetic distinctions of animal-type melanoma/pigment synthesizing melanoma. Am J Surg Pathol 2020;44(6):805–16.

35. Ward JR, Brady SP, Tada H, et al. Pigmented epithelioid melanocytoma. Int J Dermatol 2006;45(12):1403–5.

36. Vezzoni GM, Martini L, Ricci C. A case of animal-type melanoma (or pigmented epithelioid melanocytoma?): an open prognosis. Dermatol Surg 2008;34(1):105–10.

37. D'Souza P, Barr EK, Thirumala SD, et al. Pigmented epithelioid melanocytoma: a rare lytic bone lesion involving intradural extension and subtotal resection in a 14-month-old girl. J Neurosurg Pediatr 2020;1–4. https://doi.org/10.3171/2020.1.PEDS19359.

38. Bax MJ, Brown MD, Rothberg PG, et al. Pigmented epithelioid melanocytoma (animal-type melanoma): an institutional experience. J Am Acad Dermatol 2017;77(2):328–32.

39. Kirschner LS, Carney JA, Pack SD, et al. Mutations of the gene encoding the protein kinase A type I-alpha regulatory subunit in patients with the Carney complex. Nat Genet 2000;26(1):89–92.

40. Stratakis CA, Carney JA, Lin JP, et al. Carney complex, a familial multiple neoplasia and lentiginosis syndrome. Analysis of 11 kindreds and linkage to the short arm of chromosome 2. J Clin Invest 1996;97(3):699–705.

41. Carney JA, Ferreiro JA. The epithelioid blue nevus. A multicentric familial tumor with important associations, including cardiac myxoma and psammomatous melanotic schwannoma. Am J Surg Pathol 1996;20(3):259–72.

42. O'Grady TC, Barr RJ, Billman G, et al. Epithelioid blue nevus occurring in children with no evidence of Carney complex. Am J Dermatopathol 1999;21(5):483–6.

43. Bahrami A, Lee S, Wu G, et al. Pigment-synthesizing melanocytic neoplasm with protein kinase C Alpha (PRKCA) Fusion. JAMA Dermatol 2016;152(3):318–22.

Mucosal Melanoma
A Review Emphasizing the Molecular Landscape and Implications for Diagnosis and Management

Robert V. Rawson, BCom, MBBS, FRCPA[a,b,c],
James S. Wilmott, BSci, PhD[a,b],
Richard A. Scolyer, BMedSci, MBBS, MD, FRCPA, FRCPath[a,b,c],*

KEYWORDS

• Mucosal melanoma • Molecular • Mutations

Key points

- Mucosal melanomas are rare aggressive tumors with distinct biological, clinical, and histopathologic features with important treatment implications.

- They most frequently occur in the head and neck, vulvovaginal, and anorectal locations.

- Recent whole-exome sequencing and whole-genome sequencing have clarified the molecular landscape of these tumors and indicate that mucosal melanomas show considerable heterogeneity based on their mutation profile, mutation signatures, and chromosomal structural rearrangements.

- Site-specific, genetic, and geographic location factors appear to play a role in the pathogenesis of mucosal melanomas.

- Most mucosal melanomas harbor well-established driver mutations, which raise hope that they may be susceptible to targeted therapies.

ABSTRACT

Mucosal melanomas are rare, often aggressive tumors that can arise at any mucosal site but most frequently occur in the head and neck, vulvovaginal, and anorectal regions. They have distinct biological, clinical, and histopathologic features, which have important management implications. Recent whole-genome sequencing studies have led to a greater understanding of the molecular landscape of mucosal melanomas and uncovered oncogenic drivers that could potentially be susceptible to therapeutic manipulation. The authors provide a brief overview of epidemiologic, clinical, and histopathologic features of mucosal melanoma, with particular emphasis on recent advances in understanding, which have arisen from analyzing their molecular landscape.

OVERVIEW

Melanomas are malignant tumors that arise from melanocytes. Most melanomas arise at cutaneous locations; however, less frequently, they can also arise at extracutaneous sites, including the uveal tract, within the central nervous system, and on mucosal surfaces. Approximately 1% of all melanomas arise from mucosal surfaces, most commonly the upper respiratory, gastrointestinal, and urogenital tracts. These mucosal melanomas

---

[a] Melanoma Institute Australia, The University of Sydney, North Sydney, New South Wales, Australia; [b] Sydney Medical School, The University of Sydney, Sydney, New South Wales, Australia; [c] Tissue Pathology and Diagnostic Oncology, Royal Prince Alfred Hospital, NSW Health Pathology, New South Wales, Australia

* Corresponding author. Tissue Pathology and Diagnostic Oncology, Royal Prince Alfred Hospital, Missenden Road, Camperdown, Sydney, New South Wales 2050, Australia.

E-mail address: richard.scolyer@melanoma.org.au

Surgical Pathology 14 (2021) 293–307
https://doi.org/10.1016/j.path.2021.01.005
1875-9181/21/Crown Copyright © 2021 Published by Elsevier Inc. All rights reserved.

have distinct biological, clinical, and pathologic features and management considerations, compared with their cutaneous counterparts. In this review, the authors provide a comprehensive review of mucosal melanomas, with a particular emphasis on the recent advances in understanding of the molecular landscape of these rare tumors, which has provided crucial information on the mechanisms of disease pathogenesis and highlight possible treatment opportunities for the future.

BIOLOGY AND EPIDEMIOLOGY

Melanocytes arise in the neural crest and migrate from this embryologic structure primarily to the epidermis and the dermis.[1] However, smaller numbers of melanocytes are found at other locations, including the uveal tract, leptomeninges, and mucosal membranes, including those of the head and neck, gastrointestinal, and urogenital systems.[2] Although at cutaneous sites it is well known that melanocytes play a crucial role in protection against UV radiation (UVR), the role of melanocytes at UVR-protected sites is poorly understood and may relate to errors in migration from the neural crest or possibly because they perform an immunologic function locally at these sites.[3]

Mucosal melanoma accounts for approximately 1% of all melanomas in those populations whereby melanomas are common, such as in the United States and Australia; however, in darker-skinned populations, mucosal melanomas account for approximately 25% of all melanomas.[4] Overall, there does not appear to be racial predilection for the development of mucosal melanoma. The most common primary sites of mucosal melanomas are the head and neck region (31%–55%), female genital tract (18%–43%), and anorectal region (16%–24%).[5] They appear to arise in an older population with a median age of 70 years compared with 55 years for cutaneous melanoma. They more frequently occur in women,[6] which is most likely related to the higher incidence of involvement of the vulva and vagina as a primary site, compared with the male genitalia.

The cause of mucosal melanomas is very poorly understood. In the past, reports have linked viral exposures, including human papilloma virus[7] and human herpes virus,[8] as well as exposure to formaldehyde,[9] as possible risk factors. However, these are not generally considered important causes of mucosal melanoma. Recent studies reporting the molecular profile of these tumors, and their implications regarding disease cause, are discussed in Molecular landscape of mucosal melanoma.

CLINICAL FEATURES

Mucosal melanomas frequently present at an advanced stage, often because of their poorly visualized primary site, which leads to a delayed presentation and diagnosis. Therefore, compared with cutaneous melanomas, which show involvement of the locoregional lymph node basin in 9% of cases at diagnosis, regional lymph nodes are involved in around 60% of cases of anorectal melanoma, and 20% to 25% of cases with head and neck or vulvovaginal melanoma at primary diagnosis.[10] In addition, distant metastatic disease is present in 23% of cases[11] at presentation. However, even when accounting for this higher stage at primary diagnosis, mucosal melanomas have a poorer prognosis than cutaneous melanoma. It is known that patients with metastatic mucosal melanoma respond more poorly to immunotherapy compared with their cutaneous counterparts. Furthermore, BRAF mutations are less common in mucosal melanomas, and hence, BRAF and MEK inhibitor therapies are rarely an option for mucosal melanoma patients. Other factors that could contribute to poorer outcomes include difficulty in achieving a surgical excision with clear margins, the rich lymphovascular supply at these sites, and other biological features that are unique to mucosal melanoma.

Because of this delayed presentation of disease, patients presenting complaints are often those of an obstructing lesion or bleeding, which is often occult. **Table 1** outlines the clinical features and sites of disease of the main sites of mucosal melanoma.[2,12–17]

MICROSCOPIC FEATURES

Histopathologically, mucosal melanomas show many features in common with their cutaneous counterparts (**Figs. 1** and **2**). The invasive component usually consists of sheets and nests of atypical epithelioid, spindled, and/or nevoid cells with expansile growth. There is absent or incomplete maturation in the deeper portion of the lesion and usually readily identifiable mitoses.[18–20] The lesional cells may be pigmented or amelanotic. A desmoplastic melanoma component is not a frequent finding, but multiple foci of invasion underlying an extensive in situ component are frequently encountered, as is angioinvasion.[18]

Although in cutaneous melanoma, a preexisting nevus is identified in the surrounding tissue in approximately 30% to 40% of melanomas,[21]

Table 1
Sites or involvement and gross appearance of mucosal melanoma

	Head and Neck	Vulvovaginal	Gastrointestinal
Sites involved and frequency	SN (>55%) Oral (~40%) Laryngeal (rare)	Vulva (>75%): Most common in glabrous skin compared with hair-bearing skin. Second most common malignancy at this site following SCC Vagina (~20%)	Anorectal (>75%) Esophagus (~8%) Stomach, small bowel (rare, metastases at these sites are more common) Large bowel (rare) Gallbladder (rare)
Age	SN: Generally older (>60 y) Oral: Can occur in younger population	>60 y, postmenopausal	>60 y, often >70 y
Locations	SN: Nasal cavity, paranasal sinuses Oral: Hard palate, maxillary gingiva	Vulva: Clitoral, labia majora, labia minora Vagina: Lower third, anterior wall	Rectum and anal canal approximately equal Majority within 6 cm of anal rim
Presentation and clinical features	SN: Bleeding, nasal obstruction Oral: Pigmented lesion detected clinically with change, bleeding	Bleeding, mass, discharge, pain	Bleeding, pain, mass, pruritus
Gross appearance	SN: exophytic, polypoid, ulcerated Oral: Pigmented lesion with irregular borders, asymmetry, bleeding	Amelanotic tumors more common on glabrous skin but rare on hair-bearing skin and vaginal lesions Polypoid mass, bleeding	~30% amelanotic, ulcerated polypoid mass

Abbreviations: SCC, squamous cell carcinoma; SN, sinonasal.

they are only rarely identified in association with mucosal melanoma,[17] which could be in part due to their advanced stage at presentation. An in situ component or radial growth phase (RGP) is often present in the overlying and adjacent mucosa, which is a helpful finding favoring a primary lesion over a metastatic deposit from a distant site. The pattern of the in situ melanoma, in around 60% of cases, shows similar features to acral melanoma, another type of melanoma arising in a sunprotected site. It is characterized by an atypical junctional melanocyte proliferation arranged in a predominant lentiginous single-cell pattern. Upward spread may be present, but is rarely present in early lesions.[17,22] Similarly, nesting of junctional melanocytes is often not seen, particularly in the early stage of the disease.[18] However, other subtypes of melanoma, including a more nested superficial spreading melanoma subtype, is present in 4% to 15% of cases, whereas a minor or completely absent RGP (nodular type) is seen in around 20%[17,22] of cases. In larger tumors, a preexisting in situ component may be absent because of extensive ulceration or destruction of the surrounding tissue by the melanoma. A sometimes patchy, but often prominent lymphoplasmacytic infiltrate is often present in the superficial stroma underlying the in situ component.[23] This feature is also frequently present in acral melanoma, can be very helpful, and can assist the histopathologist in distinguishing between an early in situ melanoma and a benign nevus or lentigo.

Mucosal melanoma usually stains positive for the standard melanocytic immunohistochemical markers S100, SOX10, Melan A, and HMB45.[24] Because the atypical junctional component can be very subtle, particularly at the advancing edge of the lesion, the use of immunohistochemistry (in the authors' experience, a nuclear marker, such as SOX-10 or MiTF, is easiest to interpret) is helpful to assess for the presence of an increased density of junctional melanocytes, often indicating a subtle melanoma in situ, and the relationship of the RGP to the surgical margin.

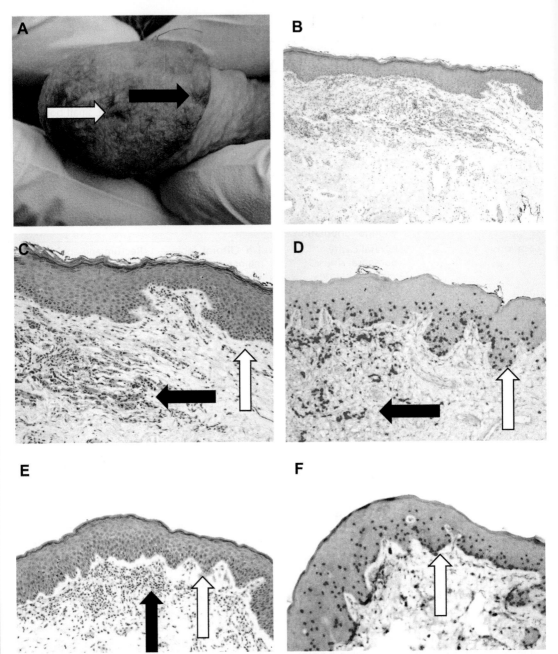

Fig. 1. Penile melanoma in a 70-year-old man. (*A*) Clinical image of melanoma arising on the glans penis. The invasive focus was slightly raised and more heavily pigmented (*white arrow (B-D)* indicating previous biopsy site). Surrounding this, there was ill-defined irregular pigmentation, and several punch biopsies were taken to characterize the extent of melanoma in situ (*black arrow*). (*B*) Scanning-power view of invasive melanoma (hematoxylin-eosin, original magnification ×10). (*C, D*) High-power view of invasive melanoma. Invasive focus consists of atypical pigmented epithelioid cells (*black arrow - (E-F)*) with occasional mitoses. Subtle associated melanoma in situ within mucosa consisting of increased numbers of mildly atypical melanocytic cells with near confluence and upward spread (*C*: hematoxylin-eosin, original magnification ×20; *D*: SOX-10 stain, original magnification ×20). (*E, F*) High-power view of ill-defined melanoma in situ, proximal to invasive focus. Prominent lymphoplasmocytic infiltrate in superficial submucosa (*black arrow*), increase in single lentiginous cells with mild atypia showing confluence and upward spread (*white arrows*), best visualized on the SOX-10 stain (*E*: hematoxylin-eosin, original magnification ×20; *F*: SOX-10 stain, original magnification ×20).

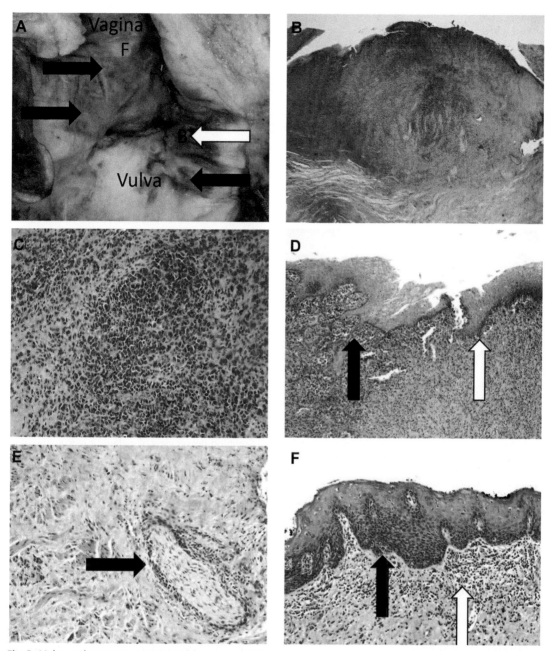

Fig. 2. Vulva melanoma in a 68-year-old woman. (*A*) Clinical image of pelvic exenteration specimen showing melanoma arising on the vulva and extending into the vagina. The invasive focus was raised and nodular with more prominent heavy pigmentation (*white arrow*). Surrounding this, there is an extensive broad ill-defined irregular and heterogeneously pigmented area of melanoma in situ (*black arrows*). (*B*) Scanning-power view of invasive melanoma (hematoxylin-eosin, original magnification ×2). (*C*) High-power view of invasive melanoma showing atypical nevoid cells with readily identifiable mitoses (hematoxylin-eosin, original magnification ×20). (*D*) Medium-power view of florid melanoma in situ and underlying invasive melanoma. The melanoma in situ consists of nests (*black arrow*) and single lentiginous cells (*white arrow*) (hematoxylin-eosin, original magnification ×10). (*E*) High-power view of advancing edge of invasive melanoma showing extensive perineural invasion (*black arrow*) (hematoxylin-eosin, original magnification ×20). (*F*) High-power view of melanoma in situ in vaginal mucosa, more than 5 cm distant from invasive focus, consisting of scattered atypical lentiginous cells (*black arrow*) associated with a moderate lymphoplasmocytic infiltrate within the superficial submucosa (*white arrow*) (hematoxylin-eosin, original magnification ×20).

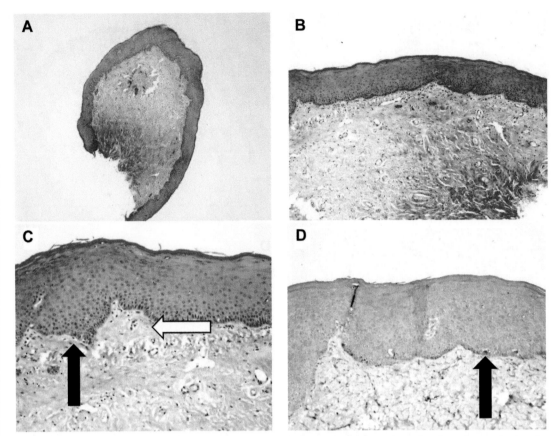

Fig. 3. Melanotic macule on a lip of a 32-year-old woman. (*A*) Scanning-power view of melanotic macule showing lip mucosa and underlying stroma (hematoxylin-eosin, original magnification ×4). (*B*) Medium-power view (hematoxylin-eosin, original magnification ×10). (*C*) High-power view showing pigmentation of basal squamous cells in mucosa (*black arrow*), with very subtle focal pigment incontinence and melanophages within superficial submucosa (*white arrow*) (hematoxylin-eosin, original magnification ×20). (*D*) High-power view demonstrating no increase in junctional melanocytes with only occasional cells identified (*black arrow*) (SOX-10 stain, original magnification ×20).

The more recently described Preferentially Expressed Antigen in Melanoma (PRAME) antibody has also been shown to stain positive in most mucosal melanoma, with a high expression score predicting poorer prognosis.[25]

DIFFERENTIAL DIAGNOSIS

A reasonably sized, well-orientated biopsy of a large mucosal melanoma does not usually pose significant diagnostic problems because of the prominent atypical features described above and the advanced stage of presentation. However, in specific locations, some entities can cause diagnostic challenges.

Melanotic Macule (Mucosal Melanosis)

Melanotic macules, a nonspecific term that incorporates mucosal lentigo, melanosis, and melanoacanthoma,[26,27] are often encountered on the lips,

within the oral cavity, or on the vulvar, penis, nail matrix, acral skin, or mammary areolar. They are small, well-demarcated, and circumscribed pigmented lesions and microscopically consist of pigment within the basal mucosal epithelium.[28] There is no, to a very minimal, increase in junctional melanocytes with some dermal melanophages but no dermal melanocytic component present (**Fig. 3**). The pathologist must differentiate a melanotic macule from a very early, subtle form of melanoma in situ. Usually this does not pose significant difficulties; however, a very mild increase in junctional melanocytes in a pigmented lesion at these sites should trigger very careful examination of deeper levels, possibly supplemented by immunohistochemical stains and careful clinical correlation (mucosal melanomas are usually large, irregular, variably pigmented macules or plaques). When there is an increase

Table 2
Clinical and microscopic features of mucosal melanoma and benign counterparts

	Melanoma	Atypical/Benign Nevus
Clinical features	Recent change in size or color Asymmetrical growth Bleeding Irregular borders Heterogeneous Size >5 mm	Clinically stable in appearance over time No recent change Even borders Uniform Generally smaller lesions
Low-power microscopic features	Asymmetry of pigment distribution, silhouette of lesion Expansile or sheetlike growth	Symmetric No expansile or sheetlike growth
High-power microscopic features	Mitoses, particularly deep Lack of maturation Cytologic atypia, uniform throughout	No or only occasional mitoses Maturation in deep portion of lesion No significant atypia
In situ component	Ill defined Pagetoid spread Confluence Cytologic atypia Associated lymphoplasmocytic infiltrate within superficial submucosa	Well demarcated Upward spread allowed, generally toward center of lesion No sustained confluence Minimal to no associated inflammatory infiltrate within submucosa

in junctional melanocytes within a melanotic macule, it is usually mild with the melanocytes showing minimal cytologic atypia and spaced equidistant from one another, with no confluence, near confluence, or upward spread. Importantly, the presence of lymphoplasmacytic infiltrate within the superficial dermis is a concerning feature for a subtle melanoma in situ over a melanotic macule.

Mucosal Nevi

Melanocytic nevi only rarely occur at mucosal sites, but when they do, they are often very challenging. Mucosal nevi most frequently are located at conjunctival, oral, and genital sites.

Oral melanocytic nevi are usually reasonably well-demarcated pigmented and flat or raised lesions that are found more frequently in women and on the buccal mucosa or hard palate. Like their cutaneous counterparts, they are classified according to which component of the tissue is involved (junctional, compound, submucosal). Conventional nevi are the most frequently observed; however, blue nevi and occasionally Spitzoid nevi are also encountered. Similar diagnostic criteria are used to distinguish mucosal nevi from melanoma (**Table 2**) as those used at cutaneous sites, and as always, careful clinicopathologic correlation is essential.

Genital nevi are most frequently found on the vulva in premenopausal women and may involve both cutaneous and mucosal sites. Occasionally, the male genitalia is involved. A small percentage, up to 5% of cases in some reports,[29] of benign genital nevi may show atypical clinical and histologic features. Atypical genital nevi are regarded as a nevus of a special site, which also includes atypical nevi occurring around the ear, breast, scalp, and at acral sites.[30] Clark and colleagues[31] defined these lesions when they occur in genital sites as atypical melanocytic nevus of genital type (AMNGT). The dermal component of AMNGT may appear more cellular with sheetlike growth with generally mild to moderate cytologic atypia. The presence of larger nests extending into the deeper portion of the lesion is also a reported feature. A prominent fibrotic stroma is also frequently present, which gives rise to the concerning dermoscopic finding of shiny white streaks. Occasional mitoses are observed but are normally confined to the superficial portion of the lesion.[32] The junctional component is frequently nested but also lentiginous with often large junctional nests that efface the epidermis in areas. Upward spread is also seen but is usually confined to the lower half of the epidermis. However, in AMNGT, both the larger junctional nests and the upward spread are seen toward the center of

Table 3
Differential diagnosis of mucosal melanoma according to anatomic location

Site		Differential Diagnosis
Head and neck	Sinonasal	Sinonasal undifferentiated carcinoma High-grade lymphoma Olfactory neuroblastoma Ewing sarcoma Nasopharyngeal undifferentiated carcinoma Poorly differentiated carcinoma Poorly differentiated sarcoma, for example, rhabdomyosarcoma Metastatic melanoma
	Oral	Melanotic macule Oral nevi Amalgam tattoo High-grade lymphoma Poorly differentiated carcinoma Metastatic melanoma
Vulvovaginal		Atypical genital nevus Pigmented epidermal lesions (basal cell carcinoma, seborrheic keratosis, vulval intraepithelial neoplasia) High-grade lymphoma Poorly differentiated carcinoma Poorly differentiated sarcoma, for example, rhabdomyosarcoma Metastatic melanoma
Anorectal		Hemorrhoids or condyloma Nevi High-grade lymphoma Poorly differentiated carcinoma Metastatic melanoma

the lesion and not toward the periphery. Symmetry and maturation are usually preserved, which assist in distinguishing these atypical lesions from melanoma.

Other Poorly Differentiated Malignancies

One of the frequent causes for misdiagnosis of a mucosal melanoma is a failure to consider its possibility within the differential diagnosis. Misdiagnosis is more likely to occur when the lesion is amelanotic or occurs in a younger population or in an unusual location. Because melanoma has an extremely varied histologic appearance; it can mimic most poorly differentiated malignancies (**Table 3**). Fortunately, the use of appropriate immunohistochemistry rapidly makes, or excludes, the diagnosis.

Distinguishing from Metastatic Melanoma Deposit

As noted in **Table 3**, metastatic melanoma from a distant, often cutaneous, site must always be considered in the differential diagnosis of a primary mucosal melanoma. Distinguishing between

these 2 scenarios has significant prognostic and treatment implications for the patient. Careful clinicopathologic correlation usually assists in making the diagnosis (**Table 4**). The application of knowledge gleaned from the recent increased understanding of the molecular landscape of these tumors (see Molecular landscape of mucosal melanoma) may also assist in making the distinction between these 2 diagnostic possibilities.

MOLECULAR LANDSCAPE OF MUCOSAL MELANOMA

Knowledge of the molecular landscape of cutaneous melanoma has increased significantly over the past decade (**Table 5**). The initial epidemiologic observations that cutaneous melanoma occurs more frequently in those with fair skin and in those exposed to more UVR has been confirmed with the identification of a dominant UVR signature (C>T or CC>TT) in most cutaneous melanomas on whole-genome sequencing (WGS).[33] In addition, the discovery of driver mutations, particularly in the mitogen-activated protein kinase (MAPK)

Table 4
Practice points to assist in distinguishing between a primary mucosal melanoma and a deposit of metastatic melanoma at a mucosal site

Careful History and Examination	Particular Emphasis on Previous or Existing Cutaneous Melanocytic Lesions
Serum lactate dehydrogenase	If significantly elevated, may indicate presence of metastatic disease
Histopathologic features	If present, an associated atypical junctional component in the overlying and surrounding mucosa would favor a primary tumor
	However, the absence of such an atypical junctional component does not exclude a primary lesion, as a significant portion of primary melanomas lack one
Radiological correlation	Extensive involvement of nodal basin, such as the groin or axilla, with associated in-transit metastasis, could favor a metastatic cutaneous melanoma from that limb
Molecular features	See Current systemic treatment options and the future

pathway, has been crucial to the understanding of the pathogenesis of cutaneous melanoma. Initially, NRAS mutations were identified in the 1980s, which was followed by the discovery of various BRAF mutations, particularly the V600E mutation, and mutations in NF1, which are the 3 most common driver mutations identified in cutaneous melanoma. As a result, The Cancer Genome Atlas Network (TCGA)[34] recently proposed a classification of cutaneous melanomas into 4 subgroups that harbor different driver mutations: BRAF, NRAS, NF1, and "triple wild-type" (tumors lacking any of the 3 common driver mutations). Most (94%) have been found to harbor one of these 3 main MAPK-activating mutations. The discovery of these driver mutations has also been essential to the development of targeted therapies, such as those targeted against BRAF/MEK for patients in whom their tumor harbors a BRAF mutation, which have shown remarkable clinical efficacy, albeit frequently short lived.

Because of the rare occurrence of mucosal melanomas, compared with their cutaneous counterparts, the molecular landscape of mucosal melanomas has not been fully characterized until recently. However, whole-exome sequencing (WES) and more recent comprehensive WGS have provided greater insight and understanding of the molecular features of mucosal melanoma and uncovered potential oncogenic drivers that may facilitate targeted treatments for aggressive tumors.

POINT MUTATION BURDEN AND MUTATIONAL SIGNATURES

Mucosal melanomas have been shown to have a low point mutation burden with both low single-nucleotide variant (SNVs) and insertion/deletion (indel) mutation burden per tumor when compared with cutaneous melanomas[33,35–37] (see **Table 5**). In the authors' recent study, an average of 2.7 mutations per megabase in mucosal melanomas were identified,[36] which compares to an average of 49.17 mutations per megabase found in cutaneous melanoma in their earlier study.[33] Similar findings have been reported in the other large WGS study of mucosal melanomas.[37] The increased point mutation burden of cutaneous melanoma is associated with UVR exposure, with typical ranges of 70% to 95% of all mutations related to the UVR signature 7, identifiable as C>T or CC>TT nucleotide transition.[33] The authors recently showed more than 50% contributions from the UVR signature present in some mucosal melanomas of the head and neck (conjunctival, nasal and oral cavity, nasal sinuses); however, these cases showed an overall mutation burden, structural variations (SV), and copy number aberrations (CNA) more in keeping with other mucosal melanomas compared with those from cutaneous sites. These findings indicate that in some mucosal melanomas in this anatomic location, indirect or reflected UVR may play a role in carcinogenesis. No such UVR signature was identified in the vulvovaginal or anorectal melanomas of this study. They also showed that although a significant proportion of vulvar melanomas occurs in hair-bearing skin, they show similar molecular features as those arising on vulvar mucosal surfaces and at vaginal sites and should therefore be staged and managed as mucosal in origin and not from a cutaneous site.

Interestingly, all such patients with a dominant UVR signature of the head and neck were of East

Table 5
Summary of mutational landscape of melanomas arising at different anatomic sites, with particular emphasis on mucosal melanomas

	Cutaneous (n = 140)		Mucosal								Acral (n = 90)		Uveal (n = 103)	
			Nasal (n = 17)		Oral (n = 17)		Anorectal (n = 12)		Genitourinary (n = 15)					
	Median	*Range*	*Median*	*Range*	*Median*	*Range*	*Median*	*Range*	*Median*	*Range*	*Median*	*Range*	*Median*	*Range*
Mutations per megabase	49.17	(0.71–260)	2.35	(1.43–5.15)	2.86	(0.59–6.69)	2.6	(0.5–7.13)	1.55	(1.02–4.04)	2.1	(0.68–34.9)	0.5	(0.1–14)
Structural arrangements	101	(3–1123)	93	(21–1017)	262	(35–1299)	191	(51–511)	139	(49–950)	283	(32,1,251)	13	(0–213)
Driver mutations (SNV/indel)	*% mutated*		*% mutated*		*% mutated*		*% mutated*		*% mutated*		*% mutated*		*% mutated*	
BRAF	46		6		18		25		20		24		0	
NRAS	31		41		12		8		7		18		0	
CDKN2A	29		0		12		0		0		3		0	
PLCB4	22		0		0		0		0		1		5	
TP53	21		6		12		17		7		2		0.02	
NF1	16		24		6		0		27		11		0.02	
PTEN	16		0		0		0		0		8		0	
KIT	4		6		18		17		27		11		0	
CYSLTR2	0.02		0		0		0		0		0		2	
TYRP1	0.01		0		0		0		0		8		0.02	
SF3B1	5		6		0		17		33		0		14	
EIF1AX	0.03		0		0		0		0		1		19	
GNA11	0.01		0		0		0		0		0		46	
GNAQ	1		0		0		8		0		1		50	
BAP1	0.01		0		0		0		13		0		75[a]	

Note. Data are gathered from the authors' recent publications, where the anatomic location was assigned by careful clinicopathologic correlation.

[a] Germline and somatic.

Data from Refs.[33,36,48]

Asian ancestry. A mutation signature 17 (unknown cause) was only found in melanomas in patients of the same ethnic background. In addition, signature 1 was found to provide a greater contribution to the mutational burden of vulvovaginal/anorectal melanomas compared with those from the head and neck across all patients. These findings indicate possible genetic or location-specific factors playing a role in the development of mucosal melanoma. Other mutational signatures have been identified in mucosal melanoma (signature 3-like, 5, 17), which have no known cause, and therefore, more research needs to be performed in this area to try to discover what drives these mutational processes, which contribute to mucosal melanoma. An understanding of the drivers will likely provide insights into the causes of mucosal melanoma at specific sites and enable prevention strategies to be instigated.

Also of clinical significance, mucosal melanomas harbor a relatively low mutational burden, which is one of the hypothesized reasons for the much poorer response to immunotherapy, when compared with cutaneous melanoma.[38] The response rate of mucosal melanoma to anti-PD-1 immunotherapy is 23%, which is comparable to a 17% response rate observed in acral melanoma, but significantly less than the 41% reached in cutaneous melanoma.[38]

SIGNIFICANTLY MUTATED GENES

Common Mitogen-Activated Protein Kinase Mutations

Compared with the 94% of cases of cutaneous melanoma that harbor an activating MAPK pathway mutation in *BRAF*, *NRAS*, or *NF1*,[34] a recent meta-analysis has found that across all studies to date, only 28% of mucosal melanomas harbors these mutations.[39] In *BRAF* mutations, which are present in 52% of all cutaneous melanomas in the TCGA, of these, 46% was in the well-documented 600 codon, 39% being mutations in V600E. In contrast, 6% of mucosal melanomas have a proven *BRAF* V600 mutation; however, an increased number of less frequently encountered, or noncanonical, BRAF mutations, such as S432X, G469A, and V168L,[40] have been found. These noncanonical mutations are less reliant on signaling via the MEK/ERK pathway as those mutations at codon 600 and have been associated with a lower response rate to BRAF inhibitors.[41] *BRAF* fusions have been reported in mucosal melanoma, and these have been shown to be sensitive to targeted therapy[42]; however, these events are rare and occur in less than 5% of cases.[43] *NRAS* mutations most frequently occur

in human malignancies that cluster at exon 1 (G12/13) and exon 2 (Q61),[44] and these mutations are significantly lower in mucosal melanoma (8%–17%) when compared with their cutaneous counterparts (28%).[34,39] *NF1* is the third most frequent driver mutation found in cutaneous melanoma in the TCGA (14%),[34] and on recent meta-analysis, a similar rate has been found in mucosal melanoma.[39] However, *NF1* is susceptible to large-scale chromosomal or structural rearrangements, which are not detectable using targeted or exome sequencing, and may require WGS to detect. *NF1* mutations are more common in mucosal melanoma once structural variants are included.

Other Significant Mutations

Mutations in *KIT*, a transmembrane receptor tyrosine kinase, have frequently been reported in acral and mucosal melanomas and interestingly in those with significant chronic UVR exposure but not intermittent UVR exposure.[45] In cutaneous cases, *KIT* mutations have been shown in 13% of all triple-negative melanomas, or around 2% of overall cutaneous melanoma,[34] whereas in mucosal melanoma, around 13% of all cases have been reported to harbor a mutation.[39] A similar rate of *KIT* mutation has been reported in the same meta-analysis across different anatomic locations. Interestingly, a significantly higher rate of mucosal cases (32%) found comutation of *KIT* and *NF1* in one of the larger series.[40]

SF3B1 (splicing factor 3B subunit 1), which makes up part of the spliceosome and plays a significant role in RNA splicing,[46] has previously been reported as one of the frequent mutations in uveal melanoma,[47,48] blue nevus-like melanomas, and also a subset of solid organ and hematological malignancies.[49] The authors initially reported it in their large (n = 183) WGS across all subtypes of melanoma, including mucosal (n = 8), where 3 cases of vulvovaginal origin harbored the mutation. The authors and others have subsequently confirmed these results with more in-depth analysis of mucosal melanoma, where *SF3B1* mutation has been found in 13%,[36] 22%,[50] and 37%[40] of all mucosal melanoma cases and was almost exclusively found in cases from vulvovaginal and anorectal sites and not in the head and neck. Little overlap has been noted between MAPK mutations and those of *SF3B1*,[36] and the prognostic implications of this mutation have been variable across the different studies.[39]

SPRED1 has also recently been reported as a driver mutation in mucosal melanoma in 7% to 26% of cases.[36,51] It acts as a tumor suppressor gene by recruiting NF1 to the plasma membrane where it inhibits RAS-GTP signaling, and therefore, loss of this inhibitory effect can cause an increase in MAPK signaling. Although in cutaneous melanoma, most NF1 and SPRED1 mutations are found concurrently,[52] in mucosal melanoma, most mutations identified in both of the studies that identified SPRED1 mutation found the 2 mutations to be mutually exclusive.[36,51]

In addition, single cases have been found by WGS to harbor further hotspot mutations associated with the MAPK pathway, including MAP2K1, GNAQ, and KRAS.[36] The authors have also recently reported 6% of mucosal melanoma cases with mutations in the WNT signaling pathway (CTNNB1).[36]

STRUCTURAL VARIATIONS AND COPY NUMBER ALTERATIONS

Mucosal melanomas have been shown to have a higher number of SV and CNA compared with cutaneous melanomas.[33] Structural rearrangements targeting 5p, 11p, and 12p have been identified that frequently lead to amplification of oncogenes, including, among others, MDM2, TERT, and CDK4, which may be important in the carcinogenesis of melanoma.[36,37,53] To support this finding, amplification has also been found in 5p (containing TERT) and 12q (containing CDK4) in studies using WES.[53] Most of these changes have been found at oral sites and in those of East Asian ethnicity. In addition, patients with these chromosomal changes between 5p and 12p have been shown to have worse clinical outcomes.[37]

Our latest in-depth WGS study of mucosal melanomas has highlighted the significant diversity of SVs in this group of tumors. Many of these involve well-known melanoma drivers, including CDKN2A, PTEN, and TERT; however, overall, 391 predicted fusion events affecting 657 genes were identified, but no events occurred across multiple cases.[36]

SUMMARY AND CLINICAL IMPLICATIONS

These recent studies of the molecular landscape of mucosal melanoma have highlighted the significant heterogeneity of the mutational processes that occur within this broad group of tumors. There appear to be distinct anatomic or site-specific, geographic, and ethnic factors that interact in the pathogenesis of melanomas arising at mucosal sites.

In the authors' recent large study (n = 67), they demonstrated that all but 1 case had a well-established driver mutation, which highlights the potential for new treatment options, targeting these driver events, may be effective for patients with these aggressive tumors.[33] Of interest, 70% of cases contained mutations, such as those to CDK4, CCND1, and CDKN2A, which have the potential to respond to CDK4/6 inhibitors, such as palbociclib, the clinical benefits of which are still being studied.[37]

CURRENT SYSTEMIC TREATMENT OPTIONS AND THE FUTURE

For localized mucosal melanoma, a local excision of the primary lesion, possibly including any involved locoregional lymph nodes, is considered standard care. In clinically localized cutaneous melanoma, an involved sentinel lymph node biopsy has been proven to be the most important prognostic feature. However, in mucosal melanoma, only small numbers of cases have reported the utility of this procedure at sites, including vulvovaginal,[54] and those from mucosal sites in the head and neck,[55] and therefore, the role of this procedure in the staging and management of mucosal melanoma is not clear. As previously discussed, at presentation, the melanoma is frequently locally advanced, making definitive surgical excision of the lesion difficult. In addition, there is frequent lymph node involvement or distant metastatic disease identified at presentation.[56] Therefore, radiotherapy can be considered when surgical margins are involved or if the primary lesion is surgically unresectable. Although improvements in locoregional control have been reported with adjuvant radiotherapy, no significant improvements in survival have been demonstrated.[57]

Given the frequent advanced stage of presentation, effective systemic disease is often required in this aggressive disease. Unfortunately, to date, the search for an effective systemic treatment, which can show sustained clinical response, has been disappointing. Use of tyrosine kinase inhibitors in KIT mutant mucosal melanoma has shown a response rate of more than 35% in some trials; however, the median progression-free survival is still often within a few months.[58] Although there has been significant improvements in progression-free survival and overall survival with the use of immunotherapy agents, which provide immune checkpoint blockade against CTLA4 and PD1 in cutaneous melanoma, the objective response rate for combination therapy is considerably lower at 37% in mucosal melanoma (compared with 60% in cutaneous melanoma).[38] The reasons for this significant difference in response rates are poorly understood; however, it is hypothesized that the lower mutational burden and immune activation as seen by the lower levels of PD-L1 expression[38] in mucosal melanomas compared with those arising at cutaneous sites are possible explanations. However, a more promising phase 1B trial, combining anti-PD1 inhibitors with a VEGF receptor inhibitor, in 29 mucosal melanoma patients, achieved a response rate of 48%.[59] In addition, unfortunately, because of the low frequency of BRAF V600 mutation in these tumors, the use of combined BRAF/MEK-targeted treatment is of limited utility.

Therefore, there is a current unmet necessity for further effective treatments of these mucosal melanomas. Excitingly, it is the recent in-depth clarification of their molecular landscape that the authors have described, which will foster ongoing further research into more effective targeted treatments of these aggressive tumors into the future.

CLINICS CARE POINTS

- The consideration of melanoma at any mucosal site is essential when a histopathologist assesses a poorly differentiated malignancy arising at these locations.

- An immunohistochemical panel, including S100, SOX-10, Melan A, and HMB45, can rapidly exclude or make the diagnosis.

- A nuclear immunohistochemical stain, such as SOX-10, can assist in accurately highlighting the density in junctional melanocytes, which may enable more accurate assessment of surgical margin clearance and melanoma in situ to be distinguished from its benign mimics.

- PRAME immunohistochemical stain may also assist in distinguishing mucosal melanoma from benign mimics and may also provide prognostic information.

- The mutational landscape of mucosal melanoma has been clarified recently, which has highlighted potential oncogenic targets for further research.

- From a mutation standpoint, mucosal melanoma is a heterogeneous group of tumors with site-specific, ethnic, and geographic factors playing a part in their carcinogenesis.

- In general, a low rate of MAPK driver mutations and overall mutation burden, with a higher rate of CNA and SV, characterize mucosal melanoma. A dominant UVR signature has been identified in some melanomas from the head and neck.

ACKNOWLEDGMENTS

The authors gratefully acknowledge the assistance of their colleagues at Melanoma Institute Australia and the Department of Tissue Pathology and Diagnostic Oncology at the Royal Prince Alfred Hospital, Sydney, Australia.

DISCLOSURE

R.V. Rawson is supported by a Clinical Researcher Scholarship from Sydney Research. R.A. Scolyer is supported by the National Health and Medical Research Council Fellowship program. R.A. Scolyer has received professional services fees from Merck Sharp Dohme, Bristol-Myers Squibb Novartis, GlaxoSmithKline, Myriad, and NeraCare (not related to this work). All other authors declare no competing interests.

REFERENCES

1. Dupin E, Le Douarin NM. Development of melanocyte precursors from the vertebrate neural crest. Oncogene 2003;22(20):3016–23.
2. Mihajlovic M, Vlajkovic S, Jovanovic P, et al. Primary mucosal melanomas: a comprehensive review. Int J Clin Exp Pathol 2012;5(8):739–53.
3. Mackintosh JA. The antimicrobial properties of melanocytes, melanosomes and melanin and the evolution of black skin. J Theor Biol 2001;211(2):101–13.
4. McLaughlin CC, Wu XC, Jemal A, et al. Incidence of noncutaneous melanomas in the U.S. Cancer 2005; 103(5):1000–7.
5. Patrick RJ, Fenske NA, Messina JL. Primary mucosal melanoma. J Am Acad Dermatol 2007;56(5):828–34.
6. Hahn HM, Lee KG, Choi W, et al. An updated review of mucosal melanoma: survival meta-analysis. Mol Clin Oncol 2019;11(2):116–26.
7. La Placa M, Ambretti S, Bonvicini F, et al. Presence of high-risk mucosal human papillomavirus genotypes in primary melanoma and in acquired dysplastic melanocytic naevi. Br J Dermatol 2005;152(5):909–14.
8. Lundberg R, Brytting M, Dahlgren L, et al. Human herpes virus DNA is rarely detected in non-UV light-associated primary malignant melanomas of mucous membranes. Anticancer Res 2006;26(5b): 3627–31.
9. Holmstrom M, Lund VJ. Malignant melanomas of the nasal cavity after occupational exposure to formaldehyde. Br J Ind Med 1991;48(1):9–11.
10. Chang AE, Karnell LH, Menck HR. The National Cancer Data Base Report on cutaneous and noncutaneous melanoma: a summary of 84,836 cases from the past decade. The American College of Surgeons Commission on Cancer and the American Cancer Society. Cancer 1998;83(8):1664–78.

11. Lian B, Cui CL, Zhou L, et al. The natural history and patterns of metastases from mucosal melanoma: an analysis of 706 prospectively-followed patients. Ann Oncol 2017;28(4):868–73.

12. Patel SG, Prasad ML, Escrig M, et al. Primary mucosal malignant melanoma of the head and neck. Head Neck 2002;24(3):247–57.

13. Dauer EH, Lewis JE, Rohlinger AL, et al. Sinonasal melanoma: a clinicopathologic review of 61 cases. Otolaryngol Head Neck Surg 2008;138(3):347–52.

14. Clifton N, Harrison L, Bradley PJ, et al. Malignant melanoma of nasal cavity and paranasal sinuses: report of 24 patients and literature review. J Laryngol Otol 2011;125(5):479–85.

15. Brady MS, Kavolius JP, Quan SH. Anorectal melanoma. A 64-year experience at Memorial Sloan-Kettering Cancer Center. Dis Colon Rectum 1995; 38(2):146–51.

16. Sugiyama VE, Chan JK, Shin JY, et al. Vulvar melanoma: a multivariable analysis of 644 patients. Obstet Gynecol 2007;110(2 Pt 1):296–301.

17. Ragnarsson-Olding BK, Kanter-Lewensohn LR, Lagerlöf B, et al. Malignant melanoma of the vulva in a nationwide, 25-year study of 219 Swedish females: clinical observations and histopathologic features. Cancer 1999;86(7):1273–84.

18. Saida T, Kawachi S, Takata M, et al. Histopathological characteristics of malignant melanoma affecting mucous membranes: a unifying concept of histogenesis. Pathology 2004;36(5):404–13.

19. Merkel EA, Gerami P. Malignant melanoma of sun-protected sites: a review of clinical, histological, and molecular features. Lab Invest 2017;97(6):630–5.

20. Dodds TJ, Wilmott JS, Jackett LA, et al. Primary anorectal melanoma: clinical, immunohistology and DNA analysis of 43 cases. Pathology 2019;51(1): 39–45.

21. Duman N, Erkin G, Gököz Ö, et al. Nevus-associated versus de novo melanoma: do they have different characteristics and prognoses? Dermatopathology (Basel) 2015;2(1):46–51.

22. Kato T, Takematsu H, Tomita Y, et al. Malignant melanoma of mucous membranes. A clinicopathologic study of 13 cases in Japanese patients. Arch Dermatol 1987;123(2):216–20.

23. Prasad ML. Update on pigmented lesions of the sinonasal tract. Head Neck Pathol 2007;1(1):50–4.

24. Prasad ML, Jungbluth AA, Iversen K, et al. Expression of melanocytic differentiation markers in malignant melanomas of the oral and sinonasal mucosa. Am J Surg Pathol 2001;25(6):782–7.

25. Toyama A, Siegel L, Nelson AC, et al. Analyses of molecular and histopathologic features and expression of PRAME by immunohistochemistry in mucosal melanomas. Mod Pathol 2019;32(12):1727–33.

26. Sexton FM, Maize JC. Melanotic macules and melanoacanthomas of the lip. A comparative study with census of the basal melanocyte population. Am J Dermatopathol 1987;9(5):438–44.

27. Elder DE, Scolyer RA. WHO classification of skin tumours. 4th edition. Lyon (France): IARC; 2018.

28. Gondak RO, da Silva-Jorge R, Jorge J, et al. Oral pigmented lesions: clinicopathologic features and review of the literature. Med Oral Patol Oral Cir Bucal 2012;17(6):e919–24.

29. Christensen WN, Friedman KJ, Woodruff JD, et al. Histologic characteristics of vulvar nevocellular nevi. J Cutan Pathol 1987;14(2):87–91.

30. Hosler GA, Moresi JM, Barrett TL. Nevi with site-related atypia: a review of melanocytic nevi with atypical histologic features based on anatomic site. J Cutan Pathol 2008;35(10):889–98.

31. Clark WH Jr, Hood AF, Tucker MA, et al. Atypical melanocytic nevi of the genital type with a discussion of reciprocal parenchymal-stromal interactions in the biology of neoplasia. Hum Pathol 1998;29(1 Suppl 1):S1–24.

32. Gleason BC, Hirsch MS, Nucci MR, et al. Atypical genital nevi. A clinicopathologic analysis of 56 cases. Am J Surg Pathol 2008;32(1):51–7.

33. Hayward NK, Wilmott JS, Waddell N, et al. Whole-genome landscapes of major melanoma subtypes. Nature 2017;545(7653):175–80.

34. Cancer Genome Atlas Network. Genomic classification of cutaneous melanoma. Cell 2015;161(7):1681–96.

35. Furney SJ, Turajlic S, Stamp G, et al. Genome sequencing of mucosal melanomas reveals that they are driven by distinct mechanisms from cutaneous melanoma. J Pathol 2013;230(3):261–9.

36. Newell F, Kong Y, Wilmott JS, et al. Whole-genome landscape of mucosal melanoma reveals diverse drivers and therapeutic targets. Nat Commun 2019;10(1):3163.

37. Zhou R, Shi C, Tao W, et al. Analysis of mucosal melanoma whole-genome landscapes reveals clinically relevant genomic aberrations. Clin Cancer Res 2019;25(12):3548–60.

38. D'Angelo SP, Larkin J, Sosman JA, et al. Efficacy and safety of nivolumab alone or in combination with ipilimumab in patients with mucosal melanoma: a pooled analysis. J Clin Oncol 2017;35(2):226–35.

39. Nassar KW, Tan AC. The mutational landscape of mucosal melanoma. Semin Cancer Biol 2020;61: 139–48.

40. Hintzsche JD, Gorden NT, Amato CM, et al. Whole-exome sequencing identifies recurrent SF3B1 R625 mutation and comutation of NF1 and KIT in mucosal melanoma. Melanoma Res 2017;27(3):189–99.

41. Menzer C, Menzies AM, Carlino MS, et al. Targeted therapy in advanced melanoma with rare BRAF mutations. J Clin Oncol 2019;37(33):3142–51.

42. Kim HS, Jung M, Kang HN, et al. Oncogenic BRAF fusions in mucosal melanomas activate the MAPK pathway and are sensitive to MEK/PI3K inhibition

or MEK/CDK4/6 inhibition. Oncogene 2017;36(23): 3334–45.

43. Botton T, Talevich E, Mishra VK, et al. Genetic heterogeneity of BRAF fusion kinases in melanoma affects drug responses. Cell Rep 2019;29(3): 573–88.e577.

44. Bos JL. ras oncogenes in human cancer: a review. Cancer Res 1989;49(17):4682–9.

45. Gong HZ, Zheng HY, Li J. The clinical significance of KIT mutations in melanoma: a meta-analysis. Melanoma Res 2018;28(4):259–70.

46. Darman RB, Seiler M, Agrawal AA, et al. Cancer-associated SF3B1 hotspot mutations induce cryptic 3' splice site selection through use of a different branch point. Cell Rep 2015;13(5):1033–45.

47. Furney SJ, Pedersen M, Gentien D, et al. SF3B1 mutations are associated with alternative splicing in uveal melanoma. Cancer Discov 2013;3(10):1122–9.

48. Johansson PA, Brooks K, Newell F, et al. Whole genome landscapes of uveal melanoma show an ultraviolet radiation signature in iris tumours. Nat Commun 2020;11(1):2408.

49. Papaemmanuil E, Cazzola M, Boultwood J, et al. Somatic SF3B1 mutation in myelodysplasia with ring sideroblasts. N Engl J Med 2011;365(15):1384–95.

50. Quek C, Rawson RV, Ferguson PM, et al. Recurrent hotspot SF3B1 mutations at codon 625 in vulvovaginal mucosal melanoma identified in a study of 27 Australian mucosal melanomas. Oncotarget 2019; 10(9):930–41.

51. Ablain J, Xu M, Rothschild H, et al. Human tumor genomics and zebrafish modeling identify SPRED1

loss as a driver of mucosal melanoma. Science 2018;362(6418):1055–60.

52. Krauthammer M, Kong Y, Bacchiocchi A, et al. Exome sequencing identifies recurrent mutations in NF1 and RASopathy genes in sun-exposed melanomas. Nat Genet 2015;47(9):996–1002.

53. Lyu J, Song Z, Chen J, et al. Whole-exome sequencing of oral mucosal melanoma reveals mutational profile and therapeutic targets. J Pathol 2018;244(3):358–66.

54. de Hullu JA, Hollema H, Hoekstra HJ, et al. Vulvar melanoma: is there a role for sentinel lymph node biopsy? Cancer 2002;94(2):486–91.

55. Stárek I, Koranda P, Benes P. Sentinel lymph node biopsy: a new perspective in head and neck mucosal melanoma? Melanoma Res 2006;16(5):423–7.

56. Yentz S, Lao CD. Immunotherapy for mucosal melanoma. Ann Transl Med 2019;7(Suppl 3):S118.

57. Owens JM, Roberts DB, Myers JN. The role of postoperative adjuvant radiation therapy in the treatment of mucosal melanomas of the head and neck region. Arch Otolaryngol Head Neck Surg 2003;129(8): 864–8.

58. Kim KB, Alrwas A. Treatment of KIT-mutated metastatic mucosal melanoma. Chin Clin Oncol 2014; 3(3):35.

59. Sheng X, Yan X, Chi Z, et al. Axitinib in combination with toripalimab, a humanized immunoglobulin G_4 monoclonal antibody against programmed cell death-1, in patients with metastatic mucosal melanoma: an open-label phase IB trial. J Clin Oncol 2019;37(32):2987–99.

Leukocytoclastic Vasculitis and Microvascular Occlusion
Key Concepts for the Working Pathologist

Christine J. Ko, MD[a,b,*], Jeff R. Gehlhausen, MD, PhD[a],
Jennifer M. McNiff, MD[a,b]

KEYWORDS

- Vasculitis • Vasculopathy • Microvascular occlusion • Leukocytoclastic • Leukocytoclasia

---

Key points

- Leukocytoclastic vasculitis (LCV) is a reaction pattern that may have no clear trigger, be secondary to drugs or infection, or represent a manifestation of systemic disease (eg, IgA vasculitis).

- Histopathologic involvement of either small, deep dermal vessels or medium-sized vessels should be noted, because this may be associated with other organ involvement (eg, antineutrophil cytoplasmic antibody–associated vasculitis).

- Microvascular occlusion may be secondary to fibrin thrombi (eg, hypercoagulability) or immune deposits (eg, monoclonal cryoglobulinemia) as well as embolism.

- Thrombi in vessels within the fat can be seen in the setting of calciphylaxis.

ABSTRACT

Although clinicians often put vasculitis and microvascular occlusion in the same differential diagnosis, biopsy findings often are either vasculitis or occlusion. However, both vasculitis and occlusion are present in some cases of levamisole-associated vasculopathy and certain infections. Depth of dermal involvement and vessel size should be reported, because superficial and deep small vessel leukocytoclastic vasculitis and/or involvement of medium-sized vessels may be associated with systemic disease. Microvascular occlusion of vessels in the fat should prompt consideration of calciphylaxis. Clues to ultimate clinical diagnosis can be garnered from depth of involvement, size of vessels affected, and presence of both vasculitis and occlusion.

OVERVIEW

On a simplistic level, leukocytoclastic vasculitis (LCV) and microvascular occlusion easily are distinguished microscopically. Vasculitis, as suggested by the "-itis," is inflammatory, whereas typical cases of microvascular occlusion are noninflammatory. This clear-cut distinction often is blurred in everyday practice, when real-world examples may not follow typical textbook findings and broad, sometimes imprecise clinical

---

[a] Department of Dermatology, Yale University, 333 Cedar Street, PO Box 208059, New Haven, CT 06520, USA;
[b] Department of Pathology, Yale University, 310 Cedar St, New Haven, CT 06511, USA
* Corresponding author.
E-mail address: Christine.ko@yale.edu

Surgical Pathology 14 (2021) 309–325
https://doi.org/10.1016/j.path.2021.01.006
1875-9181/21/© 2021 Elsevier Inc. All rights reserved.

terminology is employed. Consider these examples: (1) certain disorders have findings of both vasculitis and luminal occlusion, like levamisole-associated vasculitis/vasculopathy and meningococcemia; (2) disease nomenclature can lead to confusion: even *vasculopathy*, often used synonymously with *microvascular occlusion*, literally means any kind of vascular damage (inflammatory or not). This review article deconstructs vasculitis and microvascular occlusion to a practical level directed at the working pathologist, with emphasis on relevant tips and clues.

DEFINITIONS

For the purposes of this article, certain terms are defined in **Box 1**.

BACKGROUND

NATURE OF THE PROBLEM

In the authors' experience, petechial (<4-mm) or purpuric (>4-mm) lesions on the lower legs often are submitted to a pathologist with a differential diagnosis of vasculitis versus pigmented purpuric dermatosis/eruption versus vasculopathy (or sometimes with no clinical information). In these cases, microscopic findings generally include extravasated erythrocytes around superficial small vessels accompanied by either perivascular lymphocytes or neutrophils with leukocytoclasia, corresponding to pigmented purpuric eruptions or LCV, respectively. There are many variants of pigmented purpuric eruptions, listed in **Table 1**; because there is not histopathologic vascular damage in these diseases, they are not addressed further. **Box 2** lists clinical diseases that can have histopathologic findings of LCV.

When considering the diagnoses in **Box 2**, the easy separation of LCV from microvascular occlusion becomes blurred. Some diseases (marked with asterisks) can exhibit simultaneous findings of LCV and microvascular occlusion, whereas others manifest as either LCV or microvascular occlusion, depending on the particular clinical scenario. For example, lupus erythematosus has protean clinical presentations in the skin, including dependent palpable purpura corresponding to LCV or dependent branching purpura corresponding to microvascular occlusion and antiphospholipid antibodies. Therefore, although it may be difficult for a practicing pathologist at the microscope to visualize the clinical presentation, flexible but robust mental representations of classic clinical morphology and distribution of typical cases of LCV versus microvascular occlusion are useful.

EVALUATION AND ASSESSMENT

Morphology—Papular versus Branching

A key clinical distinction is papular morphology versus branching morphology (**Figs. 1** and **2**). The prototype of papular purpura is palpable purpura. Pink to red to purple-black circles that are slightly elevated and circular in shape are the primary lesion; lesions that are 1 day to 2 days old should blanch partially with pressure. Early lesions may be macular (<1 cm, flat, and not elevated). Unlike the circular lesions of papular purpura, branching purpura is inclusive of netlike outlines, solid polygons with broken-up or irregular linear margins (retiform purpura), or gangrene of the toes (which may be a sign of advanced disease). Prototypes of branching purpura, which correspond to vascular occlusion, are sepsis-associated disseminated intravascular coagulation, calciphylaxis (especially early lesions), and antiphospholipid syndrome.

Although classic morphology and histopathologic findings differ, as discussed previously, vasculitis and microvascular occlusion often are in the same clinical differential diagnosis or case discussion.[1] A reason for this is the variability of lesional morphology that can be seen in a given patient. Papular lesions can display pseudo-branching, in which papules link and overlap to form confluent areas larger than 1 cm with interconnecting, darker centers[2]; such pseudobranching is best distinguished from true branching by the presence of circular 4-mm to 9-mm papules of purpura in close proximity but outside the central area (**Fig. 3**). Even as papular purpura can mimic branching purpura, patients with true branching purpura also can have, on other body sites, additional macular, papular, and patch/plaque purpuric lesions. Branching lesions also can be subtle (see **Fig. 2A**) and represent the minority of lesions on a particular patient.

Distribution

At the least, pathologists generally are given a body site, providing a clue as to distribution (**Table 2**). Dermatologists often avoid sampling cosmetically sensitive areas, like the face, and also sites that are more painful or slow to heal, like hands/feet and lower legs. Thus, if face, volar surfaces, or lower legs are biopsied, it suggests that the skin findings predominantly affect those sites, precluding other sites from being chosen instead. In general, papular purpura (ie, palpable purpura and LCV) tends to affect dependent sites, including the feet; branching purpura often is acral, involving small–medium vessels of the digits, but also can be generalized.[1,3] Certain disorders, like

Box 1
Definitions of important terms used when describing leukocytoclastic vasculitis and microvascular occlusion

Acral

- Hands, feet, ears, nose; sometimes penis, elbows, knees, buttocks, breasts, cheeks

Branching (retiform) purpura

- Netlike interconnecting purpura (livedoid, see later)

or

- Solid pink-purple-black papule/plaque centrally with intermittently jagged borders like that of a maple leaf

or

- Livedo racemosa (see later)

or

- Peripheral symmetric digital gangrene

Dependent

- Body sites that are lowest for most of the day, for example, feet/legs if standing/sitting; posterior legs/back if lying down

Generalized

- Affecting different and many parts of the body

Leukocytoclastic vasculitis (LCV)

- Perivascular neutrophil-predominant infiltrate
- Minimum criteria
  - Perivascular neutrophils
  - Some leukocytoclasia (may be subtle)
  - Some vessel wall damage (may range from fluffy swelling of wall to severe fibrin cuffing)

Livedo racemosa

- Fixed, irregular broken-up netlike pattern, violaceous to red or blue, not reversible with warming the skin; necrosis may be associated

Livedo reticularis

- Unbroken, netlike pattern of violaceous to red-blue mottling of the skin, not reversible with warming of the skin
- Livedo racemosa is considered by some to be a subtype of livedo reticularis.

Livedoid

- Imprecise term that is variably used to refer to a pattern either resembling livedo reticularis or livedo racemosa or a nonspecific branching pattern

Lymphocytic vasculitis

- Perivascular lymphocyte-predominant infiltrate with subtle vessel wall damage
- True vascular damage with fibrinoid necrosis is unusual
- Diseases that traditionally fall under this category (eg, pityriasis lichenoides et varioliformis acuta) are not discussed in this article

Medium-sized vessel vasculitis

- Inflammation within the wall of medium-sized vessels, defined as those located at the junction of the dermis and subcutis or within the subcutis
- Vessels should be at least twice the size of small vessels in the papillary dermis and may have smooth muscle in their walls
- See discussion in text, Medium vessel vasculitis.

(Continued)

Box 1
Definitions of important terms used when describing leukocytoclastic vasculitis and microvascular occlusion (*continued*)

Microvascular occlusion

- Filling of the lumen of a vessel by fibrin thrombi, immunoglobulins including cryoglobulins, or other materials
- Vasculopathy often used as a synonym in clinical practice

Palpable purpura

- Purpura that is generally composed of papules, which are less than 1 cm in diameter, raised, and partially blanchable
- Papules may overlap and form larger, confluent areas

Pseudobranching

- Interconnection and confluence of papular purpura into plaques with darker interconnecting centers

Purpura

- Extravasation of erythrocytes into the skin

Retiform purpura

- See Branching, previously
- Sometimes used exclusively to refer to purpura/necrosis in solid polygonal to stellate shapes with irregular linear/jagged borders

Small vessel vasculitis

- LCV affecting small vessels of the dermis and sometimes subcutis

Vasculitis

- Inflammation and damage of the vascular wall

Vasculopathy

- In its broadest definition, damage to vessels and, therefore, would encompass both vasculitis and microvascular occlusion
- In the clinical setting, often used more narrowly as a synonym of microvascular occlusion

---

antineutrophil cytoplasmic antibody (ANCA)-associated vasculitis or calciphylaxis, also can be pauci-random, displaying fewer lesions in no obvious pattern.[3,4]

RELEVANT CLINICAL CONSIDERATIONS

LEUKOCYTOCLASTIC VASCULITIS

LCV is defined in **Box 1**, and, in well-developed lesions, there is fibrinoid necrosis of vessels (seen as fibrin cuffing around damaged vessels) with leukocytoclasia and extravasated erythrocytes intermingling with intact perivascular neutrophils. Early lesions may be subtle without obvious fibrin (see **Fig. 1**B). Late lesions may be relatively pauci-neutrophilic (see **Fig. 1**F).[5,6]

The depth of involvement of LCV is important. LCV involving the superficial vascular plexus alone (see **Fig. 1**B, F) is more likely to be limited to the skin compared with LCV that involves superficial

and deep vessels (see **Fig. 1**D).[7] The deeper vessels that are involved may be small vessels or larger and considered medium-sized (for the skin).[8] Deep involvement more commonly is seen in association with systemic disease.[7,9]

LCV has been described as the primary histopathologic pattern for urticarial vasculitis,[10] acute hemorrhagic edema of infancy[11] (also termed, postinfectious cockade purpura), and hypergammaglobulinemic purpura of Waldenström[12] (also termed, recurrent macular vasculitis in hypergammaglobulinemia).[13] Although early lesions of LCV can be subtle and eventually develop more obvious fibrin cuffing over time, urticarial vasculitis generally does not seem to progress further than early LCV and may lack well-developed fibrin cuffing.[5,14] Acute hemorrhagic edema of infancy has findings of perivascular neutrophils and leukocytoclasia with or without fibrinoid necrosis.[11,15] Histopathologic findings of hypergammaglobulinemic

Table 1
Variants of pigmented purpuric eruptions[a]

Disease Name	Histopathologic Differences	Clinical Morphologic Differences
Schamberg disease[b]	PEEL	• Lower legs • Yellow-brown patches with superimposed petechiae resembling sprinkled cayenne pepper
Purpura annularis telangiectodes of Majocchi[e]	PEEL	• Trunk, thighs • 1–3 cm annular plaques with petechiae and telangiectasia in border
Eczematid-like purpura of Doucas and Kapetenakis[c]	PEEL plus spongiosis	• Lower legs • Associated pruritus • Scaly macules, papules, patches with hemorrhage
Pigmented purpuric lichenoid dermatitis of Gougerot and Blum	LEE	• Lower legs • Schamberg-like lesions plus lichenoid/purpuric papules
Lichen aureus[d]	LEE	• Lower extremity • Unilateral • Golden to purple patch
Granulomatous	Granulomatous inflammation with extravasated erythrocytes	• Lower legs • Brown patches with purpuric papules
Linear pigmented purpura	PEEL	• Extremities • Unilateral • Schamberg-like or lichen aureus–like

Abbreviations: LEE, lichenoid infiltrate with extravasated erythrocytes; PEEL, perivascular extravasated erythrocytes and lymphocytes.
[a] Synonyms include pigmented purpuric dermatosis, capillaritis, purpura pigmentosa chronica, purpura simplex, and Majocchi-Schamberg disease
[b] Synonyms include Schamberg purpura, progressive pigmentary dermatosis of Schamberg, and purpura pigmentosa progressive
[c] Synonyms include itching purpura and eczematoid purpura
[d] Synonym includes lichen purpuricus
[e] Synonym includes Majocchi disease

purpura of Waldenström (secondary to hyper-IgG or hyper-IgA) are variably described as those of LCV or a lymphocytic vasculitis.[12,16] It is possible that early lesions show LCV and later lesions are lymphocyte-predominant. Changes of LCV also may be seen in diseases with a more diffuse pattern of dermal neutrophils, like Sweet syndrome (in which the LCV changes are considered secondary to the neutrophil-rich inflammatory infiltrate),[5] erythema elevatum diutinum,[5] and early palisaded neutrophilic granulomatous dermatitis (which some investigators report begins as LCV).[17]

Medium Vessel Vasculitis

Medium vessel vasculitis are addressed briefly, because certain systemic vasculitides (eg, ANCA-associated vasculitis and vasculitis in the setting of other connective tissue disorders) involve both small-sized and medium-sized vessels.[5] Note that true medium-sized vessels, if defined as the size of a renal artery, are not present in the skin. In the skin, however, it is acceptable to define medium-sized vessels as larger vessels at the junction of the dermis or subcutis or within the subcutis, generally twice the size of the papillary dermal small vessels.[8] Clinically, involvement of cutaneous medium-sized vessels is suggested by the presence of livedo racemosa, nodules, cutaneous ulcers, and/or digital gangrene.[1] LCV of both small-sized and medium-sized vessels in the same biopsy generally corresponds to palpable purpura.

Box 2
Key differential diagnosis of leukocytoclastic vasculitis or microvascular occlusion as the major histopathologic finding

Leukocytoclastic vasculitis (LCV)

  Cutaneous single-organ small vessel vasculitis

  IgA vasculitis

  Mixed cryoglobulinemia[a]

  ANCA-associated vasculitis (including palisaded neutrophilic granulomatous dermatitis, early)

  Rheumatic vasculitis[b]

  Infections[b] (eg, meningococcemia[a] and sepsis[b])

  Levamisole-associated vasculitis[a,b]

Both LCV and microvascular occlusion

  Levamisole-associated vasculitis

  Certain infections (eg, meningococcemia)

  Monoclonal or mixed cryoglobulinemia[26]

  Leukemic vasculitis

Microvascular occlusion

  Examples secondary to coagulopathy

    Sepsis-associated (eg, in setting of septic shock and disseminated intravascular coagulation)

    Hereditary or acquired deficiencies in coagulation

    Calciphylaxis

    Warfarin-associated

    Heparin-associated

    Thrombocythemia

  Examples secondary to vascular occlusion by material other than/in addition to fibrin

    Antiphospholipid syndrome

    Monoclonal cryoglobulinemia

    Angioinvasive fungal organisms

    Intravascular B-cell lymphoma

    Cholesterol emboli

    Oxalosis

    Intravascular metastatic cancer (eg, inflammatory carcinoma of the breast)

    Hydrophilic polymers (iatrogenic)

[a]Also may have concomitant vascular occlusion. [b]Also may present with microvascular occlusion alone.

Polyarteritis nodosa (PAN), a medium vessel vasculitis that affects arteries of the kidney, heart, gastrointestinal system, and other organs, occasionally can present in the skin. PAN, as a term, creates confusion because there are 2 other diseases with similar names—benign cutaneous PAN (although the "benign cutaneous" often is neglected and dropped) and microscopic polyangiitis. These 3 diseases typically are distinct (**Table 3**),[1] although all 3 overlap in their cutaneous manifestations of medium vessel vasculitis. Microscopic polyangiitis, distinctively of the 3, can affect small vessels with corresponding glomerulonephritis, pulmonary capillaritis, and cutaneous small vessel vasculitis.[1]

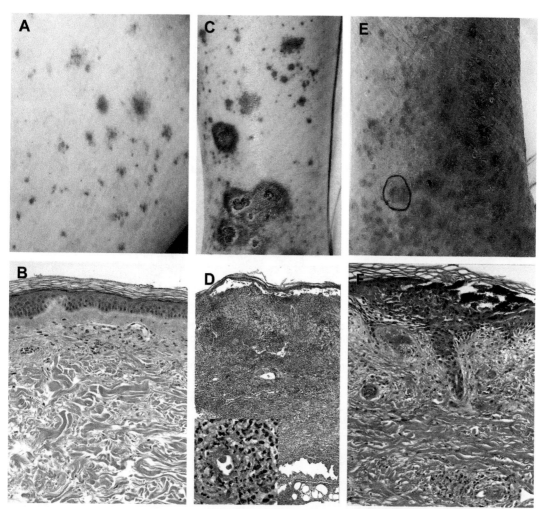

Fig. 1. (A, C, E) Papular purpura is a term used for a range of lesions, ranging from macules to lesions with central ulceration. Clinically, such lesions are termed, palpable purpura, and typically are seen on dependent sites (eg, legs and feet) as dark pink to bright red to purple macules and papules. (A) Very early lesions that may blanch to some degree with pressure, with (B) corresponding sparse perivascular neutrophils with very subtle leukocytoclasia and minimal vascular damage. (C) Well-developed lesions; this patient has a range of lesions from macular to papular to ulcerated, with typical microscopic findings of (D) fibrin cuffing, leukocytoclasia, neutrophils, and extravasated erythrocytes. (B, E) Involvement of superficial vessels is more common than (D) superficial and deep involvement. (E) Late lesions have dull red-brown erythema, and neutrophils can be the minority of the mixed infiltrate with lymphocytes; and (F) there can be foci of luminal occlusion. (B, D, F) Hematoxylin and eosin, original magnifications ×100.

Superficial thrombophlebitis (inflammation of a medium-sized vein) can be difficult to distinguish from cutaneous PAN, particularly in samples from the lower leg, where veins may develop thicker, muscular walls. A well-developed internal elastic lamina can support that a medium-sized vessel is an artery, but that structure may be destroyed by vasculitis.[18] It has been suggested that the pattern of smooth muscle deposition in vessels walls may be more reliable than the presence of internal elastic lamina, with a continuous wreath muscular pattern favoring arteries and a bundled muscular and collagen pattern favoring veins.[19]

Microvascular Occlusion

Fibrin thrombi are the most common cause of occlusion. The color of fibrin varies by laboratory, but generally it is a deeper pink than surrounding dermal collagen. Thrombi may be difficult to find and can be limited to occasional small vessels in the superficial dermis or the fat; not all vessels may be involved in a given specimen. Involvement of small vessels in the fat is not specific but has been described most commonly in cases of calciphylaxis.[20]

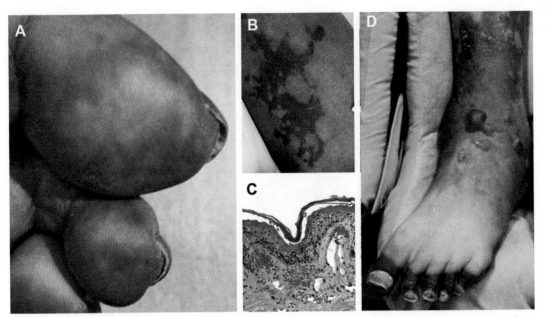

Fig. 2. Branching purpura includes a nonblanchable netlike vascular pattern ([A] livedoid) to solid areas of purpura with radiating jagged, interrupted lines ([B] retiform purpura) to solid purpura with irregular borders ([D] shin) to digital gangrene ([D] toes). There can be blisters or associated necrosis. (C) Branching purpura corresponds to microvascular occlusion. (C) Hematoxylin and eosin, original magnification ×200.

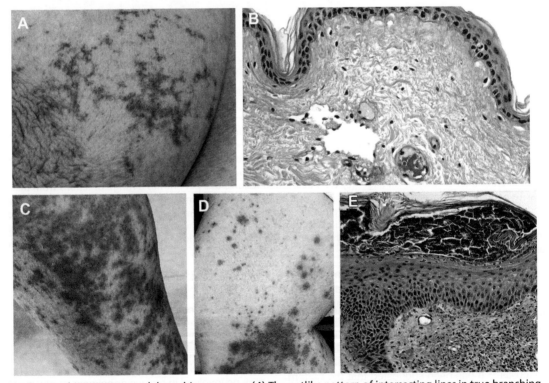

Fig. 3. Branching versus pseudobranching purpura. (A) The netlike pattern of intersecting lines in true branching, which is due to (B) microvascular occlusion can be confused with (C, D) pseudobranching. Pseudobranching is the result of interconnecting circles of purpura that often have central darker accentuation. Lesions with central change (C) correspond to LCV with epidermal changes (eg, [E] superficial crusting). (C, D) A clue for pseudobranching is the presence of discrete 0.4-cm to 0.9-cm–diameter circular lesions outside of interconnecting foci. Pseudobranching is a suggestive of IgA vasculitis. (B) Hematoxylin and eosin, original magnification ×200.

Table 2
Most characteristic distribution of purpura in selected disorders

Distribution	Disorders with Vasculitis	Disorders with Microvascular Occlusion
Dependent	Cutaneous single-organ small vessel vasculitis IgA vasculitis Mixed cryoglobulinemia	Antiphospholipid syndrome Monoclonal cryglobulinemia Calciphylaxis Livedoid vasculopathy
Pauci-random	ANCA-associated vasculitis	Infections (eg, angioinvasive fungal in immunosuppressed) Calciphylaxis
Acral[a]	Levamisole-associated vasculitis Mixed cryoglobulinemia ANCA-associated vasculitis (eg, digital gangrene)	Sepsis-associated Levamisole-associated vasculopathy Monoclonal cryoglobulinemia Antiphospholipid syndrome Other emboli, for example, cholesterol
Generalized	Single-organ cutaneous small vessel vasculitis IgA vasculitis	Sepsis-associated Levamisole-associated vasculopathy Calciphylaxis Catastrophic antiphospholipid syndrome
Over fatty areas (eg. breasts, abdomen, thighs)		Calciphylaxis Levamisole-associated Warfarin necrosis Antiphospholipid syndrome[b]

[a] Here, acral refers to concentration of lesions on acral sites without major involvement of forearms/lower legs
[b] More typically involves dependent areas

Table 3
Polyarteritis and polyangiitis—three different diseases with similar names

Disease Name	Major Systemic Features	Major Cutaneous Features Related to Medium Vessel Vasculitis	Major Cutaneous Features Related to Small Vessel Vasculitis
Classic PAN[a]	Fever, fatigue, weight loss, muscle/joint pain. neuropathy, hypertension, renal and gastrointestinal involvement, myocardial infarction or failure, scleritis, testicular infarction	0.5–2 cm nodules or ulcers Livedo racemosa	
Benign cutaneous PAN (cutaneous PAN)	Neuropathy, fever, malaise Absence of renal, pulmonary, gastrointestinal involvement	Like classic PAN	
Microscopic polyangiitis[b]	*Necrotizing glomerulonephritis* *Pulmonary capillaritis*	Like classic PAN	*Palpable purpura*

Manifestations of small vessel involvement are in italics.
[a] Deficiency of adenosine deaminase 2 (small vessel vasculitis and medium vessel vasculitis that affect the skin, brain, gastrointestinal tract, kidneys; mutation of adenosine deaminase 2 [*ADA2*], previously known as *CECR1*, with low plasma levels of ADA2 and IgM) is in the differential diagnosis.
[b] Also can have urticarial lesions.

In addition to fibrin, vessels can be occluded by other materials. Monoclonal cryoglobulinemia generally shows occlusion of small vessels by bright pink, smooth material (reminiscent of a wash of watercolor paint). Intravascular histiocytosis and intravascular B-cell lymphoma have intravascular histiocytes or atypical B cells, respectively. Infectious processes, especially fungal organisms, may occlude and destroy vessels (**Fig. 4**A), particularly in neutropenic patients. For any of these disorders, there may be variable amounts of intravascular fibrin.

Direct Immunofluorescence Testing

According to the European League Against Rheumatisms criteria for IgA vasculitis (Henoch-Schönlein purpura), in the setting of dependent palpable purpura, just 1 more of 4 criteria needs to be fulfilled. These criteria include (1) predominant IgA deposition in any biopsy, (2) diffuse abdominal pain, (3) renal involvement (hematuria or proteinuria), and (4) acute joint pain.[21] Given these criteria, direct immunofluorescence testing of the skin (or kidney) can be useful to establishing the diagnosis.

Although IgA is the predominant immunoreactant in superficial vessels of the dermis of Henoch-Schönlein purpura, C3 and other immunoglobulins may be detectable as well.[22] Deposition of immunoreactants, including IgA, is not specific to IgA vasculitis, and some studies have described nonspecific deposition in the lower legs manifesting in a variety of different clinical diseases, including stasis dermatitis as well as erythema nodosum.[22] Thus, deposition of IgA or other immunoreactants should be interpreted in the context of the patient presentation as well as histopathologic findings.

Other diseases with vascular damage may have positive direct immunofluorescence. Cryoglobulinemia or rheumatic vasculitis (associated with connective tissue disease) may have IgM deposits, and urticarial vasculitis may have deposits of C3.[23] The lupus band, continuous granular deposition of C3 and immunoglobulins along the basement membrane zone, may be detected.[23]

DISCUSSION: SELECTED DISEASES WITH LEUKOCYTOCLASTIC VASCULITIS OR MICROVASCULAR OCCLUSION

CUTANEOUS SINGLE-ORGAN SMALL VESSEL VASCULITIS

Synonyms for cutaneous single-organ small vessel vasculitis are cutaneous leukocytoclastic angiitis, localized cutaneous vasculitis, hypersensitivity vasculitis, and primary cutaneous small vessel vasculitis.

The most common presentation is palpable purpura on the legs and feet (dependent sites). Lesions also may involve the trunk (especially lower abdomen) or arms. Early lesions may be macular (flat, <1 cm), whereas confluence of lesions may produce larger plaques. The centers of lesions can become necrotic, blister, or ulcerate. Generally, lesions are asymptomatic. Histopathologic findings are those of LCV (discussed previously; see **Box 1**), generally concentrated around superficial vessels, although deep involvement does not exclude this diagnosis.

Some patients may have systemic symptoms including fever or joint pain.[24] If the latter is accepted for an isolated single-organ cutaneous small vessel vasculitis, distinction from IgA vasculitis becomes less clear.[24] Many cases of isolated cutaneous small vessel vasculitis are idiopathic.[7] Other cases can be presumed secondary to infection (eg, *Streptococcus*), medication reaction (eg, antibiotics), connective tissue disease, or malignancy (eg, hematologic).[7] Importantly, IgA vasculitis can present clinically in much the same way.

IgA VASCULITIS

Clinically, IgA vasculitis and isolated cutaneous small vessel vasculitis can be indistinguishable, with palpable purpura corresponding to LCV (superficial more often than superficial and deep involvement; discussed previously); IgA vasculitis represents the vast majority of small vessel vasculitis in pediatric patients. A minority of cases may have patterning of the purpura, with a pseudo-branching pattern (see **Fig. 3**).[2] The classic tetrad involves palpable purpura, renal involvement (eg, hematuria and proteinuria), gastrointestinal involvement (eg, emesis and diarrhea), and joint pain.

Direct immunofluorescence testing (discussed previously) and evaluation for gastrointestinal, joint, and renal involvement are necessary to make this diagnosis. Different criteria have been proposed for IgA vasculitis,[22] but ,at their simplest, criteria include dependent palpable purpura plus 1 more of the following: predominant IgA deposition in skin or kidney and diffuse abdominal pain, acute arthritis/arthralgias of any joint, and/or hematuria/proteinuria.[21]

URTICARIAL VASCULITIS

Urticarial vasculitis may be associated with systemic lupus erythematosus, Sjögren syndrome,

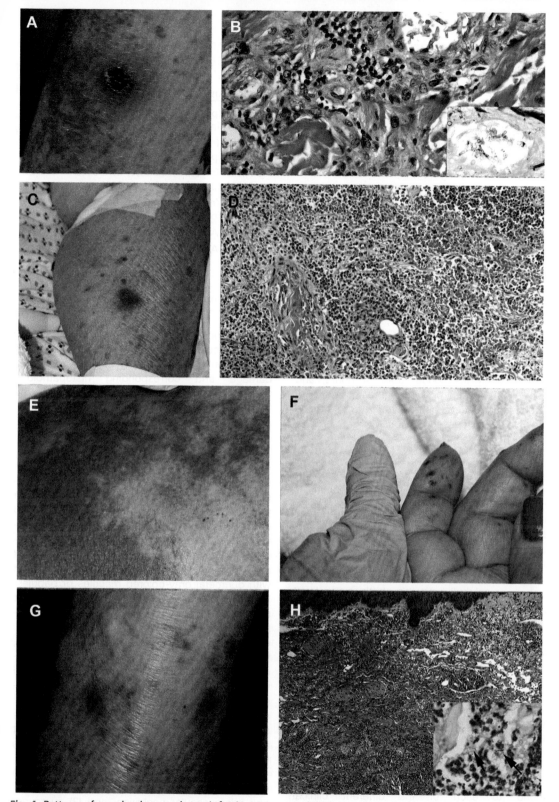

Fig. 4. Patterns of vascular damage due to infectious processes. (*A*) Ulcerated papule due to (*B*) angioinvasive fungal organisms occluding and destroying small vessels ([*inset*] Gomori methenamine silver staining). (*C, D*) Papular purpura (*C*) corresponding to LCV (*D*) in a patient with sepsis and disseminated intravascular coagulation. (*E*) Septic shock with associated purpura fulminans and disseminated intravascular coagulation corresponding to microvascular occlusion. Note solid areas of purpura bordered by irregular branching. (*F*) Purpuric papules on the fingers; this morphology can correspond to septic emboli (vascular occlusion with detectable bacteria and some degree of vasculitis). (*G, H*) Purpuric papules on the right leg only (*G*) with a neutrophil-rich infiltrate and scattered atypical mycobacteria ([*H, inset*] acid-fast bacterial stain). (*B*) Hematoxylin and eosin, original magnification ×400. (*D*) Hematoxylin and eosin, original magnification ×200. (*H*) Hematoxylin and eosin, original magnification 100×.

Table 4
Antineutrophil cytoplasmic antibody–associated diseases.[1]

Disease	Typical Antineutrophilic Cytoplasmic Antibody
Granulomatosis with polyangiitis	c-ANCA (proteinase-3) in ~70% p-ANCA in ~25%
Eosinophilic granulomatosis with polyangiitis	p-ANCA (myeloperoxidase) in ~70% c-ANCA (proteinase-3) in ~10%
Microscopic polyangiitis	p-ANCA (myeloperoxidase) in ~60% c-ANCA (proteinase-3) in ~30%
Classic PAN	p-ANCA (myeloperoxidase) in ~20% c-ANCA (proteinase-3) in ~10%
Levamisole-associated vasculitis/vasculopathy	Atypical ANCA[a]
Other (eg, inflammatory bowel disease, chronic active hepatitis, rheumatoid arthritis, systemic lupus erythematosus)	Atypical ANCA[a]

[a] Atypical ANCA is present in both the cytoplasm and perinuclear areas and this pattern is detectable only with ethanol or acetone fixation; antigens vary but include neutrophil elastase.

and/or hypocomplementemia.[25,26] Clinical lesions are urticarial, edematous plaques that are a deeper red compared with urticaria. Lesions may burn, typically last longer than 24 hours, and resolve with bruising or hyperpigmentation.[10] Histopathologic features generally are at most those of early LCV (discussed previously).[5,14]

MIXED CRYOGLOBULINEMIA

Mixed cryoglobulinemia, or types II and III cryoglobulinemia, generally is secondary to hepatitis C infection. Type II cryoglobulinemia also can be associated with autoimmune connective tissue disorders (eg, systemic lupus erythematosus) and type III with lymphoproliferative disorders. As opposed to monoclonal cryoglobulinemia, in which there is only monoclonal IgM>>IgA>IgG, type II cryoglobulinemia has both monoclonal IgM>>IgA>IgG with rheumatoid factor activity and polyclonal IgG. Type III cryoglobulinemia has circulating polyclonal IgM>>IgA>IgG (sometimes with rheumatoid factor activity) and polyclonal IgG.

The lower legs typically are affected by purpuric macules and papules; there also may be involvement of the trunk and upper extremities.[27] Histopathologic findings are those of LCV, either affecting superficial vessels only or superficial and deep vessels; there may be associated microvascular occlusion.[27]

ANCA-associated diseases include those in Table 4. Different histopathologic findings correspond to each of the different clinical manifestations (Table 5).

RHEUMATIC VASCULITIS

Rheumatic diseases that can cause palpable purpura include lupus erythematosus, rheumatoid arthritis, and Sjögren syndrome. Lupus erythematosus is a complex connective tissue disease that has different cutaneous manifestations of vascular damage and corresponding histopathology (Table 6).

INFECTIONS (EG, MENINGOCOCCEMIA AND SEPSIS)

Clinical manifestations of infectious diseases, with corresponding vasculitis or microvascular occlusion, have different morphologies.[28] Ulcerated papules, sometimes with a purpuric border and often with associated eschar, are a typical manifestation of ecthyma gangrenosum and angioinvasive fungal organisms in immunosuppressed patients (Fig. 4A, B).[28] Neisseria are associated with gunmetal gray-colored macules or papules; lesions may expand into large areas of confluent necrosis.[29] When sepsis is secondary to a bacterial nidus (eg, vegetations on the heart valves), emboli may lodge in small vessels of the skin, with corresponding papular, purpuric lesions typically on the hands (Fig. 4F).[30,31] Sepsis associated with disseminated intravascular coagulation presents with branching purpura on acral sites[31] and/or symmetric peripheral gangrene[31]; sepsis subsequently can manifest rapidly with confluent areas of skin necrosis with jagged borders (Fig. 4E).

Three different vascular patterns may be evident: (1) LCV alone (Fig. 4C, D), (2) mixed LCV and microvascular occlusion, and (3) microvascular occlusion alone.[13,28,31] These 3 patterns may or may not contain detectable organisms in the same cutaneous tissue sections; they are not specific to any particular infectious process, although certain infections have been described

Table 5
Pathologic correlate of typical manifestations of antineutrophil cytoplasmic antibody–associated vasculitides

Histopathology	Clinical Correlate
Granulomatosis with Polyangiitis (Pulmonary Lesions, Sinusitis)	
LCV	Palpable purpura
Medium vessel vasculitis	Digital gangrene Subcutaneous nodules Ulcerations
Palisaded granulomatous and neutrophilic dermatitis[a]	Papulonodules, characteristically on the elbows, sometimes umbilicated/ulcerated
Granulomatous inflammation	Strawberry gums
Eosinophilic granulomatosis with polyangiitis (asthma, allergic rhinitis, eosinophilia [blood and tissue])	
LCV	Palpable purpura
Eosinophils and neutrophils	Urticaria
Palisaded granulomatous and neutrophilic dermatitis[a]	Papulonodules characteristically on the scalp and extremities
Microscopic polyangiitis (necrotizing glomerulonephritis, pulmonary capillaritis)	
LCV	Palpable purpura
Medium vessel vasculitis	Livedo racemosa, nodules

Three major antineutrophil cytoplasmic antibody–associated vasculitides are granulomatosis with polyangiitis, eosinophilic granulomatosis with polyangiitis, and microscopic polyangiitis.

[a] Centers of palisade may be bluer in GPA and more pink-red in EGPA; PNGD also may be associated with other connective tissue disorders (eg, lupus erythematosus).

more with 1 pattern than another. For example, *Neisseria* infections have features of mixed LCV and occlusion.[29,31,32] Septic shock can have associated coagulopathy and derangements in protein C and protein S, leading to disseminated intravascular coagulation and microscopic findings of vascular occlusion of small vessels.[32] Classic septic emboli, which also may be associated with positive blood cultures, often contain detectable organisms, with or without vascular occlusion and/or associated inflammation.[33] Similarly, angioinvasive fungal organisms destroy and

Table 6
Lupus erythematosus: cutaneous manifestations with vascular damage

Vascular Pathology	Clinical Correlate
LCV	Palpable purpura
Early LCV[a]	Urticarial vasculitis
Thickened, pink walls of superficial vessels, sometimes with PAS-positive material in lumina	Atrophie blanche[b] Livedoid vasculopathy[b]
Microvascular occlusion	Livedo reticularis or livedo racemosa, often with associated antiphospholipid syndrome[b] CAPS
Palisaded neutrophilic and granulomatous dermatitis[c]	Papulonodules, sometimes umbilicated

Lupus erythematosus can present with skin lesions due to vasculitis or occlusion.

[a] Without well-developed fibrinoid necrosis of vessels.

[b] Also can be a manifestation of lupus erythematosus or idiopathic/primary.

[c] Also can be associated with other diseases (eg, granulomatosis with polyangiitis).

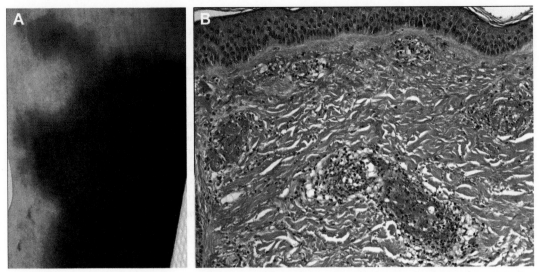

Fig. 5. Mixed LCV and microvascular occlusion in levamisole-associated vasculopathy. The bright red, branching border surrounding a dark center is characteristic of levamisole-associated vasculopathy (*A*). This pattern (*B*) also can be seen with certain infectious processes like meningococcemia. (*B*) Hematoxylin and eosin, original magnification ×200.

occlude vessels with variable inflammation.[34] Other infectious organisms also may cause papular purpura (eg, atypical mycobacteria [**Fig. 4**G, H]).

LEVAMISOLE-ASSOCIATED VASCULOPATHY

Levamisole is an antihelmintic drug that is tasteless and of a white, powdery consistency that is used as a cutting agent for cocaine. Levamisole alone, which was used to treat nephrotic syndrome in children, or levamisole-adulterated cocaine, can cause branching purpura that most typically is on acral sites (characteristically the ear) but may become generalized.[35,36] Clinical lesions can be extensive or limited with a typical dark purple-black center and bright red border.

As with infectious processes, 3 different vascular patterns can be seen—LCV alone, mixed LCV and microvascular occlusion (**Fig. 5**), and microvascular occlusion alone.

ANTIPHOSPHOLIPID SYNDROME

Clinical criteria for antiphospholipid syndrome include detection of anticardiolipin antibodies, lupus anticoagulant, or anti-β_2-glycoprotein I antibodies on 2 separate occasions, at least 12 weeks apart. These need to be present in the setting of vascular thrombosis in any organ or pregnancy morbidity.[37] Histopathologic findings, when diagnostic,[37] are those of microvascular occlusion.

The most common cutaneous finding is fixed netlike lesions (a livedo pattern) on dependent sites and/or the trunk, either continuous (livedo reticularis) or coarser and broken up (livedo racemosa).[37,38] The interconnecting rings that make up the netlike pattern are of variable diameter, usually 1 cm to 4 cm. This size is dependent on the body site and is related directly to the surface area of skin supplied by an individual arteriole. Other cutaneous lesions include ulcerations, digital gangrene, atrophie blanche–like lesions, splinter hemorrhage, and anetoderma.[37,38] Nonspecific purpuric macules and papules can be present and resemble lesions of LCV (palpable purpura).[9]

Two particular clinical presentations of note include Sneddon syndrome and catastrophic antiphospholipid syndrome (CAPS) (also known as Asherson syndrome). Sneddon syndrome is the combination of livedoid lesions with labile hypertension and cerebrovascular disease, often in young women[38]; a subset of Sneddon syndrome patients have deficiency of adenosine deaminase 2 (see **Table 3**).[39] CAPS, in terms of skin findings and associated triggers, can present much like purpura fulminans, with extensive purpura and necrosis, often including digital gangrene.[38] Systemic involvement of kidneys, lungs, brain, and heart is common. Triggers are similar to purpura fulminans and include infections, obstetric complication, trauma, and medication reactions. CAPS may be associated with systemic lupus erythematosus.

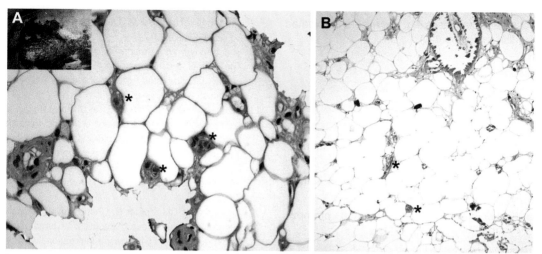

Fig. 6. Calciphylaxis. [*Inset*] Eschar with branching borders. (*A*) So-called pannicular thrombosis often is evident (*asterisks*), and, although not fully diagnostic, calciphylaxis can be suspected on the basis of this finding alone. The initial biopsy in this patient showed only focal thrombi in small vessels in the fat. Such pannicular thrombosis, although not fully diagnostic, should raise suspicion for calciphylaxis in the correct clinical setting. (*B*) An incisional biopsy 1 week later was typical of calciphylaxis with calcified vessels, interstitial calcium, and microvascular occlusion (*asterisks*). (*A*) Hematoxylin and eosin, original magnification ×200. (*B*) Hematoxylin and eosin, original magnification ×100.

LIVEDOID VASCULOPATHY

Synonyms for livedoid vasculopathy are livedo reticularis with summer ulcerations, segmental hyalinizing vasculitis, livedo vasculitis, hypersensitivity-type vasculitis, and painful purpuric ulcers with reticular pattern of the lower extremities (PURPLE).[38]

Narrowly defined, livedoid vasculopathy refers to a clinical presentation of branching purpura, generally on the feet/ankles, with interspersed shallow ulcers that heal as approximately 1-cm porcelain-white stellate scars. Ideally, the white scars have associated peripheral telangiectasia; these scars are termed, *atrophie blanche*. Atrophie blanche can be present in individuals as an isolated finding without associated purpura or systemic findings.[38]

Both livedoid vasculopathy and atrophie blanche have similar histopathologic findings with hyalinization of superficial vessels with fibrin in the walls and sometimes thrombi within lumina.[5]

MONOCLONAL CRYOGLOBULINEMIA (TYPE I CRYOGLOBULINEMIA)

Monoclonal cryoglobulinemia is secondary to circulating monoclonal IgM>IgG>>IgA that precipitates with cold, particularly affecting small vessels in acral sites where body temperature is lower. Monoclonal cryoglobulinemia may be secondary to a hematologic abnormality. Acral involvement (eg, hands, feet, and ears) is typical.[27]

Typical cases of monoclonal cryoglobulinemia have findings of microvascular occlusion (discussed previously). Inflammation generally is absent.[27]

CALCIPHYLAXIS

Early lesions of calciphylaxis typically affect the thigh with branching purpura. Later lesions of calciphylaxis are classically ulcerated with dark black adherent eschar; a bright red border may be present.

Although the most diagnostic finding of calciphylaxis is deposition of calcium in the intimal layer of vessels of the subcutaneous, microvascular occlusion of small capillaries in the fat, which has been termed, *pannicular thrombosis*, is characteristic (**Fig. 6**),[20] especially in the setting of branching purpura on the thigh with extreme pain.[40] Other findings that may be present include interstitial calcification of the dermis or subcutis, necrosis, calcification around eccrine glands,[40] and a neutrophilic infiltrate in the dermis or subcutis. The combination of vascular calcification and thrombosis in the same biopsy is highly suggestive of calciphylaxis.[41]

SUMMARY

Comprehensive analysis of vasculitis and microvascular occlusion includes depth of involvement and reporting of medium-sized vessel involvement if present. Presence of both vasculitis and occlusion affecting the same vessels also is suggestive of particular diagnoses (eg, levamisole-associated vasculitis/vasculopathy).

DISCLOSURE

The authors have nothing to disclose. There are no funding sources for this article.

REFERENCES

1. Piette WW. Primary systemic vasculitis. In: Sontheimer RD, Provost TT, editors. Cutaneous manifestations of rheumatic disease. 2nd edition. Philadelphia, PA: Lippincott Williams and Wilkins; 2004. p. 159–76.
2. Stone MS, Piette WW. A cutaneous sign of IgA-associated small dermal vessel leukocytoclastic vasculitis in adults (Henoch-Schönlein purpura). Arch Dermatol 1989;125:53–6.
3. Piette WW. The differential diagnosis of purpura from a morphologic perspective. Adv Dermatol 1994;9:3–23.
4. Wetter DA, Dutz JP, Shinkai K, et al. Cutaneous vasculitis. In: Bolognia JL, Schaffer JV, Cerroni L, editors. Dermatology. 4th edition. China: Elsevier; 2018. p. 409–39.
5. Carlson JA. The histological assessment of cutaneous vasculitis. Histopathology 2010;56:3–23.
6. Zax RH, Hodge SJ, Callen JP. Cutaneous leukocytoclastic vasculitis. Serial histopathologic evaluation demonstrates the dynamic nature of the infiltrate. Arch Dermatol 1990;126:69–72.
7. Sanchez NP, Van Hale HM, Su WP. Clinical and histopathologic spectrum of necrotizing vasculitis. Report of findings in 101 cases. Arch Dermatol 1985;121:220–4.
8. Yen A, Braverman IM. Ultrastructure of the human dermal microcirculation: the horizontal plexus of the papillary dermis. J Invest Dermatol 1976;66:131–42.
9. Gehlhausen JR, Wetter DA, Nelson C, et al. A detailed analysis of the distribution, morphology, and histopathology of complex purpura in hospitalized patients: a case series of 68 patients. J Am Acad Dermatol 2020; S0190-9622(20):30771–4.
10. Sanchez NP, Winkelmann RK, Schroeter AL, et al. The clinical and histopathologic spectrums of urticarial vasculitis: study of forty cases. J Am Acad Dermatol 1982;7:599–605.
11. Ince E, Mumcu Y, Suskan E, et al. Infantile acute hemorrhagic edema: a variant of leukocytoclastic vasculitis. Pediatr Dermatol 1995;12:224–7.
12. Yamamoto T, Yokoyama A. Hypergammaglobulinemic pupura associated with Sjögren's syndrome and chronic C type hepatitis. J Dermatol 1997;24:7–11.
13. Sunderkötter CH, Zelger B, Chen K, et al. Nomenclature of cutaneous vasculitis: Dermatologic addendum to the 2012 revised international Chapel Hill consensus conference nomenclature of vasculitides. Arthritis Rheum 2017;70:171–84.
14. Hodge SJ, Callen JP, Ekenstam E. Cutaneous leukocytoclastic vasculitis: correlation of histopathological changes with clinical severity and course. J Cutan Pathol 1987;14:279–84.
15. Legrain V, Lejean S, Taïeb A, et al. Infantile acute hemorrhagic edema of the skin: study of ten cases. J Am Acad Dermatol 1991;24:17–22.
16. Finder KA, McCollough ML, Dixon S, et al. Hypergammaglobulinemic purpura of Waldeström. J Am Acad Dermatol 1990;23:669–76.
17. Chu P, Connolly MK, LeBoit PE. The histopathologic spectrum of palisaded neutrophilic and granulomatous dermatitis in patients with collagen vascular disease. Arch Dermatol 1994;130:1278–93.
18. Hall LD, Dalton SR, Fillman EP, et al. Re-examination of features to distinguish polyarteritis nodosa from superficial thrombophlebitis. Am J Dermatopathol 2013;35:462–71.
19. Dalton SR, Fillman EP, Ferringer T, et al. Smooth muscle pattern is more reliable than the presence or absence of an internal elastic lamina in distinguishing an artery from a vein. J Cutan Pathol 2006;33:216–9.
20. El-Azhary RA, Patzelt MT, McBane RD, et al. Calciphylaxis: a disease of pannicular thrombosis. Mayo Clin Proc 2016;91:1395–402.
21. Ozen S, Ruperto N, Dillon MJ, et al. EULAR/PReS endorsed consensus criteria for the classification of childhood vasculitides. Ann Rheum Dis 2006;65:936–41.
22. Helander SD, De Castro FR, Gibson LE. Henoch-Schönlein purpura: clincopathologic correlation of cutaneous vascular IgA deposits and the relationship to leukocytoclastic vasculitis. Acta Derm Venereol 1995;75:125–9.
23. Goesser MR, Laniosz V, Wetter DA. A practical approach to the diagnosis, evaluation, and management of cutaneous small-vessel vasculitis. Am J Clin Dermatol 2014;15:299–306.

24. Arora A, Wetter DA, Gonzalex-Santiago MD, et al. Incidence of leukocytoclastic vasculitis, 1996 to 2010: a population-based study in Olmsted County, Minnesota. Mayo Clin Proc 2014;89:1515–24.

25. Valentin DO, Alzghouls B, Urbine D. Hypocomplementemic urticarial vasculitis: a rare cause of emphysema. J Thorac Imaging 2012;27(3):W50–1. https://doi.org/10.1016/j.chest.2019.08.1163.

26. Aydogan K, Karadogan SK, Adim SB, et al. Hypocomplementemic urticarial vasculitis: a rare presentation of systemic lupus erythematosus. Int J Dermatol 2006;45:1057–61.

27. Cohen SJ, Pittelkow MR, Su WPD. Cutaneous manifestations of cryoglobulinemia: clinical and histopathologic study of seventy-two patients. J Am Acad Dermatol 1991;25:21–7.

28. Georgesen C, Fox LP, Harp J. Part I: retiform purpura: a diagnostic approach. J Am Acad Dermatol 2019. https://doi.org/10.1016/j.jaad.2019.07.112.

29. Hill WR, Kinney TD. The cutaneous lesions in acute meningococcemia; a clinical and pathologic study. J Am Med Assoc 1947;134:513–8.

30. Martinez-Mera C, Fraga J, Capusan Tm, et al. Vasculopathies, cutaneous necrosis and emergency in dermatology. G Ital Dermatol Venereol 2017;152: 615–37.

31. Tomasini C. Septic vasculitis and vasculopathy in some infectious emergencies: the perspective of the histopathologist. G Ital Dermatol Venereol 2015;150:73–85.

32. Lucas S. The autopsy pathology of sepsis-related death. Curr Diagn Pathol 2007;13:375–88.

33. Alpert JS, Krous HF, Dalen JE, et al. Pathogenesis of Osler's nodes. Ann Intern Med 1976;85:471–3.

34. Berger AP, Ford BA, Brown-Joel Z, et al. Angioinvasive fungal infections impacting the skin: diagnosis, management, and complications. J Am Acad Dermatol 2019;80:883–98.

35. Rongioletti F, Ghio L, Ginevri F, et al. Purpura of the ears: a distinctive vasculopathy with circulating autoantibodies complicating long-term treatment with levamisole in children. Br J Dermatol 1999;14: 948–51.

36. Walsh NMG, Green PJ, Burlingame RW, et al. Cocaine-related retiform purpura: evidence to incriminate the adulterant, levamisole. J Cutan Pathol 2010;37:1212–9.

37. Miyakis S, Lockshin MD, Atsumi T, et al. International consensus statement on an update of the classification criteria for definite antiphospholipid syndrome (APS). J Thromb Haemost 2006;4:295–306.

38. Weinstein S, Piette W. Cutaneous manifestations of antiphospholipid antibody syndrome. Hematol Oncol Clin North Am 2008;22:67–77.

39. Santo GC, Baldeiras I, Guerreiro R, et al. Adenosine deaminase two and immunoglobulin M accurately differentiate adult Sneddon's syndrome of unknown cause. Cerebrovasc Dis 2018;46:257–64.

40. Dutta P, Chaudet KM, Nazarian RM, et al. Correlation between clinical and pathological features of cutaneous calciphylaxis. PLoS One 2019;14:e0218155.

41. Ellis CL, O'Neill WC. Questionable specificity of histologic findings in calcific uremic arteriolopathy. Kidney Int 2018;94:390–5.

Updates on the Pathology and Management of Nail Unit Tumors and Dermatoses

Mohammed Dany, MD, PhD[a], Andrew S. Fischer, MD[a],
Susan Pei, MD[a], Adam I. Rubin, MD[a,b],*

KEYWORDS

• Nail unit • Dermatopathology • Nail tumors • Nail dermatosis

Key points

- A honeycomb pattern on nail clipping with cavities less than 0.10 mm in diameter should prompt a biopsy of the matrix to assess for a malignant lesion.
- Onychocytic matricoma (OCM) and subungual seborrheic keratosis (SK) are now considered to belong to the same spectrum of disease, known as nail unit longitudinal acanthoma.
- Dermoscopy of the nail plate free edge is a helpful tool as onychopapilloma (OP) has a characteristic subungual keratotic mass at the distal nail edge and hyponychium.
- Conservative surgery is considered the treatment of choice for in situ or minimally invasive nail melanoma ($\leq$0.5 mm).

ABSTRACT

Nail unit pathology is indispensable to reach an accurate diagnosis of nail tumors as well as inflammatory disorders. This review article provides an update from the most recently published studies on the pathology and management of nail unit tumors and inflammatory disorders. Recent findings of nail clipping histopathology are described first, followed by discussing recent data on the diagnosis and surgical management of several types of nail unit tumors, ending with discussing the recent discoveries in selected nail unit inflammatory disorders.

NAIL PLATE HISTOPATHOLOGY

Nail clipping is a simple procedure that provides a wealth of histopathological information. **Table 1** lists nail clipping histopathologic features of several nail disorders. Nail clipping is very helpful in distinguishing psoriasis from onychomycosis. In addition to negative fungal stains, nail psoriasis contains a thicker subungual region, increased subungual parakeratosis, and onychokaryosis (retention of nuclei in the nail plate). Psoriasis also has a regular and symmetric nail transition zone, which is irregular and blurred in onychomycosis.[1] Interestingly, serous lakes and neutrophils were more frequent in onychomycosis. Nail clipping findings are also helpful in assessing the overall burden of pediatric psoriasis: nail clippings showing neutrophils and serous lakes were correlated with higher Psoriasis Area and Severity Index (PASI) scores; and nail clippings showing serous lakes were correlated with higher Nail Area and Psoriasis Severity Index (NAPSI) scores. The thickness of the nail plate, subungual thickness, or number of layers of parakeratosis were not found to correlate with the PASI or NAPSI scores.[2]

[a] Department of Dermatology, Hospital of the University of Pennsylvania, University of Pennsylvania, 3600 Spruce Street, 2 Maloney Building, Philadelphia, PA 10104, USA; [b] Hospital of the University of Pennsylvania, Children's Hospital of Philadelphia, Perelman School of Medicine at the University of Pennsylvania, University of Pennsylvania, 3600 Spruce Street, 2 Maloney Building, Philadelphia, PA 10104, USA
* Corresponding author.
E-mail address: adam.rubin@pennmedicine.upenn.edu

Surgical Pathology 14 (2021) 327–339
https://doi.org/10.1016/j.path.2021.03.006
1875-9181/21/© 2021 Elsevier Inc. All rights reserved.

Table 1
Overview of the clinical and histopathologic features on nail clipping of various nail unit disorders

Entity	Clinical Features	Histopathologic Features in a Nail Clipping
Onychomycosis	Nail plate thickening, xanthonychia, subungual hyperkeratosis, onycholysis	Demonstration of fungal elements by PAS/GMS staining; thick subungual region with numerous layers of parakeratosis, serous lakes and neutrophils[a]; NTZ is irregular; absence of bacteria
Dermatophytoma	White or yellow band with hyperkeratosis	Compact mass of fungal elements within the nail plate
Psoriasis	Nail plate thickening, subungual hyperkeratosis, onycholysis; oil spots, pitting, splinter hemorrhage	Thick subungual region with layers of parakeratosis, serous lakes and neutrophils[a]; NTZ is regular; absence of onychokaryosis; presence of bacteria
Subungual hematoma	Irregular pigment, typically not contiguous with proximal nail fold	Hemorrhage, which may be highlighted by a diaminobenzidine stain
Onychomatricoma	Acquired longitudinal pachyonychia; splinter hemorrhages; nail plate has a honeycomb appearance when viewed head-on	Thick nail plate with large circular cavities (up to 2 × 2.4 mm) and minute cavities (0.05–0.10 mm); may have cytokeratin-positive associated epithelium
Onychocytic matricoma	Acquired longitudinal pachyonychia, usually pigmented; splinter hemorrhage	Thick nail plate with multiple circular cavities (up to 0.15 × 0.40 mm) filled with serous fluid
Onychocytric carcinoma in situ	Acquired longitudinal pachyonychia	Thick nail plate with multiple circular cavities (<0.13 mm) filled with serous fluid
Melanonychia	Usually presents as a longitudinal pigmented band	Pigmentation, as highlighted by Fontana staining, in the dorsal nail plate corresponds to a lesion in the proximal matrix, whereas pigmentation of the ventral nail plate corresponds to a lesion in the distal matrix
Nail unit melanoma in situ	Variable presentations, but may include brown to black pigmented band, >3 mm in diameter, variegated borders, + Hutchinson sign	Scattered pigmented pagetoid melanocytes, highlighted by S100 (most reliably)
Amelanotic melanoma in situ	Onychodystrophy; many clinical presentations are possible, including a lichen planuslike presentation	Scattered pagetoid melanocytes, highlighted by S100 (most reliably)

Abbreviations: NTZ, nail transition zone between subungual region and nail plate; PAS/GMS, periodic acid-Schiff/Grocott methenamine silver.

[a] Thick subungual region with numerous layers of parakeratosis, serous lakes and neutrophils were found to be more prominent in onychomycosis than psoriasis.

Moreover, nail clipping helps in distinguishing onychomatrical tumors: onychomatricoma (OM), onychocytic matricoma (OCM), and onychocytic carcinoma (OC), all of which present with acquired longitudinal pachyonychia (longitudinal thickening of the nail plate), and with nail plate holes in a honeycomb pattern (**Fig. 1**). A prior study showed that the dimensions of the cavities at the distal plate can be a helpful discriminating factor. In OCM, the cavities were in the inferior two-thirds of the nail plate with a diameter larger than 0.15 mm. In OM, 2 types of cavities were observed, including those either smaller or larger than 0.1 mm. In OC, the size of the cavities was consistently less than 0.1 mm. Therefore, a honeycomb pattern on nail clipping with cavities smaller than 0.10 mm

Fig. 1. Nail clipping from a nail with OM showing the honeycomb pattern (hematoxylin-eosin, original magnification ×40).

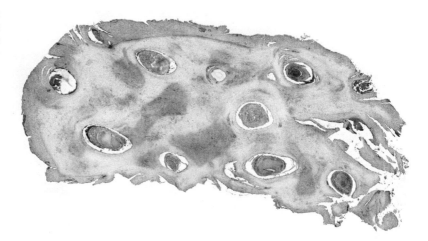

in diameter should prompt a biopsy of the matrix to assess for a potentially malignant lesion, whereas cavities greater than 0.15 mm are more reassuring of a benign process.[3]

ONYCHOMATRICOMA

OM is a benign fibroepithelial tumor that affects the nail matrix and connective tissue. Under dermoscopy, OM shows longitudinal white lines and holes at the distal margin of the nail plate. These findings are particularly helpful in distinguishing OM from onychomycosis. In many cases, the 2 conditions coexist, as channels within the nail plate may be a nidus for fungal invasion. Unlike OM, however, which shows honeycomb cavities, onychomycosis shows subungual hyperkeratosis with a "ruin appearance."[4]

Histopathologically, OM forms papillary structures lined by matrix epithelium that forms deep projections into the thickened nail plate, in addition to a subjacent CD34-positive spindle cell proliferation[5] (**Fig. 2**). A myxoid variant has been recently described in which the tumor stroma contains a prominent mucinous component[6] (**Fig. 3**). Another variant is pigmented OM, which shows hyperpigmentation of basal keratinocytes without an increase in melanocytes or the presence of melanocytic atypia.[7] While evaluating for pigmented OM, it is important to orient the specimen longitudinally to ensure all aspects of the nail unit are evaluated to reliably exclude melanoma. The histopathologic differential diagnosis also includes CD34-positive tumors such as superficial acral fibromyxoma (SAF).[8,9] Although SAF is positive for CD99, CD10, and EMA focally, OM is negative for CD99 and EMA, and expression of CD10 is limited to dermal dendritic cells in a patchy, weak distribution.

ONYCHOCYTIC MATRICOMA/LONGITUDINAL SUBUNGUAL ACANTHOMA

The term "onychocytic matricoma" was introduced in 2012 to describe an acanthoma of the nail matrix that produces onychocytes, and has overlapping histopathologic features with ungual seborrheic keratosis.[10] OCM and subungual SK are now considered to belong to the same spectrum of disease, known as "nail unit longitudinal acanthoma."[11,12]

Clinically, OCM typically presents as a localized thickening of the nail plate, known as pachyonychia, and is associated with a pigmented longitudinal band (pachymelanonychia). Hypopigmented examples also have been reported.[10] Because of its clinical features, OCM can simulate a foreign body, or nail unit pigmented lesion, including nail unit melanoma.[11,13] The clinical differential diagnosis includes subungual SK, foreign body, melanocytic nevus, onychomatricoma, onychopapilloma, and OC. Dermoscopy can be used to help distinguish these tumors: although OCM is characterized by the presence of white dots in the nail plate, subungual malignant melanoma (MM) has irregular longitudinal lines, and Bowen disease has surface scales.[3]

Microscopically, OCM appears as a benign acanthoma of the nail unit with key features that include an increased proportion of basaloid cells, the presence of spheres of prekeratogenous and keratogenous zone cells located in the basaloid compartment in the acanthotic type, and can also have distal superficial epithelial papillae[10,11] in the papillomatous type. OCM was initially classified into the following 3 variants:

- Acanthotic: characterized by acanthosis with an increased proportion of basaloid cells and

A

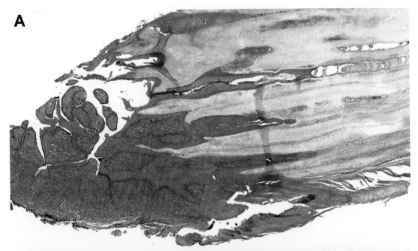

B

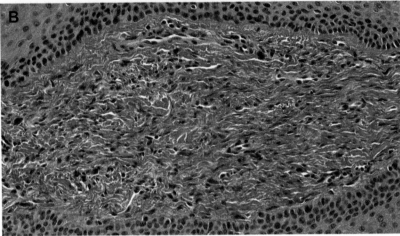

Fig. 2. (*A*) Histopathology of OM (hematoxylin-eosin, original magnification ×30). (*B*) Spindle cells in OM (hematoxylin-eosin, original magnification ×400).

the presence of spheres of prekeratogenous and keratogenous zone cells located in the basaloid compartment[10–13] (**Fig. 4**).

- Papillomatous: characterized additionally by the presence distal superficial epithelial papillae.[10,11]
- Keratogenous: characterized by a prominent keratogenous zone, presence of longitudinal parakeratosis, and distal differentiation into onychocytes.[10]

ONYCHOPAPILLOMA

Onychopapilloma (OP) is a benign neoplasm of the nail bed in which the distal matrix is characterized by a typical clinical appearance of longitudinal erythronychia and distal localized subungual keratosis[14] (**Fig. 5**). Clinically, OP presents as a painful or painless lesion on the thumb that can interfere with normal digit functioning.[15,16] OP manifests as monodactylous longitudinal erythronychia, but

can also present as longitudinal leukonychia or longitudinal melanonychia.[15–18] It was previously suggested that OP is caused by human papilloma virus (HPV); however, HPV was detected in only a few cases making this theory less likely.[16]

Examination of the nail unit head-on is essential to differentiate OP from other tumors. Dermoscopy of the free edge of the nail plate is a helpful tool, as OP has a characteristic subungual keratotic mass at the distal nail edge and hyponychium,[14,19] found in approximately 85% of the cases[15] (**Fig. 6**). **Table 2** lists the differential diagnoses with their distinguishing features. OP can be confused with other etiologies presenting with longitudinal erythronychia. Unlike Darier disease, which manifests as polydactylous longitudinal erythronychia along with longitudinal leukonychia, OP presents as monodactylous.[20] A glomus tumor presenting with longitudinal erythronychia can be distinguished by the lack of associated changes to the nail plate and a positive Love test (pain

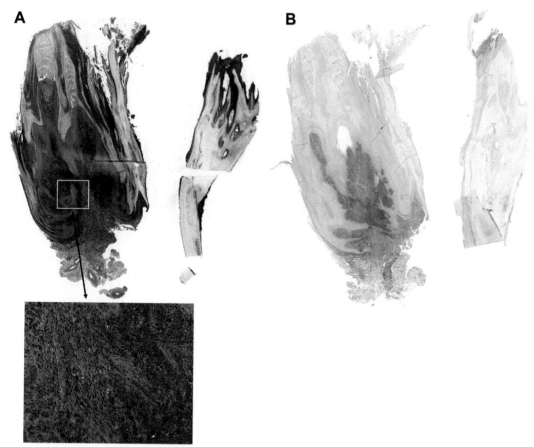

Fig. 3. (*A*) Nail unit biopsy showing myxoid variant of OM (hematoxylin-eosin, original magnification ×10) with a magnified area showing the spindle cells (hematoxylin-eosin, original magnification ×140). (*B*) Colloidal iron staining showing prominent mucin deposition (colloidal iron, original magnification ×10).

elicited with pressure on the nail) or Hildreth sign (diminished pain after insufflating a brachial cuff).[21,22] When OP presents as longitudinal melanonychia, dermoscopy would be an important diagnostic tool. OP, unlike melanocytic hyperplasia, shows a homogeneous band without lines and is associated with a subungual keratotic mass.[17]

In the clinical management of longitudinal erythronychia, observation may be a reasonable option for stable asymptomatic lesions. In cases in which a biopsy is indicated, a longitudinal excisional

Fig. 4. Histopathology of the acanthotic type of OCM (hematoxylin-eosin, original magnification ×90).

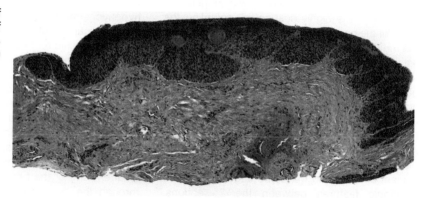

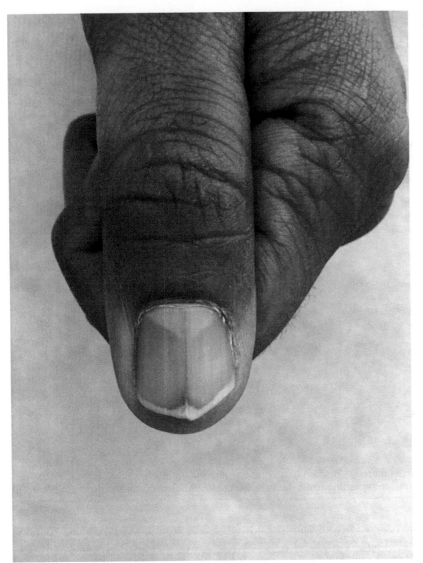

Fig. 5. Clinical presentation of OP characterized by typical clinical appearance of longitudinal erythronychia and distal localized subungual hyperkeratosis.

biopsy is advised, to ensure that lesions considered in the clinical differential diagnosis are adequately sampled. In the clinical scenario in which a glomus tumor presenting with longitudinal erythronychia is highly suspected, sampling the origin of the band of erythronychia can also establish the diagnosis without the need for a longitudinal excision.

Histopathologically, OP is characterized by papillomatous acanthosis of the nail bed with acanthosis of the distal matrix and layers of subungual hyperkeratosis and focal parakeratosis[14] (**Fig. 7**). A recent study that compared diagnosing OP using transverse versus longitudinal histologic sections reported no statistically significant difference in the percentage of detected histologic features between the 2 sections.

However, the pathologic interpretation was more difficult on transverse sections because longitudinal sections allow examination of the whole lesion from the distal matrix through the hyponychium.[16]

OP typically involves the distal matrix, nail bed, and hyponychium. Two approaches have been formally studied: a classic deep longitudinal excision or a tangential longitudinal excision.[16,23] For the classic deep approach, the longitudinal excision starts in the distal matrix and extends to the digital pulp and extends to the depth of the bone.[16] For the tangential approach, the goal is to obtain a superficial specimen, typically less than 1 mm thick by performing a delicate longitudinal shaving of the tumor from the distal matrix through the hyponychium.[16] Even though there

Fig. 6. Onychoscopy of the nail plate free edge shows a subungual keratotic mass, a characteristic finding of OP.

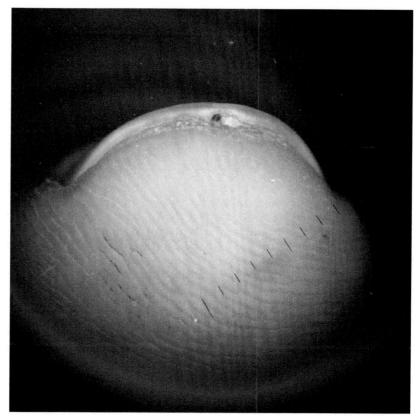

was no statistically significant difference observed in the outcomes of both approaches, there was a trend in favor of the classic deep excision, which resulted in a 14% recurrence rate, compared with a 36% recurrence rate with the tangential approach.[16]

MELANOCYTIC NAIL TUMORS

Longitudinal melanonychia (LM) refers to a dark melanocytic stripe in the nail and can be secondary to either a benign or malignant process. LM is common in the pediatric population and is

Table 2
Differential diagnosis of onychopapilloma and distinguishing features

Diagnosis	Clinical and/or Dermoscopic Features
Darier disease	Polydactylous longitudinal erythronychia and leukonychia
Haily-Hailey disease	Polydactylous longitudinal leukonychia[66]
Lichen planus	Erythronychia associated with onychorrhexis and nail plate thinning
Glomus tumor	Painful tumor; lacks distal free edge subungual keratotic mass, may present with longitudinal erythronychia
Melanocytic hyperplasia/melanoma	Longitudinal pigmented band; lacks distal free edge subungual keratotic mass
Squamous cell carcinoma in situ	May lack distal free edge subungual hyperkeratosis, may present as a warty growth or with oozing or bleeding.

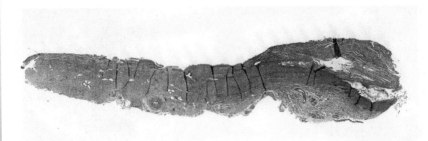

Fig. 7. Histopathology of OP characterized by papillomatous acanthosis of the nail bed with acanthosis of the distal matrix and layers of subungual hyperkeratosis and focal parakeratosis (hematoxylin-eosin, original magnification ×10).

almost always benign. In a recent large case series of pediatric patients, no nail unit melanomas were reported, even if there were clinical worrisome features for melanoma.[24,25] Interestingly, pediatric nail matrix nevi presented with LM 3.5 times wider than adults, and more often displayed nail dystrophy and "Hutchinson sign" with pigmentation extending to the nail fold or hyponychium.[24]

Nail unit melanoma exhibits several histologic features. A recent study provided reproducible criteria for the diagnosis of nail unit melanoma in situ and proposed counting the number of melanocytes per 1 mm in the basal layer of the nail unit epithelium, as well as the intervening number of keratinocytes between melanocytes.[26] An increased density of melanocytes, as well as loss of equidistance between melanocytes (unpredictable distribution), is considered worrisome. Other features were published in the largest series of subungual melanoma in situ characterized by the presence of scattered, solitary, pleomorphic, hyperchromatic nuclei, surrounded by retraction artifact, in the lower portion of the nail matrix.[27] The degree of atypia and density of melanocytes varied. In two-thirds of cases, the melanocyte density was greater than 50 melanocytes per 1 mm, but in the remaining third it was between 20 and 50 per mm. Immunohistochemical stains, including p16, HMB-45, and Ki-67/MelanA were not useful in discriminating benign and malignant nail unit melanocytic lesions.[28] Pagetoid spread is an important criterion for melanoma, but can be particularly difficult to evaluate in the nail unit, as melanocytes can normally be located in the upper layers of the nail matrix.[29] Melanocytes, however, should not reach the keratogenous zone, and the presence of single melanocytes in the nail plate may be a marker for melanoma. This clue was noted on routine nail clippings, and led to the diagnosis of melanoma when it was not suspected clinically.[28,30] The exception is nevi in children, which can show pagetoid spread of melanocytes in the nail plate.

Matrix tangential excision and matrix shave biopsy are the preferred methods for sampling pigmented lesions of the nail unit because of lower risk of postoperative dystrophy.[31] Recently, CO_2 lasers were used to create a "window" in the nail plate and a longitudinal strip nail plate 'window' to assist with obtaining a nail matrix biopsy and to potentially reduce the risk of regimentation afterward.[32,33] A recent meta-analysis demonstrated that conservative surgery is the treatment of choice for in situ or minimally invasive nail melanoma ($\leq$0.5 mm). The data from this study revealed no difference in local recurrence between conservative, functional surgery, and amputation for nail for these types of nail unit melanoma.[34]

NAIL UNIT SQUAMOUS CELL CARCINOMA

Nail unit squamous cell carcinoma (NSCC) is the most frequent nail unit malignant neoplasm (**Figs. 8 and 9**), yet its diagnosis is often delayed because NSCC can mimic benign conditions, such as onychomycosis, verrucae, and paronychia.[35] Although metastasis is rare, local destruction and bone invasion can occur.[36] There is no clear pathogenic etiology, but some of the risk factors include HPV infection, radiation, and chronic trauma.[37] A recent study assessed 136 cases of HPV-positive NSCC and found that half of the cases were associated with high-risk HPV subtypes (16 and 18).[38] Because the authors found that a quarter of the patients with NSCC had a history of other HPV-associated diseases, they hypothesized that there is a possibility for genito-digital HPV transmission and that NSCC could be a reservoir for sexually transmitted high-risk HPV.[38]

Another study reviewed clinical and histopathologic data from 40 NSCC tumors and described 2 subtypes that arise from different epithelia and have different clinical behaviors: group A was described as NSCC arising from the nail bed and presenting as a nodular or ulcerated tumor with potential for invasion; group B was described as NSCC arising from the nail fold presenting as a verrucous lesion, or hyperkeratotic bands.[39] Group A NSCC exhibited poorer histopathologic

Fig. 8. Clinical presentation of NSCC.

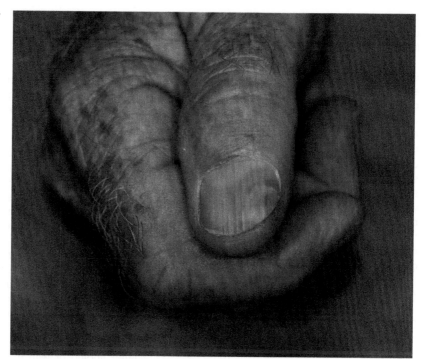

grade, occurred in an older patient population, and followed a more aggressive disease course.[39]

Mohs micrographic surgery (MMS) is considered the standard of care for NSCC because of its ability to maximize tissue preservation while achieving histologic clearance.[40] This has been supported by several case series with cure rates ranging from 78.0% to 96.5%,[41–43] and by a recent retrospective review study of 42 cases treated with

MMS with recurrence observed in only 3 cases (7.1%).[40]

ACRAL DERMATOFIBROSARCOMA PROTUBERANS

Acral dermatofibrosarcoma protuberans (DFSP) is a superficial, low-grade, infiltrative mesenchymal

Fig. 9. Nail unit SCC appearance after nail avulsion.

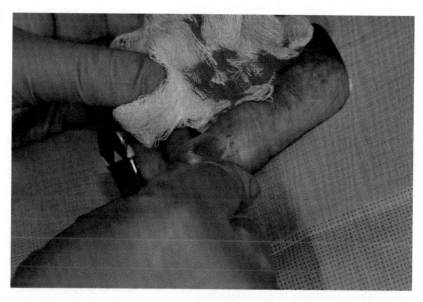

neoplasm[44] that can involve the nail unit causing diagnostic confusion and delayed therapy.[44–46] Metastases are rare and occur after repeated local recurrences.[47] A recent study reported the largest series of 27 cases of DFSP occurring at the distal extremities and acral sites.[44] Histologically, all cases showed classic storiform morphology and were all diffusely CD34 positive and uniformly positive for COL1A1-PDGFB gene fusion.[44] Based on the clinical behavior of the cases, the investigators concluded that acral DFSP clinically behaves similar to DFSP in other locations, and therefore a high index of suspicion should be present when a patient presents with slow-growing violaceous papules coalescing into multinodular plaques at acral sites.[44] These cases should be referred for MMS as the standard of care because of to the infiltrative property of the tumor.[48]

GLOMUS TUMOR

Glomus tumor is a benign vascular soft tissue neoplasm of glomus bodies.[49] It typically presents with a clinical triad of tenderness, paroxysmal pain, and cold intolerance.[50] Histopathologically, glomus tumors are characterized by small polygonal cells with pale cytoplasm and round nuclei. Rarely, atypical and malignant variants have been reported.[51] Tumors are considered malignant with a risk of metastasis if they fulfill one of the following criteria: depth and size of more than 2 cm, presence of atypical mitotic figures, or a combination of moderate-to-high nuclear grade and mitotic activity (>5 mitoses/50 high-power fields).[52] Tumors that have atypical features but do not meet the definition criteria of malignant glomus tumor are labeled glomus tumors of uncertain malignant potential.[52] Finally, tumors that show marked nuclear atypia in the absence of any other criteria for malignancy and with the absence of mitotic activity are considered benign and are referred to as symblastic glomus tumors.[53]

The traditional surgical approach for managing glomus tumors is a transungual excision, which starts by avulsion of the nail plate followed by either a transversal incision when the tumor is under the nail matrix, or a longitudinal incision when the tumor is under the nail bed.[54] The literature shows that the transungual approach results in low recurrence rates, but it has been thought that it causes high rates of nail deformities, such as longitudinal ridging and complete split nail deformities.[55] A study performed traditional direct transungual approach on 12 cases of subungual glomus tumor and found that all patients reported relief of signs and complete recovery of the nail plate,[54] without resulting in nail deformities.[56]

NAIL INFLAMMATORY DISORDERS: PSORIASIS, LICHEN PLANUS, AND ONYCHOTILLOMANIA

Nail unit psoriasis is common and can present with or without accompanying skin psoriasis.[57] Psoriasis of the nail matrix presents with pitting, leukonychia, and red spots in the lunula, whereas psoriasis of the nail bed presents with onycholysis, subungual hyperkeratosis, salmon patches, and splinter hemorrhages.[58] Histopathology can distinguish nail psoriasis from its clinical mimickers. In a series of 60 cases of nail biopsies, the most common histopathologic features of nail unit psoriasis were hyperkeratotic parakeratosis, neutrophilic infiltration of nail bed epithelium, and hypergranulosis.[58] Other features included serum exudates, melanin pigment, and acanthosis. It is important to emphasize that unlike cutaneous psoriasis, which demonstrates *hypo*granulosis, nail psoriasis demonstrated *hyper*granulosis in more than half of cases studied.

Nail lichen planus (NLP) can present as an isolated finding or with mucocutaneous lichen planus.[59] NLP involving the nail matrix presents clinically as longitudinal ridging, splitting, trachyonychia, anonychia, and pterygium. This is in contrast to NLP involving the nail bed, which presents as onycholysis and nail bed hyperkeratosis. In children, NLP presents with atypical features such as twenty-nail dystrophy, longitudinal striations, and loss of nail plate luster. Histologically, NLP is characterized by a bandlike lymphocytic infiltrate in the nail matrix and/or nail bed dermis with hyperkeratosis, hypergranulosis, and acanthosis of the nail matrix epithelium.[59] These diagnostic features of NLP can be seen at a higher rate depending on site of biopsy: 100% in nail fold biopsy, 95.5% in nail bed biopsy, and 85.5% in matrix biopsy.

Onychotillomania refers to self-induced trauma caused by nail picking.[60] It is associated with psychiatric conditions, medications such as metoclopramide and methylphenidate, spinal cord injury, congenital pain insensitivity, and genetic syndromes such as Smith-Magenis syndrome and Lesch-Nyhan syndrome.[61] Clinical findings are often nonspecific and include generalized dystrophy, transverse grooves, rough areas, brittleness, and onychoatrophy.[61,62] The periungual skin may be erythematous, edematous, eroded, or secondarily crusted. Melanocyte activation due to repetitive trauma results in nail plate pigmentation and LM.[63] Characteristically, wavy lines are seen under dermoscopy, which are uneven longitudinal white, reddish-purple, brown, or black pigmented lines appearing on different planes of the nail plate and are secondary to uneven or absent nail plate growth after repetitive trauma.[64] Histopathology of onychotillomania is variable and diagnosis requires clinicopathologic correlation. Findings analogous to lichen simplex chronicus in the skin can be seen, such as epithelial hyperplasia, acanthosis, and hypergranulosis.[61,62] To maintain a therapeutic relationship with patients with onychotillomania, care must be taken to avoid assigning the nail changes to the patient. Often patients will report that they have started a particular nail-altering behavior in an attempt to treat an underlying nail disorder. Indeed, once the nails are altered by secondary changes, it may be impossible to distinguish if a primary nail disorder was present and has since resolved.[65]

CLINICS CARE POINTS

- Mohs micrographic surgery (MMS) is considered the standard of care for nail unit squamous cell carcinoma because of its ability to maximize tissue preservation while achieving histologic clearance.

- Unlike cutaneous psoriasis, which demonstrates hypogranulosis, nail psoriasis demonstrated hypergranulosis in more than half of cases studied.

DISCLOSURE

The authors have nothing to disclose.

REFERENCES

1. Trevisan F, Werner B, Pinheiro RL. Nail clipping in onychomycosis and comparison with normal nails and ungual psoriasis. An Bras Dermatol 2019; 94(3):344–7.
2. Uber M, Carvalho VO, Abagge KT, et al. Clinical features and nail clippings in 52 children with psoriasis. Pediatr Dermatol 2018;35(2):202–7.
3. Perrin C, Cannata GE, Langbein L, et al. Acquired localized longitudinal pachyonychia and onychomatrical tumors: a comparative study to onychomatricomas (5 cases) and onychocytic matricomas (4 cases). Am J Dermatopathol 2016;38(9):664–71.
4. Kallis P, Tosti A. Onychomycosis and onychomatricoma. Ski Appendage Disord 2015;1(4):209–12.
5. Perrin C, Baran R, Balaguer T, et al. Onychomatricoma: new clinical and histological features. A review of 19 tumors. Am J Dermatopathol 2010; 32(1):1–8.
6. Stewart CL, Sobanko JF, Rubin AI. Myxoid onychomatricoma: an unusual variant of a rare nail unit tumor. Am J Dermatopathol 2015;37(6):473–6.
7. Nguyen CV, Moshiri AS, Council ML, et al. Pigmented onychomatricoma mimicking nail unit melanoma. J Cutan Pathol 2019;46(12):895–7.
8. Agaimy A, Michal M, Giedl J, et al. Superficial acral fibromyxoma: clinicopathological, immunohistochemical, and molecular study of 11 cases highlighting frequent Rb1 loss/deletions. Hum Pathol 2017;60:192–8.
9. Lee JY, Park SE, Shin SJ, et al. Diagnostic pitfalls of differentiating cellular digital fibroma from superficial acral fibromyxoma. Ann Dermatol 2015;27(4):462–4.
10. Perrin C, Cannata GE, Bossard C, et al. Onychocytic matricoma presenting as pachymelanonychia longitudinal. A new entity (report of five cases). Am J Dermatopathol 2012;34(1):54–9.
11. Baran R, Moulonguet I, Goettmann-Bonvallot S, et al. Longitudinal subungual acanthoma: one denomination for various clinical presentations. J Eur Acad Dermatol Venereol 2018;32(9):1608–13.
12. Spaccarelli N, Wanat KA, Miller CJ, et al. Hypopigmented onychocytic matricoma as a clinical mimic of onychomatricoma: clinical, intraoperative and histopathologic correlations. J Cutan Pathol 2013; 40(6):591–4.
13. Wanat KA, Reid E, Rubin AI. Onychocytic matricoma: a new, important nail-unit tumor mistaken for a foreign body. JAMA Dermatol 2014;150(3):335–7.
14. Haneke E. Review of a recently delineated longitudinal lesion of the nail: onychopapilloma. J Eur Acad Dermatol Venereol 2018;32(11):1839–40.
15. Tosti A, Schneider SL, Ramirez-Quizon MN, et al. Clinical, dermoscopic, and pathologic features of onychopapilloma: a review of 47 cases. J Am Acad Dermatol 2016;74(3):521–6.
16. Delvaux C, Richert B, Lecerf P, et al. Onychopapillomas: a 68-case series to determine best surgical procedure and histologic sectioning. J Eur Acad Dermatol Venereol 2018;32(11):2025–30.
17. Miteva M, Fanti PA, Romanelli P, et al. Onychopapilloma presenting as longitudinal melanonychia. J Am Acad Dermatol 2012;66(6):e242–3.
18. Halteh P, Magro C, Scher RK, et al. Onychopapilloma presenting as leukonychia: case report and review of the literature. Ski Appendage Disord 2017; 2(3–4):89–91.
19. Kim M, Sun EY, Jung HY, et al. Onychopapilloma: a report of three cases presenting with various longitudinal chromonychia. Ann Dermatol 2016;28(5): 655–7.
20. Cohen PR. Longitudinal erythronychia: individual or multiple linear red bands of the nail plate: a review of clinical features and associated conditions. Am J Clin Dermatol 2011;12(4):217–31.
21. Vieira FG, Nakamura R, Costa FM, et al. Subungual glomus tumor. J Clin Rheumatol 2016;22(6):331.
22. Sethu C, Sethu AU. Glomus tumour. Ann R Coll Surg Engl 2016;98(1):e1–2.

23. Tambe SA, Ansari SMM, Nayak CS, et al. Surgical management of onychopapilloma, onychomatricoma, and subungual osteochondroma: case series. J Cutan Aesthet Surg 2018;11(3):143–7.

24. Lee JH, Lim Y, Park JH, et al. Clinicopathologic features of 28 cases of nail matrix nevi (NMNs) in Asians: comparison between children and adults. J Am Acad Dermatol 2018;78(3):479–89.

25. Cho EB, Jang YJ, Lee MK, et al. Longitudinal melanonychia in adults and children: a clinical and histopathological review of Korean patients. Eur J Dermatol 2018;28(3):400–1.

26. Fernandez-Flores A. Skin biopsy in the context of systemic disease. Actas Dermosifiliogr 2019. https://doi.org/10.1016/j.ad.2019.02.012.

27. Park SW, Jang KT, Lee JH, et al. Scattered atypical melanocytes with hyperchromatic nuclei in the nail matrix: diagnostic clue for early subungual melanoma in situ. J Cutan Pathol 2016;43(1):41–52.

28. Boni A, Chu EY, Rubin AI. Routine nail clipping leads to the diagnosis of amelanotic nail unit melanoma in a young construction worker. J Cutan Pathol 2015;42(8):505–9.

29. Fernandez-Flores A, Cassarino DS. Histopathological diagnosis of acral lentiginous melanoma in early stages. Ann Diagn Pathol 2017;26:64–9.

30. Gatica-Torres M, Nelson CA, Lipoff JB, et al. Nail clipping with onychomycosis and surprise clue to the diagnosis of nail unit melanoma. J Cutan Pathol 2018;45(11):803–6.

31. Samie FH. Tangential excision of pigmented nail matrix lesions responsible for longitudinal melanonychia: evaluation of the technique on a series of 30 patients. J Am Acad Dermatol 2019. https://doi.org/10.1016/j.jaad.2019.05.038.

32. Ohn J, Jo G, Chae JB, et al. A novel window technique using CO2 laser, and a review of methods for nail matrix biopsy of longitudinal Melanonychia. Dermatol Surg 2018;44(5):651–60.

33. Zhou Y, Chen W, Liu Z ru, et al. Modified shave surgery combined with nail window technique for the treatment of longitudinal melanonychia: evaluation of the method on a series of 67 cases. J Am Acad Dermatol 2019;81(3):717–22.

34. Jo G, Cho SI, Choi S, et al. Functional surgery versus amputation for in situ or minimally invasive nail melanoma: a meta-analysis. J Am Acad Dermatol 2019;81(4):917–22.

35. Lee TM, Jo G, Kim M, et al. Squamous cell carcinoma of the nail unit: a retrospective review of 19 cases in Asia and comparative review of Western literature. Int J Dermatol 2019;58(4):428–32.

36. Li PF, Zhu N, Lu H. Squamous cell carcinoma of the nail bed: a case report. World J Clin Cases 2019; 7(21):3590–4.

37. Tang N, Maloney ME, Clark AH, et al. A retrospective study of nail squamous cell carcinoma at 2 institutions. Dermatol Surg 2016;42:S8–17.

38. Shimizu A, Kuriyama Y, Hasegawa M, et al. Nail squamous cell carcinoma: a hidden high-risk human papillomavirus reservoir for sexually transmitted infections. J Am Acad Dermatol 2019;81(6):1358–70.

39. Dika E, Starace M, Patrizi A, et al. Squamous cell carcinoma of the nail unit: a clinical histopathologic study and a proposal for classification. Dermatol Surg 2019;45(3):365–70.

40. Gou D, Nijhawan RI, Srivastava D. Mohs Micrographic Surgery as the Standard of Care for Nail Unit Squamous Cell Carcinoma. Dermatol Surg. 2020 Jun;46(6):725-732. https://doi.org/10.1097/DSS.0000000000002144. PMID: 31567588.

41. Zaiac MN, Weiss E. Mohs micrographic surgery of the nail unit and squamous cell carcinoma. Dermatol Surg 2001;27(3):246–51.

42. Dika E, Fanti PA, Patrizi A, et al. Mohs surgery for squamous cell carcinoma of the nail unit. Dermatol Surg 2015;41(9):1.

43. Dika E, Piraccini BM, Balestri R, et al. Mohs surgery for squamous cell carcinoma of the nail: report of 15 cases. Our experience and a long-term follow-up. Br J Dermatol 2012;167(6):1310–4.

44. Shah KK, McHugh JB, Folpe AL, et al. Dermatofibrosarcoma protuberans of distal extremities and acral sites. Am J Surg Pathol 2018;42(3):413–9.

45. Rabinowitz LG, Luchetti ME, Segura AD, et al. Acrally occurring dermatofibrosarcoma protuberans in children and adults. J Dermatol Surg Oncol 1994; 20(10):655–9.

46. Al-Zaid T, Khoja H. Acral dermatofibrosarcoma protuberans with myoid differentiation: a report of 2 cases. J Cutan Pathol 2017;44(9):794–7.

47. Skoll PJ, Hudson DA, Taylor DA. Acral dermatofibrosarcoma protuberans with metastases. Ann Plast Surg 1999;42(2):217–20.

48. Kricorian GJ, Schanbacher CF, Paul Kelly A, et al. Dermatofibrosarcoma protuberans growing around plantar aponeurosis: excision by Mohs micrographic surgery. Dermatol Surg 2000;26(10):941–5.

49. Lee SH, Roh MR, Chung KY. Subungual glomus tumors: surgical approach and outcome based on tumor location. Dermatol Surg 2013;39(7):1017–22.

50. Morey VM, Garg B, Kotwal PP. Glomus tumours of the hand: review of literature. J Clin Orthop Trauma 2016;7(4):286–91.

51. Kamarashev J, French LE, Dummer R, et al. Symplastic glomus tumor - a rare but distinct benign histological variant with analogy to other "ancient" benign skin neoplasms. J Cutan Pathol 2009; 36(10):1099–102.

52. Folpe AL, Fanburg-Smith JC, Miettinen M, et al. Atypical and malignant glomus tumors: analysis of 52 cases, with a proposal for the reclassification of glomus tumors. Am J Surg Pathol 2001;25(1):1–12.

53. Da Silva DR, Gaddis KJ, Hess S, et al. Nail unit glomus tumor with myxoid and symplastic change

presenting with longitudinal erythronychia. Dermatopathology 2018;5(2):74–8.

54. Jawalkar H, Maryada VR, Brahmajoshyula V, et al. Subungual glomus tumors of the hand treated by transungual excision. Indian J Orthop 2015;49(4): 403–7.

55. Madhar M, Bouslous J, Saidi H, et al. Which approach is best for subungual glomus tumors? Transungual with microsurgical dissection of the nail bed or periungual? Chir Main 2015;34(1):39–43.

56. Reinders EFH, Klaassen KMG, Pasch MC. Transungual excision of glomus tumors: a treatment and quality of life study. Dermatol Surg 2020;46(1): 103–12.

57. Rigopoulos D, Baran R, Chiheb S, et al. Recommendations for the definition, evaluation, and treatment of nail psoriasis in adult patients with no or mild skin psoriasis: a dermatologist and nail expert group consensus. J Am Acad Dermatol 2019;81(1):228–40.

58. Kaul S, Singal A, Grover C, et al. Clinical and histological spectrum of nail psoriasis: a cross-sectional study. J Cutan Pathol 2018;45(11):824–30.

59. Goettmann S, Zaraa I, Moulonguet I. Nail lichen planus: epidemiological, clinical, pathological, therapeutic and prognosis study of 67 cases. J Eur Acad Dermatol Venereol 2012;26(10):1304–9.

60. Sidiropoulou P, Sgouros D, Theodoropoulos K, et al. Onychotillomania: a chameleon-like disorder: case report and review of literature. Ski Appendage Disord 2019;5(2):104–7.

61. Reese JM, Hudacek KD, Rubin AI. Onychotillomania: clinicopathologic correlations. J Cutan Pathol 2013;40(4):419–23.

62. Rieder EA, Tosti A. Onychotillomania: an underrecognized disorder. J Am Acad Dermatol 2016; 75(6):1245–50.

63. Anolik RB, Shah K, Rubin AI. Onychophagia-induced longitudinal melanonychia. Pediatr Dermatol 2012;29(4):488–9.

64. Maddy AJ, Tosti A. Dermoscopic features of onychotillomania: a study of 36 cases. J Am Acad Dermatol 2018;79(4):702–5.

65. Magid M, Mennella C, Kuhn H, et al. Onychophagia and onychotillomania can be effectively managed. J Am Acad Dermatol 2017;77(5):e143–4.

66. Bel B, Jeudy G, Vabres P. Dermoscopy of longitudinal leukonychia in Hailey-Hailey disease. Arch Dermatol 2010;146(10):1204.

Dysplastic Nevi
Morphology and Molecular and the Controversies In-between

Katharina Wiedemeyer, MD[a,b,1],
Wolfgang Hartschuh, MD[b,2],
Thomas Brenn, MD, PhD, FRCPath[a,c],*

KEYWORDS

• Dysplastic nevus • Melanoma • Familial melanoma • Melanocytic • Neoplasm

---

Key points

- Dysplastic nevi (DN) show distinctive histopathologic features and are part of the spectrum of atypical nevi.

- DN are clinically, histopathologically, and genetically intermediate between common acquired nevi and melanoma.

- DN may be single or multiple, sporadic, or familial.

- DN are benign but rarely progress to melanoma.

- The presence of multiple DN or severely DN is associated with an increased overall melanoma risk.

- Complete excision of DN with clinically concerning features is advisable to allow for adequate histopathologic examination and diagnosis.

ABSTRACT

Dysplastic nevi are distinctive melanocytic lesions in the larger group of atypical nevi. They often are multiple and sporadic with genetic features intermediate between common acquired nevi and melanoma. Dysplastic nevi may be multiple, familial, and seen in patients with familial melanoma syndrome. Although their behavior is benign, they rarely represent a precursor to melanoma. If clinically suspicious, dysplastic nevi should be removed for adequate histopathologic examination and to exclude possibility of melanoma. Partial sampling should be avoided because reliable separation from melanoma requires visualization of the entire lesion to allow for examination of architectural histopathologic features and avoid sampling error.

OVERVIEW

Dysplastic nevi (DN) are benign melanocytic proliferations that initially were documented by Dr Wallace Clark and colleagues[1] in patients with the familial melanoma syndrome, also known as familial atypical multiple mole melanoma (FAMMM) syndrome. They belong to the broader group of

---

[a] Department of Pathology and Laboratory Medicine, Cumming School of Medicine, University of Calgary, Calgary, Alberta, Canada; [b] Department of Dermatology, University Medical Center, Ruprecht-Karls-University, Heidelberg, Germany; [c] Arnie Charbonneau Cancer Institute, Cumming School of Medicine, University of Calgary, Calgary, Alberta, Canada
[1]Present address: Diagnostic and Scientific Centre, 9-3535 Research Road NW, Calgary, AB, T2L 2K8, Canada.
[2]Present address: University Hospital Heidelberg, Im Neuenheimer Feld 440, 69120 Heidelberg, Germany
* Corresponding author. Diagnostic and Scientific Centre, Room IW-210, 9-3535 Research Road NW, Calgary, Alberta T2L 2K8, Canada,
E-mail address: thomas.brenn@ucalgary.ca

Surgical Pathology 14 (2021) 341–357
https://doi.org/10.1016/j.path.2021.01.007

atypical nevi and are intermediate between common acquired nevi and superficial spreading melanoma in terms of their clinical appearance, histopathologic features, and molecular genetics. DN may be solitary or multiple, and a majority are sporadic. They show atypical clinical presenting features and distinctive and reproducible histopathologic findings characterized by a combination of architectural and cytologic atypia. The clinical behavior is benign, but, similar to common acquired nevi, DN may be viewed as a melanoma precursor.[2] Ongoing controversies regarding DNs relate mainly to terminology, histopathologic grading, treatment, and surveillance. This review aims to provide an overview of current knowledge with a practical guide to the diagnosis and management of DN.

HISTORICAL BACKGROUND

The concept of atypical moles and their association with melanoma developed in the 1970s. In 1978, Clark and colleagues[1] documented a group of unique melanocytic nevi in patients with familial melanoma. The patients were found to have multiple (>10 to <100) of these nevi, ranging in size from 5 mm to 15 mm and showing irregular outlines with variegated appearances and a predilection for the upper trunk and extremities. Histopathologically, these nevi were found to be compound with an atypical junctional melanocytic hyperplasia composed of enlarged atypical epithelioid or spindled melanocytes, arranged singly and in irregular nests, but generally confined to the sides and tips of the rete. The melanocytes often contained finely dispersed, "dusty" cytoplasmic melanin pigment. Additional findings were delicate fibroplasia of the papillary dermis, lymphocytic infiltration, and prominent vessels of the superficial dermis. The investigators also mentioned that their use of the term, *atypical melanocytic hyperplasia*, is synonymous with *melanocytic dysplasia*, comparable to squamous dysplasia in actinic keratoses or of the cervical mucosa, and they were able to demonstrate transformation to melanoma of 2 such nevi with time. These distinctive nevi were termed, *B-K moles*, and the associated familial melanoma syndrome was termed, *B-K mole syndrome*, with B and K representing the first letters of 2 of the study patients' names.[1] A family with a similar clinical phenotype was documented in the same year by Dr Henry Lynch and colleagues,[3] who applied the term, FAMMM. Nevi with clinical and histologic features identical to the B-K mole subsequently also were identified in patients with nonfamilial melanoma, and remnants of these nevi were noted in the patients' melanoma. The investigators referred to these nevi as DN and to the clinical presentation as dysplastic nevus syndrome.[4]

TERMINOLOGY AND SYNONYMS

There has been significant controversy and debate regarding the terminology and the use of the term, *dysplastic nevus*. The term, *dysplasia*, as applied for epithelial proliferations, implies a premalignant condition with risk for progression to invasive carcinoma. Yet the concept of DN as a premalignant precursor necessary for the development of melanoma has never been proved, and it has been argued that the term, *dysplastic*, is used inappropriately in this setting.[5] To resolve issues around terminology, a 1992 consensus conference at the National Institutes of Health proposed replacing dysplastic nevus with *nevus with architectural disorder and cytologic atypia*.[6] Similar to atypical nevus, nevus with architectural disorder and cytologic atypia is a broad term and encompasses a wide spectrum of melanocytic lesions. The eponymous, *Clark nevus*, was proposed by Dr B Ackerman, but its definition lacks nuclear atypia, and, therefore, it is not synonymous with dysplastic nevus.[5] In the authors' opinion, dysplastic nevus remains the preferred terminology. Despite its flaws, it is of historic significance and most accurately refers to this unique subset of melanocytic nevi. In a 2004 survey, it also was found the preferred terminology by members of the American Society of Dermatopathology and the American Academy of Dermatology,[7] and it is the preferred terminology by the International Melanoma Pathology Study Group and the current fourth edition of the World Health Organization *Classification of Skin Tumors*.[8,9]

DYSPLASTIC NEVUS AND MELANOMA RISK

Early studies emphasized an increased melanoma risk in patients with DN and advocated to regard DN as premalignant conditions.[1,4,10] It now has become evident that DN are relatively common in the general population, and their prevalence vastly exceeds that of melanoma. A majority of DN remain stable or regress, and only a limited subset of DN shows potential to progress to invasive melanoma, with approximately 75% of melanomas arising de novo.[2,11–14] Furthermore, both common acquired nevi and DN are seen as benign melanoma precursors with approximately equal frequencies, and there does not appear to be a linear progression from common acquired nevi to

DN before transformation to outright melanoma occurs.[2,14] Although the risk of transformation to melanoma is low for individual DN, the presence of multiple clinically atypical or DN correlates with an overall increased melanoma risk.[8,15] The presence of greater than 10 clinically DN confers a 12-fold increased melanoma risk compared with a 2-fold increased melanoma risk in the presence of a solitary clinically dysplastic nevus. For comparison, increased numbers of small non-DN correlate with a 2-fold increased melanoma risk whereas large non-DN show a 4-fold increased melanoma risk.[16] The relative melanoma risk for individuals with dysplastic nevus syndrome is highest for individuals with greater than or equal to 2 family members diagnosed with melanoma and lowest for those with dysplastic nevus syndrome but no personal or family history of melanoma.[17]

CLINICAL FEATURES

Clinically, DN large are macular lesions, typically measuring greater than or equal to 5 mm in diameter. An additional central raised papular area represents the dermal growth component, giving rise to a fried egg or targetoid appearance (**Fig. 1**). Additional findings are irregular borders; variegated colors, ranging from light brown to dark brown and black; and peripheral erythema. DN typically present in adolescence and young adulthood with a decreasing prevalence with increasing age. They are most common in individuals of northern European descent with a prevalence of approximately 10% (range 7%–24%). They may be solitary or multiple and affect intermittently sun-exposed skin with a predilection for the back. DN also may be seen in patients with hereditary and nonfamilial melanoma and they are seen in up to 43% of patients with melanoma compared with 10% in the control group.[1,4,16] A majority of DN remain unchanged or regress over time, even in in melanoma-prone families.[18] The clinical presenting features also are summarized in **Table 1**.

MICROSCOPIC FEATURES

The histologic criteria for a diagnosis of DN are based on the original description by Clark and colleagues[1] and require both architectural and cytologic changes.[19,20] Histopathologically, DN are intermediate between common acquired nevi and superficial spreading melanoma with atypical architectural and cytologic features not associated with common acquired nevi but insufficient for a diagnosis of superficial spreading melanoma. A diagnosis of DN is reproducible with excellent

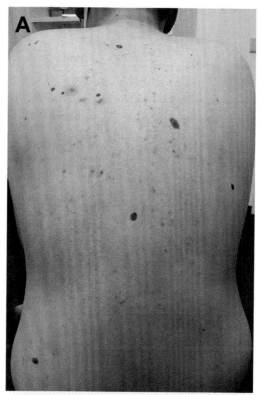

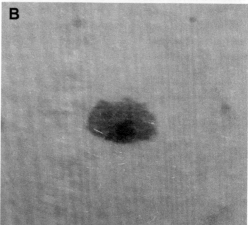

Fig. 1. This patient presents with multiple DN on the back (*A*). This dysplastic nevus is enlarged with irregular borders, color variegation, and a central raised area (*B*).

intraobserver and reasonable interobserver agreement when applying previously agreed-on histopathologic criteria.[21–23] DN may be junctional or compound. They are relatively circumscribed and symmetric but may show somewhat ill-defined radial borders with a trickling of single melanocytes toward their periphery (**Fig. 2**A, B). If present, the dermal component is shallow and centrally placed, and there is variable radial extension of the junctional component beyond the dermal

Table 1
Summary of the clinical presenting features of dysplastic nevi

Clinical Features of Dysplastic Nevi	
Sex	Equal gender distribution
Age	Adolescents, young adults
Site	Intermittently sun-exposed areas, in particular, the back
Size	≥5-mm diameter
Clinical appearance	Solitary or multiple Sporadic or familial Macular component representing junctional melanocytic proliferation Central papular growth representing the dermal melanocytic proliferation and giving rise to targetoid or fried-egg appearance Color variegation Ill-defined border Peripheral erythema
Associated syndromes	Dysplastic nevus syndrome, familial melanoma syndrome

growth (**Fig. 2**C). This phenomenon is regarded as shoulder formation. The junctional component is broad and composed of epithelioid to ovoid melanocytes in a lentiginous and nested growth pattern (**Fig. 2**D). The junctional melanocytic nests are irregularly shaped and distributed along the basilar epidermis mostly confined to the sides and tips of elongated rete, and there is fusion of junctional nests of adjacent and elongated rete ridges, referred to as *bridging* (**Fig. 3**A). In addition, there may be fusion of adjacent rete ridges (**Fig. 3**B). Focal suprabasal scatter of single melanocytes may be present, but it is confined to the lower levels of the epidermis and generally restricted to the lesional center (**Fig. 3**C). The melanocytes contain moderate amounts of cytoplasm, frequently with finely dispersed, dusty cytoplasmic melanin pigment (**Fig. 4**A). Cytologic atypia invariably is present and characterized by nuclear enlargement with variably prominent and occasionally multiple nucleoli, chromatin clumping, and nuclear hyperchromasia (**Fig. 4**B). The cytologic atypia is scattered and random rather than confluent and monotonous. Mitotic activity of the junctional component is rare. The involved epidermis shows a pronounced rete ridge pattern, and there is increased eosinophilic fibrous tissue surrounding the elongated rete ridges, known as *concentric eosinophilic fibroplasia* (**Fig. 5**A). A lamellar arrangement of connective tissue at the base of the rete ridges is referred to as *lamellar fibroplasia*. Other stromal and host response changes include a patchy lymphocytic infiltrate, increased vascularity in the superficial dermis,

and pigmented melanophages (**Fig. 5**B).[20] The dermal component appears nevic and generally lacks cytologic atypia and mitotic activity (**Fig. 6**). Due to its shallow nature, it may be difficult to assess for maturation with depth.[19–21,24] DN may show varying degrees of cytologic and architectural atypia within a lesion, and they may be present in the background of an unequivocal melanoma (**Fig. 7**).

HISTOPATHOLOGIC GRADING

Controversy remains regarding the histopathologic grading of DN and interobserver reproducibility. Traditionally, the degree of atypia in DN has been divided into mild, moderate, and severe. The use of a 2-tier system using low-grade for mild and moderate atypia and high-grade for severe atypia also has been advocated.[25] Grading may be based solely on the degree of cytologic atypia or on a combination of architectural and cytologic features.[20,26] Mild melanocyte atypia has been defined as nuclear size similar to the nucleus of basal layer keratinocytes with condensed chromatin and inconspicuous nucleoli, whereas moderate atypia shows nuclear enlargement up to 1.5 times the size of the basal layer keratinocyte nucleus, and severe atypia is characterized by nuclear size twice or greater that of basal layer keratinocyte nuclei with nuclear hyperchromasia or vesicular nuclei with prominent nucleoli.[26] The degree of architectural disorder may be of equal importance to cytologic atypia when grading DN. Architectural features indicative of severe

Fig. 2. This low-power overview is of a broad but relatively circumscribed and symmetric compound dysplastic nevus (hematoxylin-eosin, original magnification x10) (*A*). At the periphery there is a proliferation of single melanocytes (hematoxylin-eosin, original magnification x100) (*B*). The junctional melanocytic proliferation extends beyond the dermal component, also referred to as shoulder formation (hematoxylin-eosin, original magnification x100).

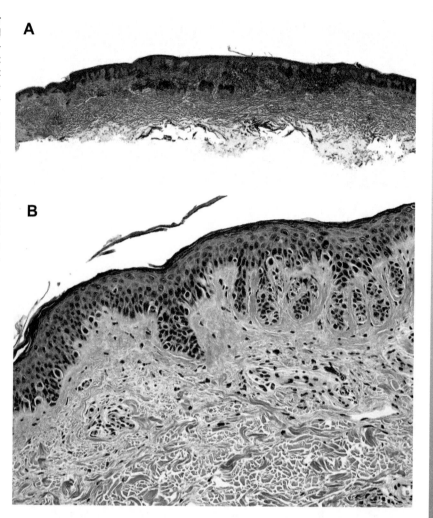

atypia include increased lesional diameter and lack of circumscription, asymmetry, an effaced rete ridge pattern, focally confluent growth of the junctional melanocytic proliferation, single cells predominating over nests, junctional mitotic activity, and low-level pagetoid spread.[20] The grading of DN is of particular importance to guide treatment because those with severe atypia show many overlapping histologic features with melanoma and may be difficult to reliably separate from early melanoma in individual challenging cases. In addition, the degree of atypia in DN correlates with a personal history of melanoma.[8] In 1 study, 19.7% of patients with severely DN were found to have a personal history of melanoma compared with 8.1% of patients with moderately DN and 5.7% with mildly DN.[27]

IMMUNOHISTOCHEMISTRY

The melanocytes in DN express S100, SOX10, Melan-A, microphthalmia-associated transcription factor (MITF), and tyrosinase (**Fig. 8**A). HMB45 staining typically is present only in the junctional and superficial dermal melanocytes but is lost in the deeper dermal component. The Ki-67 proliferative index of the dermal component is low, with less than 5% of melanocytes staining in a dermal hot spot.[28] P16 expression is preserved whereas there is lack or only focal expression of preferentially expressed antigen in melanoma (PRAME) (**Fig. 8**B).[29] Staining for Melan-A or SOX10 is of particular importance in routine daily practice to highlight confluent melanocyte growth and pagetoid spread.

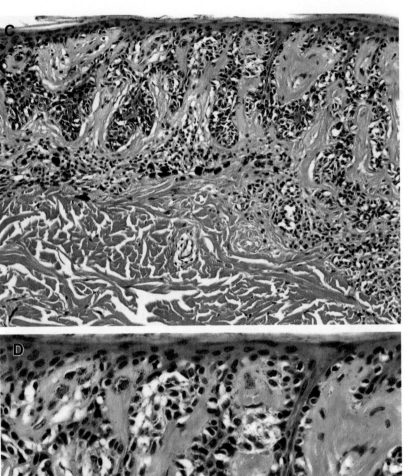

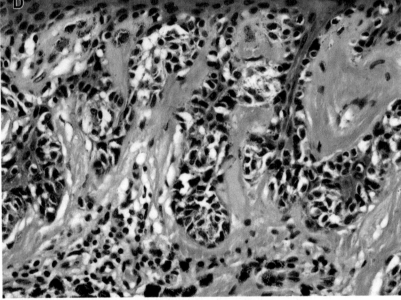

Fig. 2. (continued). (C). The rete ridges are elongated and there is a lentiginous and nested junctional melanocytic proliferation with disorderly arranged melanocytic nests (hematoxylin-eosin, original magnification x200) *(D).*

MOLECULAR AND GENETIC FEATURES

Over the past few years, knowledge of the molecular and genetic underpinnings of the various melanocytic proliferations has expanded significantly and several familial melanoma susceptibility genes now have been identified. A majority of melanoma prone families carry inherited mutations in *cyclin-dependent kinase 2A inhibitor (CDKN2A).* Other less frequently mutated genes in familial melanoma patients include *cyclin-dependent kinase 4 (CDK4), BRCA1-associated protein-1 (BAP1), MITF, telomerase reverse transcription (TERT),* and *protection of telomeres 1 (POT1).*[30] Sporadic DN have recently been shown by several methods to be genetically intermediate between common

Fig. 3. Fusion of junctional melanocytic nests across elongated rete ridges is known as bridging. Also, note the patchy chronic inflammatory infiltrate within superficial dermis (hematoxylin-eosin, original magnification x40) (*A*). Fusion of adjacent rete ridges (hematoxylin-eosin, original magnification x40) (*B*). In the center of this dysplastic nevus, there is low-level intraepidermal ascent of single melanocytes (hematoxylin-eosin, original magnification x200) (*C*).

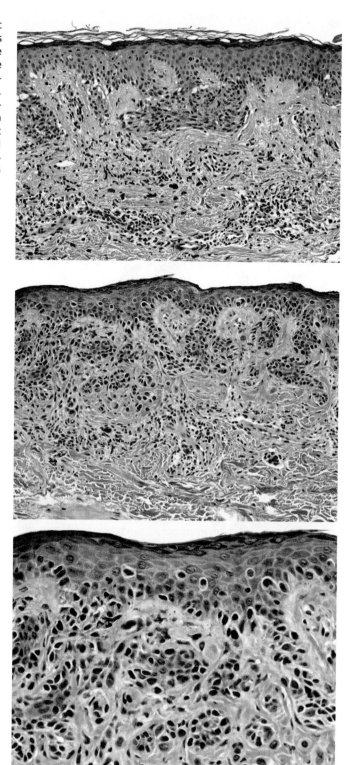

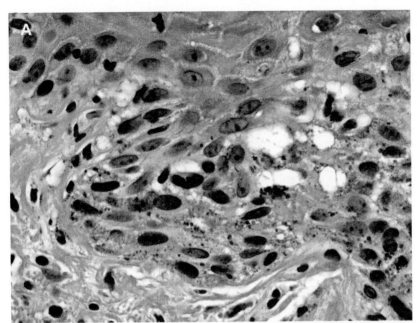

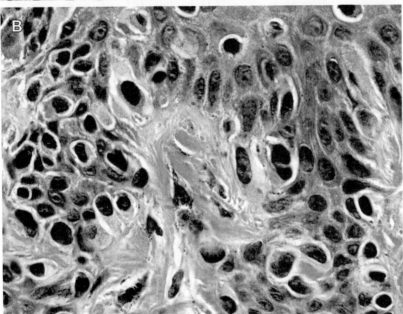

Fig. 4. Finely dispersed melanin pigment is seen in these atypical ovoid melanocytes giving rise to an olive-green, dusty appearance (hematoxylin-eosin, original magnification x400) (*A*). Marked cytologic atypia is appreciated in these melanocytes showing nuclear enlargement, nuclear hyperchromasia and prominent nucleoli (hematoxylin-eosin, original magnification x400) (*B*).

nevi and melanoma, further confirming the clinical and histopathologic impression.[31–33] Mutational analysis of melanomas and their benign precursors revealed single driver mutations in *BRAF^V600E* in common nevi whereas multiple driver mutations were observed in DN. Driver mutations resulting in activation of the *MAPK* signaling pathway, *TERT* promoter mutations and heterozygous abnormalities in *CDNK2A* were common. DN also show an overall mutational burden that is, higher compared with common nevi but lower than that observed in outright melanoma.[31–33] Similarly, studies on microRNA expression have confirmed the intermediate position of DN in the biologic spectrum form common nevi to melanoma.[34–36]

Fig. 5. Eosinophilic fibroplasia surrounds these rete ridges (hematoxylin-eosin, original magnification x200) (*A*). Pigment incontinence and prominent vessels are seen in the superficial dermis (hematoxylin-eosin, original magnification x200) (*B*).

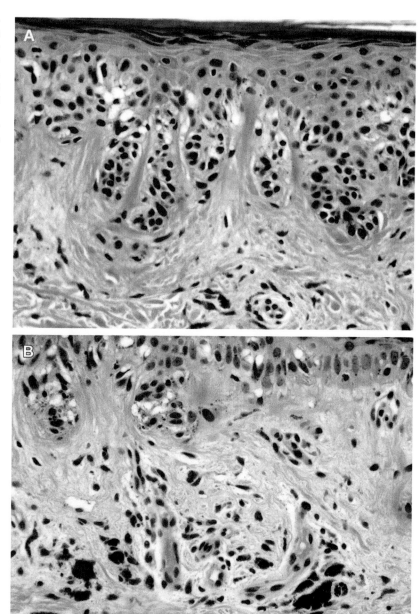

TREATMENT

DN and clinically atypical nevi require regular clinical monitoring and should be removed by excision, preferably with a 1-mm to 3-mm clinical margin, to exclude melanoma in the presence of clinically concerning findings, such as a history of recent growth, change in shape or color, increasing erythema, and itching sensation.[37,38]

It is important to avoid partial and fragmented sampling using superficial shave biopsies, small punch biopsies through the lesional center, or sampling by curettage.[39] These procedures do not allow for adequate histopathologic assessment of important architectural features necessary to separate DN from superficial spreading melanoma, such as lesional symmetry and circumscription and maturation of the dermal component with depth. Partial samples also are

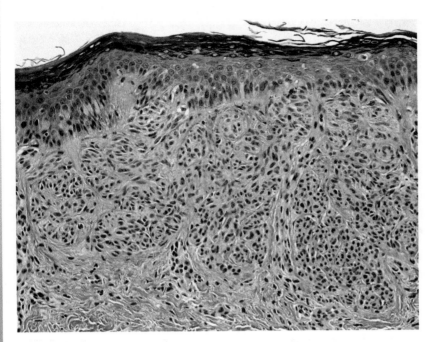

Fig. 6. The dermal component is bland and devoid of cytologic atypia or mitotic activity. Maturation with depth is preserved (hematoxylin-eosin, original magnification x40).

prone to sampling error because more concerning or outright melanomatous areas may not be represented in the original biopsy.[37] Furthermore, subsequent excisional biopsies of previously partially sampled melanocytic lesions often are difficult to assess due to distortion by the presence of a scar and the concerning features of recurrent nevus phenomenon, leading to potential for overdiagnosis as melanoma. Complete excision of clinically atypical nevi, even with narrow margins, allows for a more confident initial diagnosis and reduces the number of surgical procedures for the patient by avoiding frequent repeat biopsies and excisions of partially sampled DN. Furthermore, there is little argument for performing formal re-excisions of completely excised DN, even if severely atypical.[40] Similarly, there is no good evidence to suggest re-excisions of mildly or moderately DN even if tissue edges are only focally involved as long as the lesion is adequately sampled and represented in the biopsy and there is no evidence of residual pigmented lesion clinically.[41–43]

DIFFERENTIAL DIAGNOSES

DN can be separated from lentiginous junctional and lentiginous compound nevi by the presence of architectural and cytologic atypia.

Nevi of special sites show considerable histologic overlap with DN and reliable separation may be challenging. Nevi of special sites frequently present at anatomic sites where DN are rare, for example, acral and genital skin. Although acral nevi show worrisome architectural features, including a lentiginous junctional growth and upward scatter of single melanocytes within the epidermal layers, there is little, if any, cytologic atypia and a minimal host response in the form of fibrosis or a lymphohistiocytic inflammatory infiltrate.[44,45] Similarly, genital nevi show significant architectural atypia with a disorderly nested growth of the junctional component and focal pagetoid spread.[46] In contrast to DN, however, there is no prominent junctional lentiginous growth component, and the cytologic atypia is confluent rather than scattered and random. Genital nevi also lack the host response typical of DN. Despite their concerning histologic features, nevi of special sites are benign. They do not appear to be melanoma precursors, and they are not associated with an overall increased melanoma risk.

Most important and challenging is the separation of DN from early superficial spreading melanoma. DN show architectural and cytologic features overlapping with those of superficial spreading melanoma, and the distinction is based on the overall constellation of features and the severity of changes. It is important to understand that the border between severely DN and early melanoma may be blurred and not sharply defined; moreover, there is poor interobserver

Fig. 7. There is marked lesional asymmetry in this melanoma (right) arising in a background of a dysplastic nevus (hematoxylin-eosin, original magnification x10) (left) (A). Higher magnification of the dysplastic nevus component shows architectural disorder and scattered cytologic atypia of the junctional component and a bland, nevi dermal component (hematoxylin-eosin, original magnification x40) (B). The adjacent melanoma shows marked and confluent cytologic atypia.

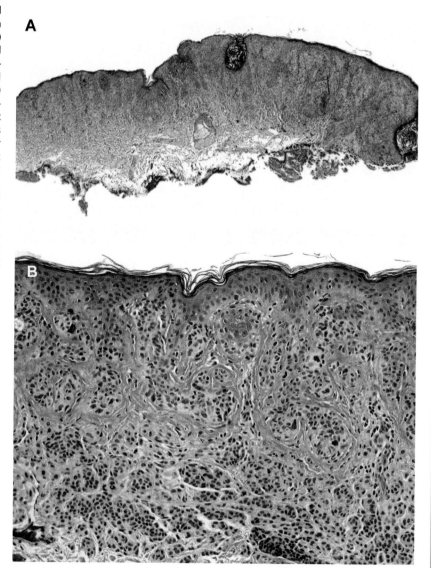

agreement in this diagnostic setting. Features in favor of a diagnosis of melanoma are large lesional size with marked asymmetry and poor circumscription and significant architectural disorder of the junctional component, resulting in contiguous growth of melanocytes with effacement and atrophy of the overlying epidermis and diffuse pagetoid spread across the lesion. Melanoma shows severe and confluent rather than scattered and random cytologic atypia and there is cytologic atypia with loss of maturation of the invasive dermal component and mitotic activity. Areas of regression, especially when present in different stages,

also are indicative of melanoma. Increased Ki-67 proliferative index greater than 5%, loss of p16 expression, and diffuse PRAME expression of the dermal components are immunohistochemical findings in support of a diagnosis of invasive melanoma.

An additional significant diagnostic dilemma is lesions variably referred to as lentiginous DN in the elderly or lentiginous melanoma.[47–50] These neoplasms show elongated rete ridges and a diffuse proliferation of epithelioid melanocytes in a disorderly single cell and nested pattern reminiscent of DN. Cytologic atypia is limited but focal

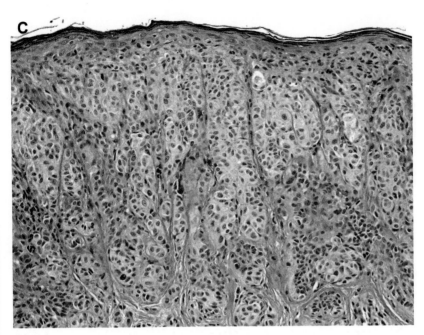

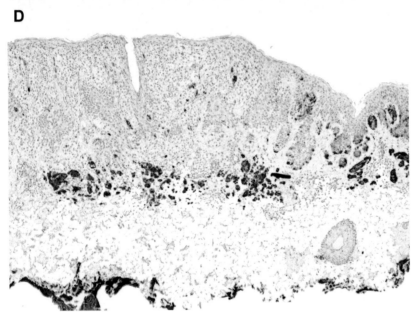

Fig. 7. (continued). (hematoxylin-eosin, original magnification x100) (*C*). P16 staining highlights the background dysplastic nevus whereas there is lack of p16 expression in the melanoma (p16, original magnification x20) (*D*).

pagetoid spread may be present. Clinically, these melanocytic tumors often are large, measuring approximately 1 cm in diameter. They present on sun-damaged skin of elderly patients in their 50s and 60s, with a predilection for the upper back, shoulder, and head and neck area. They are best regarded as early melanoma or at least a significant precursor lesion to melanoma. Familiarity with this clinicopathologic entity is important to avoid underdiagnosis as dysplastic nevus, particularly on partial samples. The histologic features of DN in contrast to those of common acquired nevi and superficial spreading melanoma are summarized in **Table 2.**

Fig. 8. Melan-A staining (*red*) highlights junctional and dermal melanocytes. The mib-1 (*brown*) proliferative index in melanocytes is low (Melan A, original magnification x40) (*A*). There is preserved p16 expression in dermal melanocytes (p16, original magnification x40) (*B*).

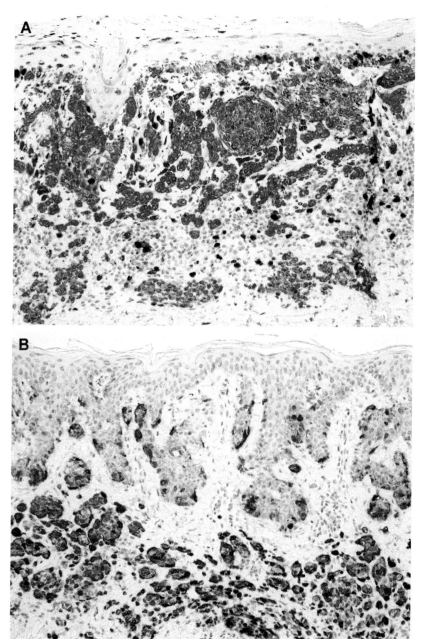

Table 2
Summary of the histopathologic findings of dysplastic nevi in comparison to common acquired nevi and superficial spreading melanoma

	Common Acquired Nevus	Dysplastic Nevus	Superficial Spreading Melanoma
Overall architecture			
Size	Small	Large (≥0.5 cm)	Large (>0.5 cm)
Symmetry	Symmetric	Mainly symmetric	Asymmetric
Circumscription	Circumscribed	Relatively circumscribed	Ill-defined
Junctional component			
Growth pattern	Mainly nested	Lentiginous and nested	Variably lentiginous and nested
Nest arrangement	Base of rete ridges	Disorderly arranged with bridging of nests	Disordered arrangement with fusion of nests
Intraepidermal ascent of melanocytes (pagetoid spread)	No intraepidermal ascent of melanocytes	Focal low-level intraepidermal ascent of melanocytes in lesional center	Prominent intraepidermal ascent of melanocytes into granular cell layer and across the entire lesion
Cytologic atypia	Absent	Scattered	Confluent
Epidermal changes	Preserved epidermal architecture	Pronounced rete ridge pattern	Epidermal atrophy with consumption of the epidermis
Dermal component (if present)			
Junctional shoulder	Absent	Present	Extensive
Cytologic atypia	Absent	Absent	Present
Maturation with depth	Preserved	Preserved	Absent
Mitotic activity	Rare	Rare	Variable
Mesenchymal changes			
Inflammation	Variable	Patchy	Variable
Fibrosis	Absent	Concentric eosinophilic and lamellar surrounding rete ridges	Diffuse

SUMMARY

DN are a distinctive clinicopathologic entity with clinical, histopathologic, and molecular features intermediate between common acquired nevi and superficial spreading melanoma. Although initially reported in patients with familial melanoma and thought to represent an important melanoma precursor, a majority of DN occur in the sporadic setting. They are benign and transformation of DN to melanoma is a rare event. The overall count of DN and increasing degrees of atypia are of importance, however, because they correlate positively with an increased overall melanoma risk in a given patient. If clinically concerning due to recent change, DN should be removed, preferably by excision, to allow adequate histopathologic examination with visualization of the entire lesion. Histopathologic grading should take into account both cytologic and architectural features. DN with severe atypia pose the main diagnostic challenge, and reliable separation from early melanoma may be difficult in individual cases. The histopathologic findings also need to be interpreted in a patient's individual clinical background, including age, extent of sun damage, localization, and medical history; and a close interaction between the treating clinician and the pathologist/dermatopathologist is necessary to guide appropriate treatment.

CLINICS CARE POINTS

When reporting DN, the following should be considered:

- Appropriate clinical information available at time of biopsy: age, anatomic site, gender, clinical and dermoscopic findings, lesional size, level of clinical concern, type of biopsy, and incisional versus excisional biopsy

- Using preferred nomenclature: lentiginous junctional/compound dysplastic nevus with mild/moderate/severe atypia

- Grading of atypia, taking into account both cytologic and architectural features

- Reporting status of margins and adequacy of excision

- Immunohistochemistry for Melan-A/SOX10, which is helpful to highlight lesional architecture of the junctional component

- Immunohistochemistry for p16, PRAME, and Ki-67, which may be useful to exclude melanoma in challenging and severely atypical tumors, but adequate interpretation relies on the presence of a significant dermal component

- Liaising with treating clinician/dermatologist to gain insight into local clinical practice and expectations and to issue treatment recommendations accordingly

- Avoiding treatment recommendations, which, in general, are not necessary for mildly DN and moderately DN

- For small, superficial, and fragmented partial samples, alerting clinician to possibility of sampling error

- Expressing level of concern and ambiguity in challenging lesions because distinction of severely DN from early melanoma is notoriously challenging

DISCLOSURE

The authors have nothing to disclose.

REFERENCES

1. Clark WH Jr, Reimer RR, Greene M, et al. Origin of familial malignant melanomas from heritable melanocytic lesions. 'The B-K mole syndrome. Arch Dermatol 1978;114(5):732–8.

2. Martin-Gorgojo A, Requena C, Garcia-Casado Z, et al. Dysplastic vs. Common Naevus-associated vs. De novo Melanomas: an observational retrospective study of 1,021 patients. Acta Derm Venereol 2018;98(6):556–62.

3. Lynch HT, Frichot BC 3rd, Lynch JF. Familial atypical multiple mole-melanoma syndrome. J Med Genet 1978;15(5):352–6.

4. Elder DE, Goldman LI, Goldman SC, et al. Dysplastic nevus syndrome: a phenotypic association of sporadic cutaneous melanoma. Cancer 1980;46(8):1787–94.

5. Ackerman AB, Magana-Garcia M. Naming acquired melanocytic nevi. Unna's, Miescher's, Spitz's Clark's. Am J Dermatopathol 1990;12(2):193–209.

6. NIH Consensus conference. Diagnosis and treatment of early melanoma. JAMA 1992;268(10): 1314–9.

7. Shapiro M, Chren MM, Levy RM, et al. Variability in nomenclature used for nevi with architectural disorder and cytologic atypia (microscopically dysplastic nevi) by dermatologists and dermatopathologists. J Cutan Pathol 2004;31(8):523–30.

8. Shors AR, Kim S, White E, et al. Dysplastic naevi with moderate to severe histological dysplasia: a risk factor for melanoma. Br J Dermatol 2006;155(5): 988–93.

9. Xiong MY, Rabkin MS, Piepkorn MW, et al. Diameter of dysplastic nevi is a more robust biomarker of increased melanoma risk than degree of histologic dysplasia: a case-control study. J Am Acad Dermatol 2014;71(6): 1257–1258 e1254.

10. Reimer RR, Clark WH Jr, Greene MH, et al. Precursor lesions in familial melanoma. A new genetic preneoplastic syndrome. JAMA 1978;239(8):744–6.

11. Elder DE. Precursors to melanoma and their mimics: nevi of special sites. Mod Pathol 2006;19(Suppl 2): S4–20.

12. Halpern AC, Guerry Dt, Elder DE, et al. Natural history of dysplastic nevi. J Am Acad Dermatol 1993; 29(1):51–7.

13. Tucker MA, Fraser MC, Goldstein AM, et al. A natural history of melanomas and dysplastic nevi: an atlas of lesions in melanoma-prone families. Cancer 2002;94(12):3192–209.

14. Bevona C, Goggins W, Quinn T, et al. Cutaneous melanomas associated with nevi. Arch Dermatol 2003;139(12):1620–4, [discussion 1624].

15. Halpern AC, Guerry Dt, Elder DE, et al. Dysplastic nevi as risk markers of sporadic (nonfamilial) melanoma. A case-control study. Arch Dermatol 1991; 127(7):995–9.

16. Tucker MA, Halpern A, Holly EA, et al. Clinically recognized dysplastic nevi. A central risk factor for cutaneous melanoma. JAMA 1997;277(18): 1439–44.

17. Slade J, Marghoob AA, Salopek TG, et al. Atypical mole syndrome: risk factor for cutaneous malignant

melanoma and implications for management. J Am Acad Dermatol 1995;32(3):479–94.

18. Bishop JA, Wachsmuth RC, Harland M, et al. Genotype/phenotype and penetrance studies in melanoma families with germline CDKN2A mutations. J Invest Dermatol 2000;114(1): 28–33.

19. Clemente C, Cochran AJ, Elder DE, et al. Histopathologic diagnosis of dysplastic nevi: concordance among pathologists convened by the World health organization melanoma programme. Hum Pathol 1991;22(4):313–9.

20. Elder DE. Dysplastic naevi: an update. Histopathology 2010;56(1):112–20.

21. de Wit PE, van't Hof-Grootenboer B, Ruiter DJ, et al. Validity of the histopathological criteria used for diagnosing dysplastic naevi. An interobserver study by the pathology subgroup of the EORTC Malignant Melanoma Cooperative Group. Eur J Cancer 1993; 29A(6):831–9.

22. Piepkorn MW, Barnhill RL, Cannon-Albright LA, et al. A multiobserver, population-based analysis of histologic dysplasia in melanocytic nevi. J Am Acad Dermatol 1994;30(5 Pt 1):707–14.

23. Rhodes AR, Mihm MC Jr, Weinstock MA. Dysplastic melanocytic nevi: a reproducible histologic definition emphasizing cellular morphology. Mod Pathol 1989; 2(4):306–19.

24. Shea CR, Vollmer RT, Prieto VG. Correlating architectural disorder and cytologic atypia in Clark (dysplastic) melanocytic nevi. Hum Pathol 1999; 30(5):500–5.

25. Duffy KL, Mann DJ, Petronic-Rosic V, et al. Clinical decision making based on histopathologic grading and margin status of dysplastic nevi. Arch Dermatol 2012;148(2):259–60.

26. Weinstock MA, Barnhill RL, Rhodes AR, et al. Reliability of the histopathologic diagnosis of melanocytic dysplasia. The dysplastic nevus panel. Arch Dermatol 1997;133(8):953–8.

27. Arumi-Uria M, McNutt NS, Finnerty B. Grading of atypia in nevi: correlation with melanoma risk. Mod Pathol 2003;16(8):764–71.

28. Vyas NS, Charifa A, Desman GT, et al. Observational study examining the diagnostic practice of Ki67 staining for melanocytic lesions. Am J Dermatopathol 2019;41(7):488–91.

29. Lezcano C, Jungbluth AA, Nehal KS, et al. PRAME expression in melanocytic tumors. Am J Surg Pathol 2018;42(11):1456–65.

30. Aoude LG, Wadt KA, Pritchard AL, et al. Genetics of familial melanoma: 20 years after CDKN2A. Pigment Cell Melanoma Res 2015;28(2):148–60.

31. Shain AH, Bastian BC. From melanocytes to melanomas. Nat Rev Cancer 2016;16(6):345–58.

32. Shain AH, Joseph NM, Yu R, et al. Genomic and transcriptomic analysis reveals incremental disruption of key signaling pathways during melanoma evolution. Cancer Cell 2018;34(1):45–55 e44.

33. Shain AH, Yeh I, Kovalyshyn I, et al. The genetic evolution of melanoma from precursor lesions. N Engl J Med 2015;373(20):1926–36.

34. Quiohilag K, Caie P, Oniscu A, et al. The differential expression of micro-RNAs 21, 200c, 204, 205, and 211 in benign, dysplastic and malignant melanocytic lesions and critical evaluation of their role as diagnostic biomarkers. Virchows Arch 2020;477(1): 121–30.

35. Torres R, Lang UE, Hejna M, et al. MicroRNA ratios distinguish melanomas from nevi. J Invest Dermatol 2020;140(1):164–173 e167.

36. Xu Y, Brenn T, Brown ER, et al. Differential expression of microRNAs during melanoma progression: miR-200c, miR-205 and miR-211 are downregulated in melanoma and act as tumour suppressors. Br J Cancer 2012;106(3):553–61.

37. Fleming NH, Shaub AR, Bailey E, et al. Outcomes of surgical re-excision versus observation of severely dysplastic nevi: a single-institution, retrospective cohort study. J Am Acad Dermatol 2020;82(1): 238–40.

38. Terushkin V, Ng E, Stein JA, et al. A prospective study evaluating the utility of a 2-mm biopsy margin for complete removal of histologically atypical (dysplastic) nevi. J Am Acad Dermatol 2017;77(6): 1096–9.

39. Elston DM, Stratman EJ, Miller SJ. Skin biopsy: biopsy issues in specific diseases. J Am Acad Dermatol 2016;74(1):1–16, quiz 17–8.

40. Engeln K, Peters K, Ho J, et al. Dysplastic nevi with severe atypia: long-term outcomes in patients with and without re-excision. J Am Acad Dermatol 2017;76(2):244–9.

41. Goodson AG, Florell SR, Boucher KM, et al. Low rates of clinical recurrence after biopsy of benign to moderately dysplastic melanocytic nevi. J Am Acad Dermatol 2010;62(4):591–6.

42. Hiscox B, Hardin MR, Orengo IF, et al. Recurrence of moderately dysplastic nevi with positive histologic margins. J Am Acad Dermatol 2017;76(3): 527–30.

43. Dickman JS, Haddad RM, Racette A. Predictive value of positive margins in diagnostic biopsies of dysplastic nevi. Dermatol Res Pract 2020;2020: 6716145.

44. Clemente C, Zurrida S, Bartoli C, et al. Acral-lentiginous naevus of plantar skin. Histopathology 1995; 27(6):549–55.

45. Kerl H, Trau H, Ackerman AB. Differentiation of melanocytic nevi from malignant melanomas in palms, soles, and nail beds solely by signs in the cornified layer of the epidermis. Am J Dermatopathol 1984; 6(Suppl):159–60.

46. Gleason BC, Hirsch MS, Nucci MR, et al. Atypical genital nevi. A clinicopathologic analysis of 56 cases. Am J Surg Pathol 2008;32(1): 51–7.

47. King R, Page RN, Googe PB, et al. Lentiginous melanoma: a histologic pattern of melanoma to be distinguished from lentiginous nevus. Mod Pathol 2005;18(10):1397–401.

48. Kossard S. Atypical lentiginous junctional naevi of the elderly and melanoma. Australas J Dermatol 2002;43(2):93–101.

49. Kossard S, Commens C, Symons M, et al. Lentiginous dysplastic naevi in the elderly: a potential precursor for malignant melanoma. Australas J Dermatol 1991;32(1):27–37.

50. King R. Lentiginous melanoma. Arch Pathol Lab Med 2011;135(3):337–41.